Crimes of violence
by mentally
abnormal offenders

Crimes of violence by mentally abnormal offenders

A psychiatric and epidemiological study
in the Federal German Republic

H. HÄFNER
Professor of Psychiatry, University of Heidelberg, and
Director, Central Institute of Mental Health,
Mannheim, Federal Republic of Germany

W. BÖKER
Professor of Psychiatry, University of Berne, and
Director, Psychiatric Hospital, Berne-Waldau, Switzerland

In collaboration with

H. Immich, C. Köhler, A. Schmitt, G. Wagner, J. Werner

Foreword by T.C.N. Gibbens

Translated by Helen Marshall
Formerly Librarian, Institute of
Psychiatry, London

CAMBRIDGE UNIVERSITY PRESS
Cambridge
London New York New Rochelle
Melbourne Sydney

Published by the Press Syndicate of the University of Cambridge
The Pitt Building, Trumpington Street, Cambridge CB2 1RP
32 East 57th Street, New York, NY 10022, USA
296 Beaconsfield Parade, Middle Park, Melbourne 3206, Australia

Originally published in Germany as Gewalttaten Geistesgestörter
by Springer-Verlag, Berlin, Heidelberg & New York in 1973 and
© Springer-Verlag 1973

First published in English by Cambridge University Press 1982
as Crimes of Violence by Mentally Abnormal Offenders
© Cambridge University Press 1982

Printed in Great Britain at the University Press, Cambridge

Library of Congress catalogue card number : 81-17974

British Library Cataloguing in Publication Data

Häfner,H.

Crimes of violence by mentally abnormal offenders.
1. Offences against the person - Germany (West)
2. Insane, Criminal and Dangerous - Germany (West)
I.Title   II.Böker,W.
III.Gewalttaten Geistesgestörter. English

364.3'8'0943   HV6133

ISBN 0 521 24136 7

CONTENTS

The greatest injustices proceed from those who pursue immoderation
and not from those who are guided by necessity
(Aristotle)

AUTHORS AND COLLABORATORS

Authors

Dr. med. Dr. phil. H. Häfner
Professor of Psychiatry, University of Heidelberg
Director, Central Institute for Mental Health, 6800 Mannheim,
Federal Republic of Germany

Dr. med. W. Böker
Professor of Psychiatry, University of Berne
Director, Psychiatric Hospital, Berne-Waldau, Switzerland

Collaborators

Dr. med. H. Immich
Professor for Medical Documentation and Statistics, University of Heidelberg
Director, Institute for Medical Documentation, Statistics and Data-Processing,
6900 Heidelberg, Federal Republic of Germany

Dr. rer. pol. C. Köhler
Lecturer for Medical Information Processing, University of Heidelberg,
Institute for Medical Documentation, Statistics and Data-Processing,
6900 Heidelberg, Federal Republic of Germany

Dr. med. A. Schmitt
Institute for Medical Examinations (IMPF), Grosse Langgasse 8, 6500 Mainz,
Federal Republic of Germany

Prof. Dr. med. G. Wagner
Director, Institute for Documentation, Information and Statistics of the
German Cancer Research Centre, 6900 Heidelberg, Federal Republic of Germany

Prof. Dr. phil. J. Werner
University of Heidelberg, Institute of Psychology, Hauptstr. 47-51,
6900 Heidelberg, Federal Republic of Germany

FOREWORD

The publication of this monograph in English translation will enable it to be read throughout the world, and will help to bring to the authors the recognition they well deserve. It is the most systematic and detailed epidemiological study yet undertaken of the extent to which the mentally abnormal are responsible for major crimes of violence.

Their sample consists of all the 533 men and women detained as legally irresponsible in the Federal Republic of Germany between 1955 and 1964 suffering from psychosis or serious degrees of subnormality after committing homicide or intended but unsuccessful homicide.

Hitherto the extensive literature on the subject has mainly dealt with individual psychiatrists' collections of patients, selected in unknown ways. In addition, all forensic research tends to be complicated by differences in the criteria of behaviour in the criminal law and the medical criteria of abnormality. Apart from this, an unknown number of violent offences are not reported or followed by detection, and many psychotic individuals may not be known to the health authorities. The authors therefore chose to study a type of offender which is probably most reliably notified and arrested, and types of mental disorder (schizophrenic, affective, or organic psychoses, and moderate to severe subnormality) about which there is a substantial agreement among psychiatrists.

In popular imagination mentally ill or subnormal patients are liable to unpredictable outbursts of dangerous violence. The representativeness of the sample enables the authors to calculate that such individuals are no more, but also no less, likely to commit homicide than the mentally healthy.

The detailed analysis of age, family, social and occupational relations, motives, symptoms, as well as the duration of illness and quality of any aftercare the offenders may or may not have received, has made it possible to point to situations or symptoms of special danger, especially for close relatives, and to suggest better policies of prevention.

The data are set out in great detail. The concluding summary chapter gives a clear impression of the main findings, and readers may find it convenient to read this first before turning to the earlier chapters on matters which especially concern them.

In supervising the translation, I should like to express my overwhelming debt to Miss Helen Marshall, for many years personal secretary to the late Professor Sir Aubrey Lewis, and later librarian of the Institute of Psychiatry, who carried out not only the initial translation but all the typing.

T.C.N. Gibbens

PREFACE

The efforts of modern psychiatry are resulting in more open treatment of the
mentally abnormal. An unknown but growing number of chronic patients suffering from mental illness and mental handicap who used to be regarded as needing
permanent institutional care are being given the chance of living in the
community. This places a greater burden upon their families and upon society,
and may also expose them to greater risks than they have been accustomed to
bear.

Those of us who took part in early attempts to introduce community
psychiatry and psychiatric rehabilitation into the Federal German Republic
know what resistances had to be overcome. How could one really reply to the
main objection that 'the mentally abnormal are unpredictable and dangerous'?
The divergent lines of thought current in our own specialty were of little
help. There was no empirical study which could supply reliable information.
The scientist's own beliefs - though highly esteemed by many - do not provide
him with a solid foundation, even if he is himself a practitioner.

If we want to encourage a society to take risks, then our knowledge of the extent of these risks must be fairly assured. If the risks are
great, involving possibly death or serious bodily harm, then the citizen has
a right to know whether he is more at risk from the violence of 'normal' men
than from the violence of the mentally abnormal. If more mentally abnormal
individuals are to live freely in the community, then we must be in a position
to identify those among them who represent a high risk. So long as this is not
possible, we must either use protective measures indiscriminately against a
large number of harmless patients, or be prepared for unknown dangers. So far
no serious consideration has been given to the development of well-aimed
preventive measures carefully directed at the criminal violence of the
mentally abnormal.

The present investigation was planned with this goal in mind: at
the same time we hoped it would contribute to the development of the research

in the field of 'psychiatric epidemiology', which has been neglected in
Germany since 1935. The empirical basis of the study is a comprehensive
epidemiological survey of all mentally abnormal offenders who committed a
violent crime in the Federal Republic between 1 January 1955 and
21 December 1964.

For methodological and practical reasons the study is limited to
violent crime committed by the mentally ill and the mentally handicapped. It
was not possible to investigate other crimes committed by the mentally
abnormal, or the criminality of those psychiatric patients who do not fall
within this diagnostic definition. This is to be regretted, particularly when
one considers the important question of 'instinctual crimes', which the project
leader (Häfner) had originally wished to include in the study when he was first
in touch with the then Federal Ministry of Health.

The risk of violent crime is nevertheless probably the most important factor in our research aims. The amount of work involved and the time
required were also considerations which helped to limit the questions we were
able to ask.

The study is essentially a collaborative effort. After a preliminary investigation by one of us (Häfner), who also developed the methodological framework of the enquiry and drew up the questions to be asked in it,
there followed a phase of planning which lasted eight months and which
covered also a pilot study, conducted jointly by the two authors and partly
by Wagner, Immich, Köhler and Schmitt. The transcription of hospital records
and police and court files onto the coded questionnaire was carried out by
A. Schmitt (343 cases) and W. Böker (130 cases). The analysis of data and
the interpretation of results was carried out by the project leader (Häfner)
supported by preparatory work done by A. Schmitt and W. Böker and by
statistical advice given by G. Köhler and J. Werner. There are several
reasons for the long time which elapsed between the actual survey and the
publication of the findings. For example, the protracted work of evaluation
was still further delayed because in the random selection of the control
population an error occurred which was discovered by the authors only after
the second draft manuscript had been prepared. We therefore had to obtain a
new control group from the admissions to another regional hospital and
repeat part of the statistical work.

The conduct of such an extensive investigation calls for the co-
operation of a large number of people and institutions, and this was admirably
forthcoming. We are indebted to the officials of the Regional Offices of
Justice, the Federal Criminal Bureau and the Regional Criminal Bureaus, to

the judges of the regional courts and to the prosecuting authorities who so readily made the necessary documents available to us. In particular we thank Dr Rangol of the Federal Statistical Bureau who responded to our many requests unfailingly, promptly and to all feasible extent.

The directors, physicians and archivists of the regional psychiatric hospitals gave us not only every support in our collection of data but also offered us friendly hospitality. We would record our special gratitude to Dr Hoffman-Steudner, Professor Heinrich and their colleagues at the regional hospitals of Wiesloch and Landeck. We also had the support of colleagues at the Institute for Documentation and Statistics at the German Cancer Research Centre, who helped in the electronic processing of data whenever we needed their co-operation.

It is not possible to name individually all those without whom this study would not have been possible. Representative mention may be made of Frau Brigitta Kroeber, documentalist, who collaborated in the collection and preparation of data, and of Hannelore Holz, Rosemarie Illgen, Christa Khalil and Stefanie Steiniger, of the secretarial staff, who tackled a mountain of manuscripts in several revisions, drew up tables and helped to calculate significant values and to prepare innumerable documents. Our thanks are finally due to the Federal Ministry of Youth, Family and Health for providing the resources which enabled us to carry out the research programme.

Before concluding we would like to make one point for the benefit of the non-specialist reader. This book sets out to present the methodology and detailed findings of a very comprehensive empirical investigation and to weigh up critically all possible adequate interpretations. Therefore its chapters on results abound in tables and in difficult textual passages. In the final chapter we have, however, tried to give a readable summary of the main findings and their practical implications. By beginning there, it is possible to obtain a general synopsis which will facilitate access to the more difficult parts of the book.

Mannheim, June 1972

Heinz Häfner
Wolfgang Böker

NOTE ON THE TRANSLATION

The English version of our book is a literal translation. This seemed
appropriate since the investigations on which the book is based are completed.
Besides, they could no longer be carried out as a consequence of the present
strict regulations for the protection of confidentiality and personal data.

Some of the terms used in the text do not fully correspond to the present
usage. The diagnostic categories and groups, for example, are not identical
with the terms used in the International Classification of Diagnoses (ICD),
9th revision. We could not correct this because a classification of diagnoses
edited by the German Association of Psychiatry and Neurology was generally
applied at the time when the diagnoses and the data-collection were made in
the GFR. However, the diagnostic groups used in our investigation correspond
to a large extent to the definitions given in the ICD 8th revision.

The translator, to whom we wish to express our deep thanks for her excellent
work, has used the terms 'mentally defective' and 'mental deficiency' for
Schwachsinnige and *Schwachsinn*. The group covered by these terms is ICD
No. 311-313 (mild to severe deficiency or retardation). The other diagnostic
groups are equivalent to the German classification scheme as well as to ICD
8th revision.

September 1981

H.H.
W.B.

1 INTRODUCTION: THE PROBLEM VIEWED IN THE LIGHT OF THE PSYCHIATRIC LITERATURE

Attitude studies by American sociologists (Star, 1955; Cumming & Cumming, 1957; Nunnally, 1961) show that the layman has basically three criteria of mental illness:

1. Breakdown of rational mental functioning
2. Loss of self-control
3. Extremely inappropriate forms of social behaviour

Studying the population of the Federal Republic of Germany (GFR), both Jaeckel & Wieser (1967) and Jaeckel found a stereotyped view in which the mentally ill (who were clearly distinguished from those with other, less severe psychological disorders) were associated with loss of reason, unaccountable behaviour and to some extent dangerousness. It may well be that the intellectual element in this stereotype was hardened by descriptions such as frequently appeared in the early literature of forensic psychiatry and criminology of particularly dramatic and horrifying acts of violence committed by the mentally ill. Even today some well-known psychiatrists still adhere to the doctrine that unpredictable acts of violence may be an early and characteristic sign of incipient schizophrenia, and this, coupled with the usual popularisation of expert opinions, may well also have contributed to the general attitude.

The intellectual content of the stereotype also has emotional and behavioural implications. In practice it means that those concerned with the mentally ill, and to some extent also with the mentally retarded, are frequently subject to uncertainty and anxiety; they tend to be too solicitous and conciliatory, or to 'give them a wide berth'. There is no doubt that the latter form of behaviour contributes to the isolation of the mentally ill. According to current knowledge such factors have an unfavourable effect on the treatment and rehabilitation prospects of a large proportion of the mentally ill and mentally retarded. It is thus highly probable that the psychological repercussions of violent crimes committed by the mentally abnormal have their effect upon the actual situation of many of those who are mentally ill. On the other hand, some people react with denial. Indeed many symptoms of illness go unnoticed or are not taken seriously by relatives and observers outside the family. This may happen even when the patient behaves in a hostile or openly aggressive manner. Serious warning signs of this kind are often observed but no attention is paid to them, or they are immediately forgotten. This lessens the chance of successful prevention of actual violence by patients at risk.

It is certainly the aim of psychiatry to demolish negative prejudices which stand in the way of successful treatment and rehabilitation of the mentally ill and mentally retarded. Such an aim cannot, however, be achieved by naively substituting a new positive stereotype for the old negative one. The denial of illness or dangerousness, which is now more or less explicit in many theological, moral, sociological or political ideologies of mental illness, can help neither the patients nor their relatives, nor the small number who are actually at risk. Such an unrealistic development would produce a counter-reaction and both the trend and the reaction to it would be harmful to the patients. If we are to have effective, enlightened health education and successful preventive measures, we must promote attitudes that are based on reality and have a solid foundation in empirically acquired facts.

If we could have reasonably reliable data about the general risk of violence on the part of the mentally abnormal, and about the degree of 'dangerousness' which is characteristic of certain groups of illnesses, this would presumably provide us with an important means of encouraging the public to adopt a realistic attitude towards the mentally ill and the mentally retarded. More comprehensive knowledge about violent tendencies and about warning signs of actual violence, combined with possibilities of preventive treatment or improved protection, would constitute an important advance. If we can recognise the danger and take adequate action, generalised fears and helplessness will gradually subside.

What is the relationship between violence and mental illness? Can we hope for an unambiguous answer to this question, or will we lose our way in a maze of qualifications, in a multifactorial aetiology which may perhaps vary from illness to illness, from syndrome to syndrome, or which may even depend on personality? The French psychiatrist Esquirol (1772-1840) thought in fact that he had discovered a typical group of mentally ill murderers (his 'homicidal monomania') who, suffering from different mental illnesses and exhibiting different modes of behaviour, were said to be compelled by a single mysterious force, a 'pure instinctive drive', to commit murder. This theory was based on the assumption of a morbid drive as the single source of the pathological violence. A second monistic theory was based on the assumption of a morbid loss of 'moral' control of normal aggressiveness, i.e. of the atavistic elements in human nature. The concept of 'moral insanity' (Pritchard, 1835) was thus extended far beyond its original content of poorly endowed individuals with poor affect and 'innate' moral defects, and made to cover a generalised explanation of violence on the part of the mentally abnormal. This idea of 'moral defect' was further developed by Kahlbaum, Binswanger, Dubitscher, Meggendorfer and others and was given a new and tendentiously monistic slant, particularly in Germany, by the doctrine of degeneration (see review by Häfner, 1959).

Schipkowensky (1938) finally attempted to provide a unitary explanation of violence by relating it to particular groups of illnesses. He regarded the majority of homicides committed by schizophrenics as the 'group of pure schizophrenic murder' and elevated this concept into a type of crime. Characteristic features of other psychiatric illnesses, such as the irritability of patients with organic cerebral disorders, the mood disorders of the epileptic, or the so-called raptus melancholicus, provided criteria for other illness-specific types of crime.

In contrast to these theories of the single or multiple aetiological associations between illness and violence, we have the concept that factors of personality and environment are just as important in causing violence, if not more important, than any psychosis which may subsequently set in. Theories of this kind cover such divergent trends as Lombroso's criminological school with its 'born criminal' and the doctrines of the social origins of crime. Any thorough empirical investigation of the problem must seek to determine the influence of factors from all three areas - genetics, environment and illness - taking account also of the motives and occasion of the crime.

The important question of the motives of violent and mentally disordered offenders points to a special problem in German psychiatry. Jaspers, proceeding from Dilthey's theory that anything that could be understood was psychological in origin, and anything that could not be understood was non-psychological in origin, based his 'phenomenological' methods on a false premise. His pupils added to the confusion of methods and theories. Gruhle (1947) declared, for example, that delusion was a condition that had no known cause and was basically not understandable: the process underlying it was therefore a physical one. If an endogenous psychosis of this kind gave rise to morbid behaviour, this too would be explicable in terms of the natural sciences, and not in terms of motivation. In its popular version this theory too has doubtless contributed to the idea that the more senseless an act of violence seems to be, the more likely it is that the violence is an expression

of a mental disorder. In the practice of forensic psychiatry this reinforced
the tendency to concede that offenders suffering from an endogenous psychosis
were not responsible for their acts, or that their responsibility was greatly
diminished, regardless of whether the acts in question were recognisably
related to the illness or not. The extent to which motivation can generally be
'understood' is an open question, in cases of psychoses as in other cases, since
even offenders who are not mentally disturbed often erect a barrier which
prevents them themselves, as well as other people, from understanding the
motive for their crime. Motivation research, and comparison of motives in
mentally abnormal violent offenders, forms a legitimate area of scientific
enquiry, however many difficulties it involves.

In 1967 the Ciba Foundation held a symposium in London on the
subject of 'The Mentally Abnormal Offender', in which psychiatrists, psycho-
logists, sociologists and criminologists from Great Britain, the USA, Denmark,
Sweden and Holland discussed violent behaviour in the mentally ill and the
mentally retarded. The papers presented dealt mainly with sensible methods of
treatment and care for abnormal offenders, but considered also hypotheses about
causes and questions of differential diagnosis and the incidence of criminally
aggressive behaviour in the mentally ill. The reviews and discussions pointed
impressively to the urgent need for more and better empirical data which would
provide a basis for a reliable assessment of 'dangerousness' in various forms
of mental illness and of the risk that mentally abnormal violent offenders may
repeat their crimes.

2 PREVIOUS STUDIES OF VIOLENCE IN THE MENTALLY ABNORMAL

2.1 General studies of the incidence of serious violent crime committed by mentally abnormal offenders

The era of typological case studies

Studies of violence in mentally abnormal offenders have been published chiefly by psychiatrists, though to some extent also by criminologists and jurists. In what follows we shall consider mainly the psychiatric studies, as they contribute most to our theme and, at least in some cases, offer opportunities of comparison with our own findings. This review of important papers selected from the vast international literature on the subject makes no claim to be comprehensive.

Our approach to the studies presented will be both methodological and historical, since we believe we can show that the formulation of the problem and the results obtained reflect a historical sequence of research concepts. From the early days of psychiatry down to some sections of current psychiatric literature, the interpretation of many research findings about the dangerousness of the mentally ill reflects contemporary concepts as well as the psychiatric theories which these concepts engendered. The agelong recognition which was accorded to some of these theories can hardly be understood without awareness of the historical implications of the manner in which certain scientific methods were applied and interpreted.

In the eighteenth and early nineteenth centuries, the dawning age of psychiatry, little if any interest was shown in the use of quantitative data to confirm relationships and predict risks of illness or violence. On the one hand hopes were pinned on the discovery of organic cerebral defects (Griesinger, Maudsley, Meynert, Wernicke), or of anomalies of skull formation (Lavater, Gall), while on the other hand the aim was to achieve an intuitive or speculative understanding of human nature (Heinroth, Carus, Ideler, and others) which would explain the causes of mental disturbances and of the abnormal behaviour of the mentally ill. Both sides used the case study method which had governed mediaeval medicine and still dominated the later medical scene. But it was not only

professional circles who were interested: there was also an informed and
sensation-hungry public, including men of letters, who in that age of change
and crisis took a lively interest in the unusual individual case. They tried
to find in the criminal a reflection of a human existence that was at once
idealised and called into question, and they looked for this reflection in
the extraordinary fate of an individual and its intricate relationship with
the social and moral conflicts of the time. The question of a clear dividing
line between mentally normal and mentally abnormal offenders was relegated by
many authors to the background. De Pitaval's *Causes célèbres et intéressantes*
(1739) and Von Feuerbach's *Merkwürdige Verbrechen* (1849) report
numerous cases of violent crimes committed by mentally ill offenders, and both
these works constitute striking examples of brilliant case analyses.

In the narrower professional field of forensic or criminal psychiatry
the influence of Lombroso's *Deliquente nato* (1876) was still in evidence.
Pinel's doctrine of monomania, which was energetically championed by Esquirol
(1831), provided an early anthropological theory of the relationship between
mental illness and violence: if due moderation was neglected, strong one-sided
passions could come to dominate life to a dangerous extent. In extreme cases
they exerted an irresistible compulsive pressure upon an individual's confused
consciousness, forcing him to commit violent acts. While this theory, conceived
around the end of the eighteenth and beginning of the nineteenth century, was soon
regarded as out of date, the conviction still persisted that violence on the part
of the mentally ill was just as immediate an outcome of the illness as, for
example, a convulsive attack in epilepsy or St Vitus' dance in chorea. At the
stage when it was still busy collecting material (in fact up to the present
day), psychiatry, fascinated by extraordinary forms of behaviour, by abnormal
experiences and by other signs of madness, compiled a catalogue of psychological phenomena which contains, alongside many important observations, a
large number of items that can more properly be classed as museum specimens.
As reports came to be increasingly restricted to the description of behaviour
and of symptoms, anthropological theories withdrew more into the background.
Theories of mental illness were increasingly based on the concurrence and
course of certain symptoms. In their extreme form (K. Schneider, 1950) such
doctrines offered no explanation or model of the inner relationships between
these symptom clusters, nor was any attempt made to verify the nosological
hypotheses by a statistical study of symptoms.

When we move from the individual case to the general question of
the incidence of violence among the mentally ill, it is not surprising that
the lack of a quantitative methodical approach showed itself clearly in ready

generalisations based on the observation of cases. In the middle of the nineteenth century Karuth published a study of the public dangerousness of the
mentally ill (1845) which affords a good example of the methods and concepts
involved. Early textbooks and handbooks of forensic psychiatry (Krafft-Ebing,
1892; Cramer, 1908; Bumke, 1912; Hübner, 1914) likewise reflect the accepted
and undisputed belief that the mentally ill were violent to a high degree.
Since mental illness - which during the scientific epoch of medicine was
assumed by most psychiatrists to be a form of cerebral disease that still had
to be identified - was at the time regarded as providing an adequate explanation for the violence, conditions were ideal for the development of a general
stereotyped view: the mentally ill, robbed of reason by a mysterious,
inexplicable disease, are unpredictable and constitute a danger to the public.

As a result of this individual case study approach, interest
turned meanwhile to the psychological and psychiatric typology of offenders
and its relationship to various clinical conditions. Examples of this are to
be found in Näcke's analysis of family murders and mental illness (1908) and
Wetzel's paper on mass murderers (1920), both of which are very much
orientated towards criminal psychology. Even Schipkowensky's case studies of
schizophrenia and murder, published in 1938 and regarded until recently as
the standard work on this theme, were still, in so far as the incidence of
violence among the mentally ill was concerned, at the level of unconfirmed
expressions of opinion: it has 'long been known that criminals, especially
murderers, include a significant percentage of individuals who are mentally
ill'.

The real significance of the case study period of research does
not lie in the development of general and authoritative assertions, which
are beyond the scope of its methodology and hypotheses, but in the pursuit of
biographical, psychodynamic and social relationships in the individual case
which later could form the basis of working hypotheses and research plans. A
notable example is provided by Gaupp's reports on the well-known case of
Headmaster Wagner (1914, 1938), who after a few excesses in sodomy, committed
while under the influence of alcohol, believed he was being persecuted and
condemned to destruction by the villagers and finally, years later, killed
nine of them in delusional self-defence.[1] Gaupp's exemplary studies of the
development of a paranoid delusion on the basis of personality, life history
and environmental situation, were of far-reaching significance so far as the
creation of hypotheses was concerned, not only in forensic psychiatry but
also in important areas of clinical psychiatry.

The era of large-scale quantitative surveys
Attempts to provide comprehensive data

The practical question of the measures and procedures required in order to achieve the 'protection of society from the public dangerousness of the mentally ill' (title of a detailed report by Aschaffenburg, 1912), has in modern times become increasingly urgent. In the end this was what led to the abandonment of case studies and typological speculation in favour of a search for empirical data. The populations in which the prevalence of violent mentally abnormal offenders could be calculated consisted of those convicted of violence and those committed to psychiatric institutions because of violent offences. Aschaffenburg, who undertook a study tour of several European countries in order to make as wide a survey as possible, came to the conclusion – a surprising one in view of contemporary beliefs – that 'out of every 50 000 inhabitants of a country, an average of at most one single mentally ill patient should be regarded as actually dangerous'. Statistical comparison of the proportion of dangerous patients in the total patient population of a few large psychiatric institutions in Switzerland, Holland, Baden and Prussia, showed similar low rates, so that Aschaffenburg concluded that the building of special institutions for dangerous abnormal criminals 'was not justified by any pressing need'.

In 1921 Rixen made an estimate of twice this rate, based on very heterogeneous and incomplete psychiatric reports and criminal statistics drawn from several European countries. Drawing attention to the higher rates found in large urban areas, he reported an average rate of 40 'dangerous mentally abnormal persons' per million of the population (Aschaffenburg's estimate was 20 per million). In fact these figures are not very different from the results obtained later using somewhat more reliable methods.

In the planning of epidemiological research programmes – and the question of the incidence of certain crimes among the mentally ill or the prevalence of a combination of mental illness and violence in the total population does fall within the sphere of epidemiological research – it has since been realised that it is necessary to maintain a clear distinction between case-finding and case identification (diagnosis, etc.). The two enquiries by Aschaffenburg (1912) and Rixen (1921), which set out to study the question of prevalence on the basis of clinical opinions, depended so far as diagnosis was concerned on hospital case records and court statistics and, so far as the violence or dangerousness of the offenders was concerned, on legal classifications of crime which to some extent reflected heterogeneous legal standards and rules of jurisprudence. The collection of data was thus affected by uncontrollable selective factors.

As mentioned, case-finding was based essentially on an unrepresentative population, namely a selection from the records of different psychiatric
hospitals and from statistics of convictions in courts whose criteria of
documentation and standards of accuracy no doubt varied. One may nevertheless
conclude that the transition from individual case studies to numerical studies
based on heterogeneous statistics represented a considerable step forward. It
led to the rejection of the idea that the mentally ill were more dangerous than
the rest of the population and to the acceptance of a much lower prevalence rate
for violent offenders. Such studies could not, however, be expected to yield
more precise epidemiological data or provide an answer to detailed questions.

*Studies of cohorts drawn from expert assessments and from
patient records in psychiatric hospitals*

Analyses of expert opinions. It was soon realised that from the
point of view of research there were enormous advantages to be gained from
using restricted samples of patients, defined by unambiguous criteria. The
criteria most commonly used for case-finding were referral for psychiatric
assessment to certain institutions within easily defined time limits, and commit-
ment to a particular psychiatric hospital under Section 42b of the German Penal
Code.[2] A further advantage of studies of this kind carried out on small numbers
is that the research findings and diagnoses have been arrived at in accordance
with relatively uniform methods and criteria, and that detailed documentation
in regard to symptoms and course of illness, as well as demographic and individual social data, make it possible to use the material for testing different
hypotheses.

Natural samples of this kind, however, particularly when they
include minor crimes, are subject to the operation of various selective processes which are of decisive importance when it comes to considering the predictive value of the findings. Bochnik *et al.* (1965), for example, regarded
their statistical analysis of the forensic psychiatric assessments made by the
University Psychiatric Clinic in Hamburg between 1946 and 1961 as throwing
'empirical light on a clinical test sample of the criminal population' and
considered that their material was absolutely 'free from selective bias'. They
overlooked the fact, however, that in the referral, acceptance and rejection
of requests for expert assessment in a particular psychiatric clinic there may
already be some selective factors at work.

In the first place it may be that the request for a psychiatric
assessment made by the prosecutor or the court authority is not based exclusively
on criteria concerned with the crime or the illness. Such requests are likely

to be affected by judicial norms, by High Court decisions, by the opinions of
the prosecuting office and of the judge, which are difficult to control, and
finally by the fact that in criminal proceedings the defence has the right to
request that a particular expert witness be called in. It cannot, moreover, be
ruled out that a request for an expert opinion may be influenced by such factors
as personality traits, social class, etc., which may be some of the factors
that are due to be correlated later with illness rates or offender rates or
other data obtained from the sample.

We have to bear in mind that the influence of such uncontrollable
selective factors may be at its strongest precisely at the point when judges or
prosecutors have to decide whether or not to ask for a psychiatric report in
cases of minor crimes and less serious mental illnesses, such as in particular
the neuroses, personality disorders (psychopathies) and similar states in which
most judges and experts usually consider that Section 51, paras 1 and 2, of the
Penal Code does not apply. We may assume that these factors have relatively
little effect when the charge is a serious one, such as an attempt upon someone's life, or when the mental illness or defect in question is severe and
obvious, as in the case of psychosis or mental deficiency, where it cannot
easily be overlooked and where by legal definition there are valid grounds for
requesting an expert opinion. It may be assumed that if both these criteria
apply, almost every prosecutor and judge will ask for a psychiatric report or
for committal. But here again samples based on assessments made by university
psychiatric clinics are not representative, since in cases of crimes committed
by individuals who are manifestly mentally ill or defective, especially if it
is a second offence, the prosecutor will often order immediate detention in a
state psychiatric hospital. The idea behind this is that any treatment or
committal arising from subsequent proceedings, or from a decision under
Section 51 para 1 that the accused is unfit to plead, can be put into effect
without a transfer being required.

It must also be remembered that the low rates for reporting and
solving certain crimes (e.g. sexual offences and offences against property)
ensure that the number of persons charged and prosecuted, and hence the
statistics of Federal convictions, forms a fairly unreliable selection of the
total number of actual offenders in the population as a whole. So far as our
own enquiry is concerned, we must bear in mind the possibility that for the
mentally ill and the mentally defective the rate for solving crimes and bringing charges may be higher than for the mentally healthy and the more
intelligent, just because our subjects are on the whole less successful in
planning crimes and covering their tracks. The only crimes in which this

objection can with some justification be ignored are those which may be
assumed to have a smaller dark figure (see note 1) and a higher rate
of detection.

In judging whether the case material of a psychiatric hospital is
representative at least of a given geographical area or judicial circuit, we
must also consider, in addition to the above objections, that requests by the
courts for psychiatric reports are often made chiefly to certain experts and
particularly to the directors of university clinics. In the selection of cases
special expertise often plays a part, as well as the reputation of the expert
in question, and this often leads to his being given the task 'in special
cases' of furnishing such reports to prosecutors, courts and counsel from
other parts of the GFR. The regional allocation of requests to university
clinics, regional mental hospitals, institutes of forensic medicine, retired
consultants or consultants attached to the courts (as, for example, in
Bavaria and the Palatinate) depends on very varying factors which are hard
to assess. In addition the normal case material of a psychiatric clinic shows
a diagnostic bias which, according to studies by Häfner, Cesarino &
Cesarino-Krantz (1967) at the Psychiatric Clinics of Freiburg and Heidelberg,
and Bochnik (1961) at the University Psychiatric Clinic of Hamburg, was at
least in these instances influenced clearly by the director of the clinic.
Reports which are countersigned personally by the director or his deputy –
a rule that applied in almost all university clinics at the time of our investigation – are likely to be more strongly affected in this way and to show a
more uniform diagnostic classification than that applied to patients who are
admitted routinely for treatment.

Studies of the case material of psychiatric clinics in the German-
speaking world include those of Maier (1931) and Brack-Kletzhändler (1954) at
the University Psychiatric Clinic in Zurich, Wanner's work (1954) at the
Institute for Psychiatric Treatment and Care at Münsingen in the canton of
Bern, and the survey by Bochnik *et al.*(1965) at the University Psychiatric
Clinic of Hamburg which we have already mentioned.

Maier's material consisted of 1247 psychiatric assessments prepared
over a quarter of a century, from 1905 to 1929, in the Zurich clinic. Among
them he found 967 mentally defective, mentally ill or psychopathic individuals
who were of diminished responsibility or unfit to plead. They included 121
offenders (86 men and 35 women) who had committed crimes 'against life and
health'. As no more precise description of the crime was given, no comparison
with our own material is possible. The proportion of mentally ill offenders
'against life and health' was 12.5% of the total number who over 25 years were
assessed as completely or partly irresponsible for their actions – a figure

which, for the methodological reasons we have already discussed, is not
representative.

The assessments prepared in the same clinic between 1942 and 1950
were studied by Brack-Kletzhändler (1954). Among 1018 mentally ill, mentally
defective or psychopathic individuals assessed for penal purposes he found 118
cases (11.6% of the total material) of 'crime against life and limb' which
included manslaughter and homicide, murder, infanticide and abortion, as well
as manslaughter resulting from negligence, bodily harm, robbery, assault and
threatening behaviour. Homicidal crimes in the narrower sense (including
attempted homicide and manslaughter as a result of negligence) was recorded
in 55 cases, or 5.4% of the total material.

Wanner (1954) examined 2482 psychiatric assessments prepared over
more than half a century, from 1896 to 1952, in the Bernese Institute for
Psychiatric Treatment and Care at Münsingen. He paid particular attention to
crimes committed by schizophrenics. Crimes against life - defined according
to Articles 111 to 126 of the Swiss Penal Code[3] - were committed by 294
offenders, of whom 29 were considered to be mentally normal. This left 265
violent offenders who were mentally ill, mentally defective or psychopathic,
representing 10.6% of the original material: unlike Brack-Kletzhändler, he did
not include robbery and threatening behaviour.

It should nevertheless be noted that the ratio of mentally ill
violent offenders to other mentally ill offenders, even defined in this
unfortunately somewhat varied and imprecise way, is of the same order in all
three Swiss studies. One reason for this presumably lies in the relatively
uniform procedures followed in Swiss legal practice so far as requests for
psychiatric assessment are concerned, another factor possibly being that the
hospitals studied had a regional monopoly of such requests.

Bochnik *et al.* (1965) carried out a statistical analysis of the
376 convicted criminals (329 men and 47 women) examined in the Psychiatric
Clinic of the University of Hamburg between 1946 and 1961. The rubric
'killing and violence', comprising murder, manslaughter and attempted homicide, extended suicide and all forms of bodily harm, applied to 69 male
offenders. This figure included none convicted of manslaughter as a result
of negligence. Sixteen were judged to have full criminal responsibility,
leaving 53 violent offenders who were mentally ill, mentally defective or
psychopathic (according to the broad definitions used in this study), that
is to say, 16.1% of the male offenders examined. Among the women the authors
found 14 violent offenders, but no details are given as to their degree of
criminal responsibility.

The study by Bochnik *et al.* is superior to most comparable investigations because its use of statistical methods reached a very much higher
standard. But the methodological problems inherent in such investigations are
still evident. Since their source material is very probably not representative
of the total population of mentally abnormal offenders, the predictive value
of their incidence rates, their risk factors and the findings obtained from
factorial analysis of their data apply strictly to their own material only.

*Studies of mentally abnormal offenders based on those committed to psychiatric
hospitals.* The second category of populations which are easily available but
incomplete consists of those mentally ill or mentally defective offenders who
are committed to regional hospitals. The material obtained in this way is
more representative, since the forensic assessments made are subject to fewer
important selective factors. The decision process leading to legal committal
is, however, open to other selective influences which are difficult to control.
Since the decision whether or not to apply the relevant Section 51, para 1 or
2, is based principally on considerations of public safety and propriety, the
judge is allowed a good deal of latitude. Here again, too, we have to remember
that when the crime is serious and the degree of mental abnormality severe,
decisions will be relatively uniform in that the offenders will be committed
at least on a temporary basis; but where the offence is more trivial and the
mental disorder less severe, many uncontrollable factors affect the decision
regarding committal and thus affect also the composition of the group of
committed offenders. In addition, and this is not least in importance, there
are some crimes, such as sexual offences, in which culture and attitudes
play a part in the assessment of their dangerousness to public safety and
morals. In the case of minor offences we frequently encountered low rates of
recording and detection, and when there were lesser degrees of abnormality
we came to expect a high rate of unrecorded illness, and discordance among
experts in regard to diagnosis and assessment. In these categories the
predictive value of findings based upon committed offenders is therefore
relatively small. Where studies are based on serious cases, in which the
committal criteria are clear, as for example in acts of violence by
individuals suffering from manifest mental illness or showing a considerable
degree of mental defect, the findings may be assumed to be much more reliable.
An example of one study of this kind is Müller and Hadamik's
(1966) investigation of 675 persons committed under Section 42b of the Penal
Code on a particular day (17 May 1964).[4] As this report was based on six
regional hospitals in the Rhineland, it is more reliable than studies based

on a single hospital, in which a stronger local selective bias is to be expected.

The authors coded their 675 subjects by age, sex and diagnosis, degree of responsibility, and previous convictions. In addition they recorded special incidents such as attempted escape and outbursts of violence during their stay in the institution: we shall be returning to this point later. The rubric 'crimes of violence' - which was not defined in detail by the authors - was assigned to 80 individuals diagnosed as mentally deficient, mentally ill or psychopathic, representing 11.8% of all those committed to hospital on that day. After discarding six cases in which the preliminary diagnosis was drug abuse or psychopathy, the authors were left with 74, or 10.9%, mentally ill or mentally defective violent offenders. Although the population on which this ratio of violent offenders was based was assembled on criteria which differed from those used in studies of forensic psychiatric assessments, the ratio is still of the same order.

Quantitative analyses of motives and comparable inter-relationships

While in earlier typological case studies interest centred on characteristic symptoms and unusual modes of behaviour, or on the significance of aetiological factors and generalisations derived from them, the works just quoted are noteworthy rather for their attempt to arrive at quantitative data about the risk of violence in the mentally ill, about risk factors attached to particular illnesses, and other similar problems. There is a third group of studies which tried to combine these two approaches.

The thorough investigation of smaller groups, accompanied by quantitative analysis of data obtained usually in free psychiatric interviews, cannot of course yield reliable results if the groups in question are too small. Many such enquiries are still of considerable value, however, because the depth of their questioning reveals possible relationships or trends from which important working hypotheses may be derived that can then be subjected to quantitative testing.

Lanzkron (1963), whose study of murder and insanity was noteworthy for the precise criteria applied to the crime, examined 150 murderers whose mental state was abnormal and who had been examined in the Psychiatric State Hospital of Matteawan, Beacon, New York, between 1956 and 1961. (The concept of 'murder' is not used here in the sense in which it is used in the German Penal Code but in a comprehensive sense that corresponds to the American Penal Code and includes all homicides committed with murderous intent.) The group was thus based on official psychiatric assessments required by the

prosecuting authorities. Lanzkron found that in the unusually high proportion
of 40% of the cases the crime was the direct result of a delusion (paranoid
group). A further 32.6% of the offenders were mentally ill persons who either
had acted from motives or under circumstances which applied also to murderers
judged to be of sound mind (for example, rage, revenge or jealousy) or had
committed murder in a 'paroxysm of insanity' which could not be clearly
distinguished from severe excitement or emotional crisis in persons of sound
mind. The remaining 27.3% of the offenders who had committed their crimes out
of revenge, anger or jealousy, or in association with motives of sex or
personal gain, did not become ill until after the crime. In these cases the
diagnosis was usually 'psychosis in psychopathic personality'. The findings
in this study reveal a contrast between various groups of motives observed
on the one hand in offenders of sound mind and some mentally ill offenders,
and on the other hand in certain groups of insane offenders. In evaluating
the findings we must bear in mind that the diagnostic criteria used by.
Lanzkron were those of the *American Psychiatric Association's Diagnostic and
Statistical Manual*,[5] which differ in some respects from the diagnostic
scales used by German workers that are based largely on the so-called Würzburg
Schema.

Psychodynamic or psychoanalytical models, with their deep
studies of personality development, motivation, personality structure and
dynamic regulation of behaviour, have naturally been used mainly with
mentally disturbed offenders who were not mentally defective or insane in
the narrower sense.

Tanay's study (1969) is one of many such comparable investigations and was carried out on 53 murderers whom he interviewed in the decade
between 1958 and 1968. They were referred to him for assessment by attorneys
and examining judges and conformed to no strict criteria of selection. The
number of insane murderers was relatively low (7) and all of them were
suffering from schizophrenic psychosis. The most interesting feature of
Tanay's enquiry concerns 37 individuals in whom he found a personality
disturbance of the 'dissociative type' and whose crimes he viewed as
'dissociative reactions'. He understood this to cover personalities which,
under normal conditions of stress, function at an adequate level of integration but which at the time of the crime had developed a state of altered
consciousness as a result of various stress factors. Using the analytical
model as an analogy, Tanay interprets this process as the result of tension
between strong instinctive desires and too powerful a super-ego - a tension
which the ego is unable to tolerate. In the dissociative reaction which

results, the instinctive desire splits off and is no longer under the control
of the ego. Tanay considered that in 36 of the 37 dissociative reactions he
described, the individual had shown a strict, excessively rigid super-ego.
Apart from the great difficulties entailed in making assessments of this kind
objectively, the criticism must be made that the advantages of differentiation
and depth that are inherent in psychodynamic hypotheses concerning criminal
behaviour and morbid processes must be lost if we limit ourselves to such
general and non-specific interpretations and stereotypes.

The epidemiological era

Empirical enquiries carried out in order to obtain reliable data
on the frequency of certain characteristics among those arrested within a
defined population, fall within the province of epidemiology. Looked at in
this way, some of the studies mentioned above and carried out in the first
decades of this century can, in terms of their research strategy, be called
epidemiological: for example the outstanding enquiries by Aschaffenburg and
Rixen. Both these investigations were, in the light of then-current knowledge,
careful and wide-ranging attempts at total coverage. The conclusions reached
are not so far removed from those of a more recent date based on methodologically
more carefully devised and more thorough studies. There is, however, one
important difference, namely that the earlier investigators did not have at
their disposal the methodological knowledge and tools which psychiatric
epidemiology has partly fashioned for itself in comprehensive field studies,
particularly in the 1950s and 1960s (e.g. Dohrenwend & Dohrenwend, 1965;
Prince, 1966; Reid, 1966; Klee *et al.* 1967; Weinberg, 1967; Adelstein *et al.*
1968; Walsh, 1969; Levy & Rowitz, 1970). Between the two eras of quantitative
investigations and epidemiological studies which we have outlined there is
therefore not a sharp division but rather a transition which has been inter-
mittent in its progress and has certainly not yet ended.

One of the most important methods of conducting epidemiological
studies in the area of psychiatry with which we are concerned is the
comprehensive survey. Such surveys cover the entire population. They must
therefore as a rule be planned as field studies in the broadest sense, and
in method and approach must first and foremost be capable of producing basic
data such as morbidity risks, prevalence rates, incidence rates, and the
overall relationships of all these to demographic data and social factors
(Mechanic, 1970). Studies of representative samples of the whole are usually
equally valuable, provided the individual categories are of adequate size.
They are especially necessary and useful when large populations are being

studied. Enquiries of this kind in the field of general psychiatric epidemiology may vary a great deal in their hypotheses and methods; examples include
studies carried out by Leighton *et al.* (1963) in Canada (Stirling County
Study), Srole *et al.* (1962) in New York (Manhattan Midtown Study), and
Juel-Nielsen & Strömgren (1962) in Denmark, to mention only a few. They
have provided information about the frequency of mental illness in the
general population of Western countries and have created at least a basis of
comparison which enables us to assess the relative frequency of mentally
abnormal violent offenders.

When epidemiological enquiries turn to the deeper problems of
identifying risk factors, or testing individual hypotheses and in particular
aetiological models, more and more precise investigations are required which
can be carried out only on smaller numbers. It is then of decisive importance
that the material studied be representative of the whole population. Comparison
of sample groups with the population as a whole and with matched groups
selected according to analogous criteria (matched pairs, etc.) and varying
only in respect of one characteristic (e.g. violent offenders who are insane
compared with non-offenders who are insane), or division of the research group
into subgroups, provide an opportunity for statistical testing of individual
hypotheses. When formulating hypotheses for testing it is, of course, very
important to consider the population from which the research group and the
control group are drawn: for example, comparison between a mentally abnormal
group who are also violent offenders and a mentally abnormal group who are
not violent offenders allows us to test hypotheses about the positive and
negative influence of various forms of illness on the risk of violence, but
would not allow us to predict the general frequency of violence among the
mentally ill.

For practical reasons general epidemiological surveys are almost
always retrospective, which is often true also of group comparisons. This
means that, starting with our index of cases, we must then obtain information from the past: details of the crime, family data, personal history,
earlier stress factors, etc. The reliability of such retrospective data
naturally varies considerably. Reliable data include those which may be
assumed to have been clearly and fully recorded, such as marriage or admission
to hospital. Data that are likely to be less trustworthy include, for
example, those which depend on memory, and particularly those which depend
entirely on the proband's own judgement. The predictive value of retrospective studies is very limited, in so far as they concern the identification
and evaluation of the risk factors that are based on such unreliable data.

Prospective studies offer one of the best ways of solving these methodological difficulties. They make it possible to examine a population at risk, using standardised techniques and methods of measurement, to formulate predictions and to test them against the findings of a subsequent investigation in which the same techniques are used. The expected risk of occurrence of the item under investigation, for example the onset of mental illness or committal of an act of violence, must be relatively high in the group that is being studied, so that it is possible to arrive at statistically significant correlations with the variables in question and so that the research plan may be kept within reasonably manageable limits. These requirements must of course be borne in mind when selecting research populations for prospective studies on our theme: Suitable groups with a high risk of violence are, for example, violent offenders who have served their sentence but have a high risk of committing further crimes, mentally abnormal individuals who have threatened violence, and so on. The number of people who meet such criteria is not, under a well-ordered legal system, high and if we are dealing with homicide the same may be said of the very small number of violent offenders who are insane and who relapse into further violence. The range of possible hypotheses that can be tested in prospective studies is therefore very limited. But their value, especially so far as the testing of aetiologically significant hypotheses is concerned, should not be underestimated.

Like retrospective studies, prospective epidemiological investigations may be exploited further by dividing the material into subgroups or by comparing it with a group that differs in respect of one or more important variables (for example by comparing a cohort of violent offenders who are mentally ill with a cohort of violent offenders who are of sound mind). Where aetiological hypotheses are concerned, the comparison of cohorts affords an invaluable opportunity of making experimental changes in individual variables. By using certain therapeutic techniques or social measures we can, for example, study their effect on the risk of violence or of relapse into violence. But given a group with a high risk of future violence it is on ethical grounds hard to imagine the possibility of obtaining a matched group of individuals showing the same risk of future violence, and withholding from them for experimental purposes some hopeful measure of prevention.

Rappeport & Lassen (1965, 1966) carried out a comparative study of psychologically disturbed and mentally ill violent offenders which used epidemiological methods in the narrow sense and came near to being a comprehensive survey. It was a retrospective longitudinal study of a representative population at risk: a group of 708 men and 639 women (all

the patients discharged from the state mental hospitals of Maryland in 1947)
and a second group of 2152 men and 2129 women (all the patients discharged
from the same institutions in 1957) were compared for 'incidence of arrest'
for murder, manslaughter, rape, robbery and serious assault of other kinds
during two five-year periods before and after discharge from hospital. The
results were compared with analogous figures for the general population of
the state of Maryland. The only crime for which the group from the psychiatric
hospitals showed a higher incidence of arrest than the general population was
that of robbery. In everything else the criminality of the men who had been
patients in mental hospitals reflected exactly the criminal trends found in
the general population. So far as the women were concerned, it was only for
'aggravated assault' that those who had been in-patients showed a higher
incidence of arrest than women in the general population.

In evaluating these findings we must remember that only a limited
proportion of the mentally ill are admitted to mental hospitals (Freming,
1947; Bremer, 1951). Since an important reason for admission into the state
mental hospitals lies in the burden, worry and danger which the patient's
behaviour is likely to cause, aggressive patients presumably stood more chance
of being sent to hospital than non-aggressive patients. The likelihood of a
mentally sick individual becoming an in-patient in a state institution under
the system of care prevailing at that time in the USA was presumably affected
to some extent by the degree of deviancy in his behaviour. Nevertheless the
authors found that, apart from the two instances already mentioned, there
were no significant differences in the incidence of arrest for other crimes
between the pre-admission period and the post-discharge period, or between
the research cohort and the general public.

A prospective study of 100 in-patients - 55 men and 45 women
aged from 11 to 83 years, of whom 95 belonged to White races - was reported by
Macdonald in 1963. The group consisted of patients admitted over a 15-month
period to the Colorado Psychopathic Hospital because of threats to commit
murder. It could be assumed that these individuals showed a high risk of
violence. Exactly half of them were classed as psychotic (functional and
exogenous psychoses), the rest as suffering from neuroses and character
disorders. There was little previous history of criminal offences, and only
one person had previously been found guilty of homicide.

The reality underlying these threats was demonstrated in 1966 when a
student from Texas translated into action the threats of which he had already
spoken to the psychiatrist treating him, climbed the tower of the university building in Austin and shot several complete strangers with a hunting

rifle. After a period of five to six years Macdonald re-examined his cohort of patients who had threatened murder, but was unable to trace 25 of the original group. Three (two men and one woman, all under 30 years of age) had in the intervening period actually killed someone. One of the men was diagnosed as a sociopath, the other as a paranoid personality, and the woman as a paranoid schizophrenic. In two of these three cases the threat had been made against the person who later was killed. Four other men from the original group (two schizophrenics aged under 25 and two brain-damaged patients aged over 65) had committed suicide. The low number of offenders in this high-risk group limits the possibilities of predictive statistical evaluation and exemplifies the great difficulties in prospective studies in our field.

In his second study (1967) Macdonald compared three samples of 20 subjects each, drawn from his research cohort, from mentally ill patients from the same hospital who had never threatened homicide, and from the inmates of a penitentiary who had been found guilty of homicide. He had already formed the impression, from his retrospective study of 100 homicidal offenders (1963), that a history of severe parental cruelty and extreme maternal 'seduction', together with a history of arson, cruelty to animals and bedwetting in childhood, increased the risk of violence. Statistical analysis of the three groups revealed a further series of factors which increased the risk of homicidal violence:

1. Male sex, and age between 20 and 40 years. Blacks had
   a higher homicidal rate than Whites.
2. Psychotic depressions, acute schizophrenic reactions
   or delirium. Sociopaths and passive-aggressive personalities with poor self-control.
3. Every form of threat to kill, especially if conditions
   were attached (for example, 'If you ever leave me, I
   will kill you').
4. Obtaining weapons beforehand, or the existence of
   carefully laid plans.
5. Previous homicidal acts.
6. Previous incidents of bodily harm or forcible restraint.
7. Unsuccessful suicide attempts.
8. Death of a near friend or relative; loss of job;
   unfaithfulness on the part of spouse or threat of
   separation from spouse; wife's pregnancy.
9. Lack of family help in crisis situations.
10. Extremely provocative behaviour on the part of the
    victim. Threats against children. Macdonald pays
    particular attention to this point of the role of the victim.

These findings should be regarded with caution, since the groups studied by Macdonald are very small and the number of cases, especially in relation to the number of categories to which they are assigned, is far too small.

Following on the increase in capital offences in the USA, Guze *et al.* (1962, 1969) carried out several studies in Washington, Missouri, on the relationship between criminal behaviour and mental disorders. The first publication (1962) arising from their prospective study described the cohorts investigated: 223 men, of whom 27% were Black, who had been found guilty of a capital offence and whose cases had come before the Missouri Board of Probation and Parole. The group was made up of 46 probationers, 75 parolees, and 102 'flat-timers' (prisoners about to be discharged). The authors considered that their study thus covered representative groups of male violent offenders who might be expected to show a relatively high risk of repeating their offence. [6]

Since the capital offences were not broken down into different categories such as criminal homicide, attempted homicide, attempted murder, etc., it is hardly possible to compare their findings with our own.

In 1969 Guze, Goodwin & Crane reported their follow-up investigation, carried out on the same cohort after a period of eight to nine years. They were able personally to interview 176 of the original 223 subjects (a success rate of 78.9%). In addition to a thorough exploration of numerous factors relating to personality, profession and family, 519 close relatives were also subjected to a similar careful study. The main finding was that sociopathy, alcoholism and drug dependence were the forms of mental disorder most frequently associated with violent crimes. On the other hand the writers found that schizophrenia, manic-depressive illness and organic cerebral disease - that is to say mental illnesses in the narrower sense - were not more frequent in capital offenders than in the general population, nor were neuroses and homosexuality.

To conclude this historical survey it seems permissible to say that in the studies reviewed a certain trend may be discerned. That is, writers of the case-study era were almost always convinced that there is a close connection between mental illness and violent crime and assumed high rates of crime among the mentally ill. But findings of quantitative and particularly epidemiological research tended more and more to show that the incidence of violent offences in the mentally ill does not differ greatly from similar incidence in those who are of sound mind. This cautious formulation is borne out by the fact that in spite of methodological differences the results of numerous studies are so much in agreement. The view that there is a close connection between mental illness and violent crime, together with the

incomplete theories which stem from this view and which we still find to
some extent represented in psychiatric teaching today, must cause us
concern: such a view is based on the widespread prejudice which was to be
found in many case studies and which is being carried forward and even re-
affirmed today.

In the sections which follow we shall try to discover whether
there exist in the literature any data about differential risks for the main
group of mental illnesses.

2.2 Relationships between individual groups of illnesses and violent crime

The schizophrenias

The group of schizophrenias, whose lifetime morbidity risk in most
regions studied is around 1% of the general population, whose prevalence (ratio of
manifest cases to the total population) in Western cultures is around 0.3%,
and which in the same countries accounts for 20-40% of all hospital bed capacity, was from early times considered to stand in a particularly close relationship with crimes of violence.

In the older textbooks of clinical psychiatry and particularly of
forensic psychiatry, the concept of the incalculable dangerousness of the 'insane'
or of patients with 'dementia praecox' (two older synonyms for the group of
schizophrenias) was usually forcefully expressed and illustrated by impressive
case reports. Even in the second edition of the treatise on forensic psychiatry
by Hoche (1934), Lange spoke of the 'dullness of affect' which characterised
even the milder cases of schizophrenia and 'made such patients liable to commit
serious crimes, especially crimes against life and limb'. Even the disturbances
and deviations of personality found among the relatives of schizophrenics, who
on the assumption that there was a uniform hereditary predisposition to schizophrenia were called schizoid or heboid, were held to be dangerous and to
constitute a high-risk group in regard to violence. If we bear in mind this
widespread doctrine in German psychiatry, which naturally was reflected in a
generalised and simplified form in the stereotyped attitudes of society as a
whole, we can well understand why so many psychiatrists and informed laymen were
prepared to support the introduction of laws that aimed at preventing the propaga-
tion of such disorders by enforcing compulsory sterilisation.

Even after Stumpfl (1935) had reported that in his family studies
(which in accordance with the psychiatric orientation of that time were called
'studies of biological inheritance') he found no quantitative or real relationship between crime and psychosis, and Birnbaum (1926, 1931) had said that

there were no good reasons for assuming that schizophrenics were basically more
likely to show higher criminal tendencies, many authors still clung to the
traditional ideas. Schipkowensky (1938), for example, in the study already
quoted, investigated 15 schizophrenic murderers and tried to develop a typology
for the schizophrenic murder. He came to the conclusion, which had far-reaching
implications, that a schizophrenic process alone can 'of itself' lead to
criminal behaviour.

Stereotyped opinions, even if they take the form of scientific
doctrine, tend to become generalised and this is usually accompanied by a shift
in interpretation and by the incorporation of material from other disciplines.
This rule of social psychology probably explains the historical development of
a subsidiary theory which was derived from the above general doctrine. From
about the turn of the century onwards, a series of psychiatric studies appeared
(for example von Wyss, 1912; Birnbaum, 1926; Mikorey & Mezger, 1936), which were
to a large extent based on the examination of violent offenders who had shown
no sign of mental illness before or at the time of their crime. Since a proportion of these offenders later developed a so-called 'prison psychosis', it was
assumed that this mental illness, which was frequently schizophrenic in nature,
had been an immediate cause of the crime. The act of violence was thus seen as
the first symptom of a smouldering psychotic process which could not be detected
at the time of the crime but which later came to full and characteristic fruition.

Wilmanns (1940) moulded this theory into a sizeable treatise on
'Murder in the Prodromal Stage of Schizophrenia', which was based on an impressive
documentation of 18 cases. To prove the validity of his thesis he quoted the
experiences of several prison medical officers (Többen, 1913; Lumpp, 1913;
Viernstein, 1914) and finally invoked the then-current argument that there was
a preponderance of schizophrenics among those convicted of violent crimes. Thus
Rüdin (1909), for example, had assumed, without seeking the confirmation of
empirical data, that the number of prisoners who developed 'manifest schizophrenia' during life imprisonment was 'abnormally high'. In support of his
opinion Wilmanns also quoted Pinto de Toledo (1934) who found 44 murderers
among 52 prisoners in Portugal who had developed prison psychoses within the
first two years of their sentence. Nearly three-quarters of the 44 were
diagnosed as schizophrenic. Wilmanns had no doubt that most of these mentally
ill prisoners had committed their crime in the prodromal stage of a schizophrenic illness.[7]

By 1941 Bürger-Prinz was already criticising Wilmanns' inadmissible
extension of the diagnosis of schizophrenia. A typical prison psychosis,
which is the most frequent form of psychosis whose first manifestation occurs

during a prison sentence, is moreover different from schizophrenia in respect
of both symptoms and course. Prison psychosis came to be regarded unambiguously
as a psychogenic psychosis and as belonging to the hysterical forms of illness
(Pauleikhoff, 1957). In evaluating the very high incidence of 'prison psychosis'
found by Pinto de Toledo we must bear in mind that his material was highly
selective and that his diagnosis of schizophrenia was extremely broad. Nor
should it be overlooked that homicidal offences are usually liable to incur
long sentences or life imprisonment. The resultant psychological stress and the
prison milieu are factors which may be assumed to increase considerably the risk
of developing a prison psychosis. We cannot either exclude, in regard to the
Portuguese study, the effect of a cultural factor and of current Portuguese
forms of punishment on the patterns of behaviour shown by the prisoners.

This view gains in probability when we look at the work of the
Swiss psychiatrists Wyrsch (1947) and Dukor (1949), though their observations
were not systematic. During three years in which he acted as consultant to the
prison service in the canton of Bern, Wyrsch found no more than 2% of prisoners
who suffered from insanity in the narrower sense - a figure which is comparable
to analogous rates for the general population. Dukor, after ten years as
consultant to the prison service of the canton of Basel, formed the impression
that it was 'on the whole rather unusual to have to declare that a detainee was
insane in the narrower sense' (quoted by Schröder, 1952).

Data on the relative frequency of schizophrenia found among limited
samples of mentally ill offenders either on forensic assessment or on committal
may be extracted from some of the studies which we have already mentioned in a
different connection.

H.W.Maier (1931), who examined the case material of the University
Psychiatric Clinic of Zurich between 1905 and 1929, found 967 patients who were
judged to be of diminished responsibility or unfit to plead. Of these 249, or
approximately 26%, were schizophrenic. Thirty-four per cent of them (25 men and
9 women), or approximately 14% of the schizophrenics, had committed crimes
against the life or health of their victims. Following the then-current opinion,
Maier concluded that the schizophrenics 'would be the most frequent criminal
offenders', a prediction which, as already explained in another context, cannot
be justified on the basis of this far from representative material. Moreover,
schizophrenia headed the list of diagnoses in Maier's material only when those
unfit to plead were considered: at that time the presence of schizophrenia made
such a forensic decision almost obligatory (cf. Schneider, 1956).

The justness of our methodological criticisms of Maier's (1931)
study, and of studies based on limited material in general, becomes clear if

we compare his results with those of Wanner's (1954) investigation carried out at the Institute for Treatment and Care, Munsingen, Bern. Among 2482 criminals, 168 or 7.7% were schizophrenic, which is less than one-third of the rate reported by Maier.[8] Wanner noted that in comparison with the other diagnostic categories the schizophrenic offenders tended to commit serious crimes of aggression (against life and limb 19%, arson about 15%) and aggressive offences in general such as defamatory attacks, abuse and threats. Attempts on life were recorded in 38 schizophrenics (35 men and 3 women): 11 were fatal, 8 were cases of attempted homicide, 18 of bodily harm, and 1 of infanticide. If we compare these figures with the figure of 18 aggressive acts by women, only three of which were 'against life', the rest being abuse or arson, the relationship between male sex and violent crimes against life becomes clear. Wanner also pointed out the relative frequency of the subgroup of 'paranoid' schizophrenics (82, or 48% of the 168 schizophrenic offenders) and their particular tendency to use threats and assaultive behaviour.

Brack-Kletzhändler (1954), studying 1018 psychiatric assessments made at the Zurich clinic, tried to arrive at the order of frequency with which different groups of patients committed different crimes: in his material schizophrenics formed the fourth largest group (100, or 9.8% of the total). Looking at cases of aggression as a whole, schizophrenics figured more frequently than in the total sample - 23% as opposed to 9.8%. In cases of criminal homicide they came third on the list, after personality disorders and mental deficiency. They ranked very low in crimes against property, but in the category of minor aggressive offences - bodily harm, assault, threats, maltreatment, robbery - they again came at the top of the list.

Ichiba (1960), who examined 56 schizophrenic criminals committed to the Psychiatric Hospital of Matsuzawa, Tokyo, found a high proportion of aggressive offenders among them (approximately 30%).

Kloek (1964) examined 500 successive admissions to the psychiatric observation centre of a Dutch penal institution.[9] In 30 cases, all of them male, schizophrenia was suspected, and in half of these the diagnosis was considered to be probable. A firm diagnosis of schizophrenia was recorded only in one case of homicide. This study, too, clearly shows that in such samples the classification of the crime, as well as the diagnosis selected, depends on local and national influences.

In their above-mentioned analysis of cases referred for assessment to the University Psychiatric Clinic of Hamburg, Bochnik *et al.* (1965) found a diagnosis of 'endogenous psychosis' in only 12 cases of mentally abnormal violent offenders: no further diagnostic breakdown is given.

H.W. Müller & Hadamik (1966) investigated 675 mentally abnormal offenders and found that schizophrenics, with 27% easily headed the list of crimes of violence (45 out of 164 in this group), but this must be viewed within the context of the special selection procedures on which samples of this kind are based and which cause serious mental illnesses to be over-represented.[10]

Some information on the risk of crime in schizophrenics, at least under the quasi-experimental conditions of a milieu that fulfils many of the criteria of a total institution in Goffman's sense (1961), is given in the study we have already mentioned by Müller & Hadamik of violent attacks by patients on hospital staff and fellow-patients. The authors found 64 patients (39% of the 164 schizophrenics committed) who had at one time or another made violent attacks against their institutional environment. The mentally defective group, compulsorily admitted because of their dangerousness to public safety or because of offensive behaviour under Section 42b of the Penal Code, was actively involved in violence within the hospital in 100 cases (32%) of the 311 relevant patients.

Stierlin (1956) reported that of 773 violent incidents recorded in psychiatric hospitals in Germany, Austria and Switzerland, 462, or approximately 60%, were committed by patients diagnosed as schizophrenic. Even these high rates of violence among schizophrenic in-patients, however, provide no reliable evidence that there is a higher risk of violence in schizophrenics than in other diagnostic groups. As Stierlin himself pointed out, the proportion of in-patients diagnosed as schizophrenic in the various institutions at the time of his investigation was of roughly the same order: his figure for München-Haar (1945, around 4000 beds) is 55% and for Basel-Friedmatt (Staehelin, 1949) 50%. It must be remembered that Stierlin set no time limit for his study and his case-finding depended mainly on the memory of the doctors interviewed, which means that the results, in so far as the involvement of schizophrenics was concerned, could be affected by selective factors beyond his control, for example by prevailing attitudes. Müller & Hadamik, who based their material on one particular day, did not make any allowance for differences in the average length of stay, which probably varied from one diagnostic group to another. Nevertheless in their study, too, the rate of aggression in schizophrenics was 39%, as against a proportion of 34% schizophrenics in the total population studied. This study may be regarded as exemplifying the difficulties of interpreting such incomplete data: the diagnostic groups in question could not be kept constant in regard to social factors affecting compulsory detention, and depending on hospital milieu, duration of committal, chances of release etc., so that

differences in modes of reaction depending on personality and age, and on
factors specific to the illness, could not possibly be detected.

If one compares a sample of patients derived from psychiatric
assessments with a sample of those committed to hospital, one finds that
violent patients diagnosed as schizophrenic are much more frequent among
those committed. The explanation for this difference, however, may lie in the
fact that schizophrenic patients are more frequently sent to mental hospitals,
whether they have committed acts of violence or not, rather than in any
assumption that violent acts are more frequent among schizophrenics than among
other groups of the mentally ill. The proportion of schizophrenic patients who
have not committed any crime and who have been admitted for treatment only to
one of the regional mental hospitals in the GFR is of a similar order, namely
between 25 and 50% of the total patient population. [11]

Thus while still within the bounds of possibility, the assumption
that schizophrenics show a more marked tendency to violence than other
diagnostic groups cannot, in the light of the empirical studies we have
mentioned, be accorded a high degree of probability.

Delusion as a special risk

Several authors (Gross, 1936; Wanner, 1954; Stierlin, 1956;
Janzarik, 1956; Mowat, 1966) still put forward the view that delusional schizophrenics tend to commit very serious and terrible capital offences, a thesis
which has its historical roots in Esquirol's 'homicidal mania' and in Krafft-
Ebing's 'delusional murderers'. Stierlin, for example, pointed out that among
the 53 premeditated and apparently unprovoked acts of violence reported in his
enquiry, 29 were committed by patients suffering from delusions. Janzarik and
Mowat, as well as earlier writers such as Stransky (1904-5) and Moravcsik
(1907-8) give impressive accounts of individual cases of deluded patients who,
after suffering for a long time from delusions of persecution or jealousy,
committed acts of violence which took everyone by surprise. The classical
example which modern psychiatrists would regard as a case of paranoid delusional
development rather than of core-schizophrenia, is that of the Headmaster
Wagner, described in great detail by Gaupp (1914).

There have been no quantitative studies which would help us to
decide whether the risk of serious and terrible crimes of violence is greater
in individuals suffering from paranoia than in the population as a whole. An
unbiased perusal of the literature of forensic psychiatry leaves one with the
impression that the more unusual and extreme cases of violent crimes by paranoid individuals, particularly if they involve multiple murders, are discussed

all over the world for decades, thus achieving undue prominence in the
literature as compared with similar crimes committed by individuals of sound
mind, which happen on the international scale with disturbing frequency and
yet seem to slip more quickly into psychiatric as well as lay oblivion.

It is still noteworthy, however, that paranoia and paranoid-
delusional schizophrenia accounted for a relatively high proportion of the
mentally abnormal violent offenders studied by various investigators. Wanner
(1954), for example, reports that in his Münsinger forensic assessments he
found 25 delusional patients out of 38 violent schizophrenics, and Lanzkron
(1963) found delusional symptoms in 40% of his mentally abnormal offenders
with various diagnoses, all of whom had committed homicide. He considered
that persistent delusions occurring in so-called involutional psychoses
indicated a particularly high risk of violence. Mowat (1966), using material
from Broadmoor in England for his retrospective study of morbid jealousy and
murder, found an association between delusional jealousy and homicide in 12%
of male and 3% of female subjects: his study refers, of course, only to a sub-
category of delusion. Even if the studies quoted are based on unrepresentative
samples and therefore cannot determine whether the syndrome of delusion,
irrespective of its association with schizophrenia, increases the risk of
violence, they nevertheless indicate that this hypothesis requires careful testing.

Affective psychoses (manic-depressive illness)
General comments on diagnosis

The estimated risk of violence on the part of depressive or manic-
depressive patients in the relevant literature ranges widely. For this there
are essentially two reasons: the relatively poor reliability of diagnosis in
depression (Zubin, 1967) and the relatively low frequency of violence among
depressed and manic patients in the populations studied.

While the diagnosis of mania is relatively reliable, at least when
the illness is at its height, the same cannot be said of the different categories of depression: it is only within the central area of the so-called
psychotic depressions, which begin with severe sleep disturbances, deep
depression, marked inner tension, anxiety, or a feeling of 'emptiness', general
inhibitedness and delusions such as those of guilt, hypochondriasis or
poverty, that the diagnosis can be to some extent reliable. In border areas,
and particularly in the differential diagnosis of subgroups of
depressive illness, the reliability of diagnosis falls at times almost to
chance levels, in so far as no allowance is made for the increased uniformity
caused by shared diagnostic attitudes, institutional bias, etc. (Häfner *et al.*
1967; Zubin, 1967; Kreitman, 1969; Kramer, 1969).

Such difficulties are reflected in the considerable number of depressive categories and diagnoses which have been proposed by German-speaking psychiatrists in the last few decades against a background of very different theoretical assumptions and based at times on diagnostic criteria that can hardly be empirically confirmed.

Kraepelin's distinction between endogenous depression - by which he meant basically the depressive phase of 'manic-depressive illness' - and the reactive depressions which follow mental stress, provided a point of orientation which clarified the diagnostic process to some extent. (Jaspers sought to strengthen this distinction by introducing his dichotomy of 'understandable' and 'not understandable', which he considered to be reliable and objective correlates of the different forms and courses of depressive illness.) Depressions arising in psychopathies, which Kraepelin described and which K. Schneider in particular systematised, and neurotic depression as described by E. Bleuler, presented greater difficulties. One of the main criteria for distinguishing between the two, namely the presumed constitutional basis of certain patterns of behaviour or reaction in 'abnormal personalities', was purely theoretical and, at least in so far as the diagnosis of psychopathy was concerned, produced no symptoms that could be objectively assessed (Häfner, 1961). For German-speaking psychiatrists these speculatively based diagnostic categories reached their climax with K. Schneider. The new diagnoses of 'underlying' and 'background' depression (1949), which he introduced to supplement depressions and the manic-depressive illnesses which he renamed cyclothymia, had no meaning in empirical research and added only misleading categories in diagnostic practice.

Later attempts to bridge the gap between his speculative guidelines and the furtherance of empirical research, such as Kielholz's classification of depression (1965) and Weitbrecht's concept of 'endoreactive dysthymia' (1952) did, it is true, restore a closer approximation to clinical experience; their value for empirical clinical work (therapeutic or prognostic) or scientific enquiry is, however, still limited, because the diagnostically relevant criteria were to a large extent insufficiently reliable and valid. The important distinction between the quantitative dimension ('severity' of the depression) and the qualitative dimension (nature of the depression, diagnosis) is here, as in most 'clinical' systems, largely ignored. This problem has so far not been satisfactorily solved.

It is still an open question, for example, which psychotic depressions represent severe forms of reactive or neurotic depression and which less severe depressive mood disorders or crises can be regarded as mild depressive phases in an 'endogenous' manic-depressive illness or cyclothymia. Traditional clinical practice has always based its differential diagnosis not only on findings at examination but also on amnestic criteria such as previous personality, earlier modes of reaction or previous manic or depressive phases, as well as on the events which have led to the onset of the illness. Since epidemiological studies have shown that patients with endogenous depression have suffered significantly more stress from loss of parents in childhood than those with neurotic depression (Munro, 1965; Winokur *et al.* 1971), and that the onset of an endogenous psychotic phase is usually preceded by stressful events (Brown & Birley, 1970), the division of depression into qualitatively different illnesses has not become easier. In attempting any such diagnostic subclassification we must accept that these illnesses may require a multi-dimensional diagnosis that corresponds to their multiple aetiology. Such diagnoses must take into account on the one hand the severity of the illness and on the other the factors of age and personality which affect the individual's mode of reaction, as well as temperament and the vulnerability of the personality, including relevant biological ramifications. This is particularly important in depressive illnesses occurring after the age of 60, where such unfavourable factors as bereavement, loneliness and poor marital relationships, as well as physical illness and lack of occupation, play a decisive role within a framework of multiple aetiology (Roth & Kay, 1956; Ciompi & Müller, 1969). In genuine affective psychoses the only worthwhile distinction is that between bipolar 'cyclothymia' or manic-depressive illnesses on the one hand and unipolar depression on the other. (The course of the illness plays a decisive role here, however, so that first attacks of depressive illness are usually not classified.)

To avoid these difficulties, at least to some extent, we shall not divide depressions into subgroups or independent categories: in any case the number of depressive offenders in our study is too low to make any such divisions useful for statistical purposes. Since the criteria we used in finding cases ensured that we admitted only those depressives who had been diagnosed as psychotic, we do not think there is any real disadvantage, so far as the interpretation of our findings is concerned, in keeping them together in one group within the framework of our enquiry.

Our group includes all psychotic depressions which were diagnosed as purely functional, the description being supplemented perhaps by such terms as 'endogenous', 'cyclothymic', 'manic-depressive' or 'climacteric'. Depressions occurring in other illnesses, for example against a background of degenerative cerebral disorders or schizophrenia, are not included in this group but are entered under the main diagnosis (see Chapter 5).

The findings for this diagnostic group are more homogeneous than for the other groups in regard to demographic data, details of the crime and its motivation, etc. - a fact which would seem to justify our including them in one category.

Mania and related syndromes

Manic phases, especially in their severe forms, may be accompanied initially by a high degree of excitement, motor unrest, irritability and increased aggressiveness. It would seem reasonable to assume that patients in this state might frequently come to commit serious acts of aggression.

Earlier writers (e.g. Claude, 1932; Lange, 1934) reported case studies along these lines. With increased nosological differentiation, particularly a more precise distinction between exogenous psychoses (states of mental disorganisation based on disorders of cerebral functioning) and so-called functional, non-organic psychoses, ideas changed. It became increasingly difficult to put the *fureurs maniaques* (Fodéré, 1832) or *états maniaques* (Vladoff, 1911), which were so often apparently associated with violent crime, or the syndrome simply diagnosed as dangerous 'mania' (Krafft-Ebing, 1892), into the same class as what is today called endogenous or cyclothymic mania. Schipkowensky (1958) pointed out, for example, that these were often not cases of genuine mania but of exogenous psychoses associated with confusion or delusional disturbances in the clinical picture of which there was indeed a manic component but which had to be regarded basically·as heterogeneous forms of illness.

Most quantitative studies have placed depressive and manic offenders in one common category, because, following Kraepelin's teaching, they were both regarded as bipolar forms of a single disorder, the so-called manic-depressive illness, or cyclothymia, to use Schneider's term. In many studies reported it is impossible to obtain adequate information either about the proportion of violent offenders who showed unipolar manic disturbance or about the proportion who were manic-depressive. The impression we have gained from reading such reports is that this category of illness is under-represented in most of the investigations that were based on individuals referred for forensic psychiatric assessment or on those committed to mental institutions.

Thus H.W. Maier (1931) found only 28 manic-depressive offenders (2.3%) among his 1247 cases referred for psychiatric assessment. Brack-Kletzhändler (1954), who examined 1018 mentally abnormal offenders, found only three manic-depressives (0.3% of his total material), only one of whom was guilty of violence (criminal homicide). Wanner (1954) found only 18 manic-depressives among his 265 mentally abnormal offenders, of whom two (0.7%) were guilty of crimes of violence. There is no mention in these studies of a distinction between manic and depressive clinical pictures.

Schipkowensky (1958) based his study of 'Mania and murder' on 600 psychiatric assessments made in the Psychiatric Clinic of Sofia, Bulgaria, between 1932 and 1936. In 45 cases (7.5% of the total material) the diagnosis was 'cyclophrenia', that is to say, a manic-depressive illness. In 30 of these cases (5% of the total material) the crime had been committed in a manic phase. Crimes of violence were committed by three patients (0.5%) diagnosed as manic, two of whom were guilty of grievous bodily harm ending in death, and one of murder. While crimes of violence were rare among the manic patients, and more routine crimes such as theft, fraud, etc., were common, all 15 depressive offenders (2.5% of the total material) had committed homicide.

Zech (1959), who studied 950 offenders referred for assessment to the Regional Psychiatric Hospital of Göttingen between 1948 and 1958, found 2% with a diagnosis of manic-depressive illness: they were guilty of various crimes, all of which had been committed in a manic phase. His material as a whole did not contain a single depressive offender. Most of those diagnosed as manic were accused of crimes against property: there were only two cases (about 0.2% of the total material) of minor bodily harm and one (approximately 0.1% of the total material) of criminal homicide.

The 675 offenders studied by H.W. Müller & Hadamik (1966) likewise included only five (0.16% of the total material) who were diagnosed as manic-depressive. Two of these had committed acts of violence. There was no evidence of violence in this category of patient during their stay in hospital up to the time of the study and although the number involved is small this finding is of interest, since it is in line with the other available facts bearing on the assessment of the risk of violence in this group.

Only Stierlin's (1956) study, which was methodologically the least controlled, reported a relatively high number (29, or 3.8%, of the 773 subjects investigated) of violent manic-depressive patients in psychiatric hospitals, nearly half of whom (13 cases) had been given a diagnosis of 'mania'.

Psychotic depressions

Violent outbursts of aggression by depressed patients, the 'raptus melancholicus' which offers such a dramatic contrast to the inhibited and rigid symptomatology that characterises depressives in general, aroused the early interest of 'case-study' observers like von Muralt (1906), Näcke (1908), Strassmann (1916), Weber (1916), Jacobi (1928) and Elsässer (1939). Because

of outbursts of this kind, psychiatrists of older days attached a fairly serious
risk of violence to depressive illness.

More recent opinions show a basic change. There is now a considerable consensus that in severe depression there is first and foremost a high risk
of suicide, the risk of violence towards others being limited almost entirely
to 'murder accompanied by suicide' or 'extended suicide' (Gruhle, 1940; Wyrsch,
1947; Popella, 1964; Schulte & Mende, 1969). Many reasons are advanced for
these impulses to destroy oneself and one's nearest associates, usually members
of the family or lovers (Dolenc, 1913; Hopwood, 1927; Jacobi, 1928; Kögler,
1940; Schipkowensky, 1963; Zumpe, 1966; Greger & Hoffmeyer, 1969). There are,
however, very few quantitative studies of the incidence or prevalence of such
acts.

For this reason Woddis (1957) in his review of the literature on
depression and crime was able on the whole only to repeat the opinions of
experienced observers on this theme. In interpreting these opinions he pointed
out the close connection between suicidal and homicidal impulses, the
frequency of dreams about the death of near relatives and the unconscious
desires on the part of depressives for punishment, and spoke of a close
relationship between the risk of homicide and the risk of suicide in such
patients. [12]

Rasch & Petersen (1965), who evaluated approximately 900 special
assessments prepared in the University Psychiatric Clinic of Hamburg between
1948 and 1963, found 45 patients (5% of the total material) in whom a
depressive mood disorder was put forward as a mitigating or absolving factor
in a criminal case. Of these, 21 were adequately documented, with a diagnosis
of 'endogenous phasic disorder'. In every case the illness had begun long
before the crime was committed. The offences were listed as homicide, attempted
homicide, and crimes against property and public morals. There was no more-
detailed classification of the crimes.

The authors formed the impression that the criminal rate in
endogenous depressions is low in relation both to the overall crime rate and
to the morbidity rate for depressives. They added the important qualification
that manic patients are more quickly aroused than is normal in our culture and
their crimes, even when relatively minor, were quickly associated with the
illness. Depression, on the other hand, may remain undetected and untreated
for a long time. Once a crime has been committed, the depression may possibly
be regarded as a reaction to the event and may therefore be underestimated
when it comes to evaluating the risk of such a crime.

Among young offenders, too, as an investigation by Shoor & Speed

(1963) suggests, criminality in depressives seems to follow normal social trends. In each of the 12 cases studied these authors report a so-called grief reaction to the death of a close relative, and the offences committed consisted only of crimes against property, sexual misconduct and vagrancy: there was no instance of violence. We have to consider the possibility that the process of internalising social norms, which leads to abnormal super-ego functioning in adults inclined to severe depressions, is often still incomplete in adolescence. The late average age of onset of psychotic depressions, in the third or fourth decade of life, may be of some relevance here.

Although there have been no representative studies of the risks of criminality in depressed patients, it may be inferred from the data quoted above that the general crime rate of these patients is low compared with that of the population as a whole. Routine crimes in particular, such as offences against property, seem to be considerably under-represented here. In mania no such trend can be said to exist. In this category of illness there seems to be a preponderance of crimes against property, indecent behaviour, and minor acts of aggression, although from the studies quoted it cannot be concluded that the rate is any higher or lower than that shown by the general population. It would seem that violence in manic patients is rare. The risk of violence in psychotic depression - not used here in the sense of our own definition - refers first to suicide, which is prominent in the statistics of causes of death for this group. The second risk, which does come within our operational criteria and which seems to be quantitatively of considerable importance, is the so-called extended suicide in which the intent to kill involves not only the self but also one's nearest associates.

The epilepsies

In earlier neurological and psychiatric literature epileptics were, like the 'insane', at times arbitrarily considered to be potentially violent and of 'amoral' character (Lombroso, 1887-90). It was not at that time possible to distinguish satisfactorily between epileptic attacks, epileptic personality changes (dementia) and psychoses associated with epilepsy (hallucinosis, twilight states). Since epilepsy was classed in this general framework of an 'endogenous psychosis', analogy with schizophrenia and manic-depressive psychosis (Kraepelin) gave rise to the idea of an 'epileptoid character', an allegedly specific epileptic personality structure existing without symptoms of epilepsy itself and comparable with the schizoid and the cyclothymic character. This group of awkward, moody personalities, prone to severe excitement, was associated by E. Kretschmer (1921), by Kretschmer & Enke (1936) and by Mauz

(1937) with an athletic body build. A tendency to aggressiveness and violence was seen as a specific attribute of the 'epileptoid' individual, often in association with a particular somatic quality.

Early neurophysiological concepts supported the association of epilepsy with violence. Under the influence of Jackson's classical description of epilepsy as a sudden excessive discharge of tension in the grey matter of the brain, it was for a long time all too easy for any impulsive outburst of uncontrolled behaviour to be seen as epileptic in origin (this was convincingly expounded by Roth at the Ciba Symposium in 1967: see Roth, 1968). The diagnosis was therefore too widely used in many senses. But as the diagnosis of all kinds of genuine epileptic disorders became increasingly precise, thanks to the development and advance of Berger's encephalograph, there was a basic change in the concept of epilepsy and many pseudo-epileptic syndromes, including the 'epileptoid' personality, fell into disuse.

Clinical and neurophysiological research concerned itself with individual epileptic syndromes and different rates of involvement in aggressive behaviour were described. Gruhle (1933), who was still clearly influenced by Jaspers' false dichotomy in which 'understandable' was regarded as synonymous with psychologically determined and 'not-understandable' with organically determined, underlined three complex forms of illness which were risk factors so far as violence was concerned: epileptic mood disorder, pathological intoxication and epileptic twilight state. Common to all three was 'a mood disorder which is clearly different from the individual's normal state and which proceeds from somatic causes, i.e. it is without motivation'. A further essential factor was the sthenic affect of the epileptic, 'in other words, an affective state in which there is a mounting pressure that is discharged from time to time in an altered state of consciousness (twilight state)'. The use of alcohol in this state led to pathological intoxication in which 'the epileptic experiences a mood disorder and is often very violent even towards people who have done him no harm: he may commit senseless and furious attacks on complete strangers'. According to Lange-Lüddeke and Wyrsch, too, epileptic mood disorders and twilight states were frequent causes of severe violence. Wyrsch (1955) considered that brain-damaged epileptics, especially those with incipient dementia, were particularly dangerous and that in them 'the likelihood of explosive discharges was particularly strong'.

A recent textbook in German on 'the epilepsies' (Janz, 1969) also mentions that in 'epileptic delirium and episodic confusional states' in psychomotor epilepsy, and in the paroxysmal twilight states of grand mal epilepsy, the patient may commit occasional acts of aggression arising from a delusional misinterpretation of his situation. Janz gives no more precise details of the relative frequency of such incidents. He puts particular emphasis on the significance of the 'psychotic episodes' in which one may see fluctuations between 'an aggressiveness directed at the external world and suicidal impulses directed against the self'.

While descriptive accounts of violence on the part of epileptics are not hard to find in the literature (e.g. Iberg, 1905-6; Campbell, 1912; Alter, 1913; Wetzel, 1920; Többen, 1932), precise data on their frequency are meagre. The analyses of forensic psychiatric assessments to which we have referred provide only a rough indication of the proportion of epileptic offenders found in the case material of individual clinics.

H.W.Maier (1931) mentions 26 epileptics (2.6% of his material), of whom seven, including one woman, had committed offences against the health and life of other persons. Wanner (1954) listed 36 epileptics on whom psychiatric reports were prepared between 1895 and 1942 and of whom five were violent offenders; between 1943 and 1952 there were 23 epileptics, of whom three were violent. Brack-Kletzhändler (1954), reporting on 118 cases of aggression (11.6% of 1018 mentally abnormal offenders), found only three epileptics (guilty of bodily harm and threatening behaviour, but not of homicide) and three further patients with a history of convulsions who were guilty of abortion. There were 15 cases of epilepsy in his total material (1.5%). Bochnik *et al.* (1965), reporting on 93 cases (30% of their total material), found 15 violent offenders belonging to the somewhat heterogeneous group of 'cerebral atrophy, epileptic attacks, residual damage'.

H.W. Müller & Hadamik (1966) found only a few convulsive patients among the mentally abnormal and mentally defective offenders who were legally committed to hospital after their crimes. Out of 675 patients committed under Section 42b of the Penal Code, only five were epileptics who had been found guilty of violent offences (0.7% of the total material). Of the 20 patients with a history of convulsions, 18 had in the course of their stay in hospital behaved aggressively towards staff and/or fellow-patients.

Stierlin (1956) estimated the percentage of epileptics among his violent offenders as 12.4% (94 cases), the proportion of epileptics among in-patients in general being significantly lower (6% at the institution in München-Haar and 3% at Friedmatt-Basel). It must be borne in mind, however, that during the long period covered (the case-finding lasted from 1940 to 1950) there were changes in the diagnosis of epilepsy. It is possible, therefore, that the proportion of epileptics in the in-patient population of large institutions was calculated on a narrow diagnostic basis as compared with the broader diagnostic categories used to classify the offenders (the institutional figures were calculated at the end of the investigation, beginning on 1 March 1955). The dates of the crimes went back to before the turn of the century.

Lennox (1943) studied a larger series of cases in Boston, Mass., examining approximately 5000 patients suffering from different types of epilepsy and enquiring into specific modes of behaviour, including crime, which could be associated with alterations in consciousness during or immediately following an epileptic attack. Though a limited number of patients showed excited and occasionally dangerous behaviour after a grand mal attack or during a psychomotor attack, there was no report of homicide or of serious injury to other persons. This report must carry considerable weight because it is based on a large sample that presumably was little affected by selection.

Hill & Pond (1952) carried out an electroencephalographic (EEG) study of 105 murderers, including six women, over a period of eight years. The subjects came from London and its environs and were selected by prison doctors because of suspected epilepsy or brain damage. In 27 cases it was considered possible that the accused had suffered from 'epileptic automatisms' at the time of their crime. Nine of these patients showed specific epileptic abnormalities in the EEG; in nine further cases convulsive potentials were absent but there was a previous history of convulsive attacks which were regarded as confirmed. The remaining nine were anamnestic and there was no sign in the EEG of any illness that might be regarded as belonging to the group of the epilepsies. The 18 subjects classified as epileptic included long-term cases complicated by personality changes, alcoholism or mental deficiency, as well as short-term, more or less typical forms of the illness. Although the association between the epileptic illness and the crime was in most cases purely conjectural, the authors concluded that there was a clear association between murder and epilepsy. They conceded, however, that a direct link between the act of murder and an epileptic attack or a confusional state following such an attack must in the light of their observations be regarded as extremely rare.

A very careful follow-up study planned on epidemiological lines and covering 897 epileptics was published in 1950 by Alström. With a view to clarifying genetic relationships as well as the clinical and social prognosis for these patients, he and several colleagues carried out between 1945 and 1950 a thorough study of patients who had been admitted for observation to the Neurological Clinic at the Karolinska Institute in Stockholm (at that time the only special clinic of its kind in Sweden) because of epileptic symptoms. They were able to trace 1216 of the 1472 patients originally examined for the first time in that period (representing all clinical forms of epilepsy except

institutional cases). Complete details were obtained about 897 of them (55%
men) in regard to social milieu, marital status, course of illness, genetic
factors, etc. For the remaining cases no such data could be collected, purely
on financial grounds (for example the cost of visiting). For this reason the
inhabitants of the city of Stockholm were over-represented.

      Alström's findings in regard to criminal behaviour were as follows.
Using a control sample of the general population of Sweden, examined in 1944
and consisting of 42 000 males aged over 25, and data obtained from the
criminal register, he found no significant difference between the two groups
in regard to rates of criminal conviction. Of the 493 male epileptics in his
study, 30 appeared in the criminal register. Analysis showed that the numerically small subgroup of epileptics who were 'mentally changed', i.e. those
with symptoms of cerebral degeneration and psychiatric complications, had a
somewhat higher rate of conviction than those who showed no such changes.
Crimes of violence were not uncommon (no detailed statistics are given) but
were mostly minor and trivial; there was no case of homicide. Alström also
found, however, that 18 of his male and 11 of his female subjects had while
in psychiatric or special institutions in Sweden been occasionally or consistently regarded as violent or dangerous, although no legal proceedings had had
to be taken against them. There was no case of homicide in this subgroup either.
The authors mentioned that much of their aggressive behaviour was associated
with alcohol.

      It may be concluded from the findings surveyed above that the risk
of aggressive or in particular of violent crimes attached to the epileptic
attack and the subsequent state of altered consciousness is not above average.
It is more a question of the psychological complications of epilepsy, in
particular the deterioration of personality that accompanies dementia and other
cerebral changes, as well as a poor tolerance of alcohol: these seem to be the
main risk factors associated with the rare acts of violence committed by epileptics. We must also bear in mind that patients with epileptic disturbances of
consciousness, such as 'confusional' twilight states as opposed to 'rational'
twilight states, which in clinical experience are at times accompanied by
excitement and considerable aggressiveness, are as a rule admitted to hospital
at an early stage of the illness. When there is a disturbance in the basic
function of orientation to reality - which is different from the disorientation
seen in most schizophrenic crises - the change in behaviour will probably be
recognised very quickly as constituting a danger, especially since previous
convulsive attacks or other symptoms will usually already have served to
identify the illness. Finally, the more severe the disturbance of consciousness

the less likely is it that a direct act of aggression or a carefully planned
crime can be carried out; this also lessens the danger inherent in twilight
states, quite apart from the possibility of their responding to therapeutic
intervention.

Attention is thus focused on the epileptic with cerebral degenerative symptoms, though his perhaps slightly high rate of criminality as compared
with the general population is probably not a characteristic of the epilepsy.
It seems to be associated rather with psychological changes in the sense of
personality disintegration: such changes could be brought about by very varied
forms of severe brain damage ranging from severe cerebral trauma to epilepsy or
to arteriosclerotic degeneration, and could lead to poor social adjustment,
violent mood swings and loss of control of aggressive impulses. [13] One of the
aims of our own study is to test these hypotheses.

Acquired cerebral damage (trauma, inflammation, intoxication)
and cerebral atrophy

Convulsive attacks may occur in basically any organic cerebral
syndrome. Because of nosological differences, as well as on the grounds of
psychiatric tradition, however, we have kept our review of the literature of
violence and acquired cerebral damage separate from that of violence in the
epilepsies.

Following on what has been said above about the epilepsies, it
would seem that in patients with cerebral damage, too, irrespective of the
cause of that damage, it is the psycho-organic symptom of dementia, with its
associated effects on the control of drives and emotions, which is of significant and basic importance in estimating the risk of violence.

Several authors have differentiated between mechanical, toxic and
inflammatory brain damage, on the one hand, and degenerative cerebral processes
on the other (senile disorder). Others speak more generally of 'organic' disorders or 'organic psychoses', without always identifying clearly which
particular disorders are involved. For this reason it is often more difficult
to compare published rates of crime or estimates of the risk of violence in
these disorders than in the other psychiatric illnesses.

Brain-damaged patients, whose high numbers make them a socially
important group, have been described by forensic psychiatrists such as
Langelüddeke (1959) as showing a tendency to commit 'in particular acts of
bodily harm, sexual offences, violent abuse, fraud and theft'. According to
Wyrsch (1955) intolerance of alcohol and general excitability are the reasons
which make such individuals liable to act violently. But here again serious

crimes of aggression seem to be rare.

Lindenberg (1954) examined the case records of 4500 brain-damaged patients in the city of Berlin and isolated 28 of them who might be called 'berserk'. Nearly all of them (26) were suffering from frontal lobe damage and up to the time of their injury had mostly (23 cases) led peaceable lives. Eighteen of these patients had traumatic epilepsy associated with considerable aggressiveness, showing irritability, frequent outbursts of blind rage, and a bellicosity that often led to bodily harm; there were 17 suicidal attempts, but no case of homicide.

Hillbom's study (1960) of 514 cases of cranial injury during the Russo-Finnish war also points to aggressiveness directed particularly against the self. In nine of his subjects (2.2% of the total) he found dementia; in severe cases the most frequent complication was a personality change in the direction of emotionally labile, unreasonable and explosive behaviour (22.2%). Criminal misdemeanours were also encountered but the author did not code these under particular offences. There is, however, no mention of homicide. The most frequent form of dangerous aggression was suicide: out of all the brain-injured patients in the population studied 37 committed suicide. A third of these had shown disturbances of personality. (Quoted by Roth.)

In the study which we have already mentioned by Pokorny (1964), the 'organic' diagnostic group (which included all chronic cerebral syndromes as well as all acute organic cerebral disorders except those associated with alcoholism) had a suicide rate which was $3\frac{1}{2}$ times greater than that of comparable age structures in the average male population (78 as opposed to 22.7 per 100 000). We must take into consideration, however, the high dark figure of unreported cases in the official statistics of suicide, which contrasts with the presumably relatively high rate of documented suicides in Pokorny's population.

There is little in the literature about violent offences committed by encephalitic patients. In Langelüddeke's opinion the forensic implications of encephalitis epidemica are slight in the acute state, though in chronic encephalitis they are of importance. Acts of violence are rare, the most frequent offences being sexual offences and theft. Isolated incidents of aggressive behaviour by encephalitic patients have been described by Stertz (1931), Lange & Boeters (1936), Wyrsch (1947) and others, but no figures have been given showing how frequently they occur.

Syphilitic syndromes, in particular general palsy, seem to feature rarely among violent offenders, and vice versa. Langelüddeke quotes Alexander & Nyssen (1929), who found only one person with a criminal record among 164 syphilitic patients receiving malarial treatment, and Jossmann (1931), who reported only eight criminal offenders among 1668 patients treated for general palsy.

In 1957 Weimann published a paper on 'paralytic patients as murderers', in which he described 21 cases of murder and referred to case reports by Krafft-Ebing and Hoche. This author, too, formed the impression that reports of such cases in the published literature are 'surprisingly rare'. If such patients do commit acts of violence, these usually arise as 'short-circuit' reactions in the initial stages of irritability and affective lability that occur in progressive paralysis.

Studies of the forensic assessments prepared in individual clinics (H.W. Maier, Wanner, Brack-Kletzhändler, Bochnik *et al.*) have classified the organic cerebral syndromes which we are discussing into diagnostic categories of varying scope (e.g. together with the epilepsies, exogenous psychoses in physical disease, puerperal psychoses, etc.), so that there seems little point in reproducing their findings.

H.W. Müller & Hadamik's results (1966) are more useful. They found that among 70 offenders committed under Section 42b of the Penal Code with a diagnosis of 'brain damage including lues of the central nervous system', there were six who were guilty of violent crimes; and in 56 offenders with 'senile disorders including involutional psychoses' they again found six who were guilty of violence. (The total number of 'organic' patients was 126, of whom 12, or 9.5%, had been committed because of violent offences.) It is interesting to note that the group of 'brain-damaged' patients had a worse record of violence in the course of their hospital stay (26 cases) than the senile group (3 cases). These findings would suggest that the group of patients whose brain damage is due to trauma or inflammatory processes (lues, epidemic encephalitis) are more likely to commit dangerous acts of violence than are the senile patients or those suffering from involutional psychoses.

In their monograph on 'age and crime' Bürger-Prinz & Lewerenz (1961) put forward the view that 'very serious crimes such as murder and manslaughter are rarely committed by offenders aged 60 and over'. If such a crime does occur in this age group, then as a rule the state of the offender is not one that the authors would attribute to physiological changes in the involutional period, but represents unambiguous disease phenomena.[14] 'Delusions of jealousy, of influence and of persecution play an essential part, as does uncontrolled excitability and exaggerated affect in morbid senile decay' (*op. cit.*, p.23).

A similar view was put forward by Roth (1968), who carried out a thorough examination of the statistics of dangerous violence on the part of elderly people as compared with the general population. His data cover those found guilty of indictable offences and are analysed according to age and sex. The percentages refer to all offenders, the rates to offences per 100 000 persons in England and Wales. Table 1 shows that dangerous acts of violence are in general very much less common in the higher age groups than in young people. Parallel with this decreased rate of crime there is, according to Roth, a sharp fall in the incidence of addictive disease (drugs and alcohol).

Table 1. *Criminal rates[a] (violent offences) in three age groups in England and Wales*

	Age groups					
	60 and over		0 - 59		0 - 29	
	%	Rate	%	Rate	%	Rate
Males						
Class I : offences against the person						
(a) endangering life	4.8	3.2	7.9	91.9	7.9	168.1
(b) sexual offences	12.2	8.2	2.8	32.6	2.2	46.1
(a) and (b)	17.0	11.4	10.7	124.4	10.0	214.2
Class II : offences against property, with violence	3.4		24.4	284.5	28.0	595.8
Class III : offences against property, without violence	75.0	50.2	62.5	730.3	60.1	1283.3
Females						
Class I : offences against the person						
(a) endangering life	1.5		2.7		2.9	
(b) sexual offences	0.0		0.1		0.0	
(a) and (b)	1.5		2.8		2.9	
Class II : offences against property, with violence	0.0		3.7		5.7	
Class III : offences against property, without violence	97.8	35.3	90,7	168.1	88.6	263.1

From Roth (1968).

[a] Rates per 100 000 of population at risk

In Roth's view it is not the normal degenerative disorders of old age which
lead to serious crimes of aggression in this age group but complex mental
disorders such as arteriosclerotic psychoses, late forms of chronic alcoholism,
paranoid syndromes, etc. The rise in the suicide rate is noteworthy and is
seen in the statistics of several countries, including the GFR, in the age
group of 60 and over, most markedly in men. One is probably justified in
speaking of an increase in self-directed aggression in this age group in the
cultures in question.

Mental deficiency

Studies of the relationship between mental defect and crimes of
violence suffer to some extent from a lack of objective assessment of the
intelligence of the offenders in question. Some authors do not even state
clearly which diagnostic criteria of mental defect have been used. Often it is
a question of general achievement in life, scholastic attainment and clinical
impressions. Mental defectives are put into the same group as those with slight
brain damage which does not affect intelligence, and those with psychopathic
personalities, in a general category of 'mental handicap' (for example in
British psychiatry, see Shapiro (1968), 'mental deficiency'). We have to take
account of such variations in criteria when we try to compare and evaluate the
following published reports.

Criminal behaviour on the part of the mentally defective raises the
urgent question whether low intelligence as such predisposes individuals to
crime, or whether there may not be more complex personality and environmental
factors involved which are much more likely to contribute to antisocial behaviour.
In the first place it must be remembered that in the most severe forms of mental
deficiency, for example in idiocy, the ability to fit oneself for practical
living is very limited. Such individuals are often in need of care and therefore
have to be committed at an early age to a permanent stay in special institutions.
Severely handicapped individuals of this kind can hardly be expected to commit
crimes of violence, since they are either incapable of planning or lack motivation for such deeds, or they are under constant supervision and control. The
disturbed, impulsive behaviour which they sometimes show can hardly be translated into purposeful acts.

For these reasons Langelüddeke (1959) and Wyrsch (1947) held that
idiocy was of no forensic importance, even if individuals in this category are
sometimes led astray by others and persuaded to commit such crimes as arson.
We would at all events suggest that even where such indirect offences are
concerned, middle-grade mental deficiency and idiocy hardly enter the question.

The less severe forms of mental defect are, however, in the view of the authors quoted, of more significance. In 1945 Werner published a short review of earlier estimates and quantitative studies of the criminality of the mentally defective as a whole. He quoted Verwaeck, who in 1939 found 184 mental defectives among 540 abnormal offenders (31%); Lange (1934), who reported 20 mental defectives among 100 criminals assessed; and Strohmeyer (1928) who diagnosed oligophrenia in 20 out of 184 offenders referred for psychiatric examination. From the USA he quoted Richmond (1931), who is reported to have found 20–25% oligophrenics among the juvenile delinquents of New York: according to the same study, 29.1% of all criminals in the state of Minnesota were mentally defective.

Strohmeyer (1928), writing in Bumke's *Handbuch*, also thought it could be safely assumed that a high proportion of juvenile delinquents were mentally defective. He considered that many oligophrenics were led under the influence of alcohol to 'commit gross misdemeanours, to resist authority, to use threats, and to commit bodily harm and damage to property'. Murder, or more rarely murder associated with rape, might also occur. Among the 184 offenders whom he examined in the University Clinic of Jena between 1921 and 1926, there were 20 mental defectives who included five murderers, one of whom had committed murder and rape.

Langelüddeke (1959), who examined 262 offenders between 1941 and 1948 who were mentally abnormal or suspected of being mentally abnormal, found among them 41 mental defectives, including two charged with homicide or physical harm.

From the analyses of forensic psychiatric assessments which we have already mentioned, the following findings emerge. W.H. Maier (Zurich) reported that out of 294 confirmed oligophrenics judged to be not responsible or of diminished responsibility, 25 (8.5%) had committed offences against life and health (20.6% of all the abnormal violent offenders in this study): they included 10 women (one violent oligophrenic woman out of the total population studied was held to be fully responsible for her actions). Brack-Kletzhändler (Zurich) found that of 1018 mentally abnormal offenders, 199 (19.5%) showed some degree of mental deficiency. They included six cases of homicide, one of infanticide, seven of bodily harm and/or threats, physical maltreatment, violence and robbery. Two were guilty of illegal abortion: when these two are excluded, there were 14 violent offenders who were oligophrenic, i.e. 12% of the 118 violent offenders of all diagnoses, and 8% of all the oligophrenic offenders referred to the Zurich Clinic for psychiatric assessment. Wanner reported on 2241 offenders assessed in Münsingen/Bern in the years between 1895 and 1952 and judged to be abnormal. Of these, 545, or 24.3%, were

oligophrenic. Only 56 mentally defective offenders had committed violent acts
that endangered the life of other persons (2.5% of all those judged to be
abnormal; 10.2% of all those judged to be mentally defective; 19% of all the
violent offenders in the population studied, irrespective of diagnosis).

Werner (1945) reported on mentally defective offenders who were
sent for psychiatric assessment to the Münsingen Institution between 1906 and
1942 and analysed the types of crime committed. They represented about a
quarter of the 1293 offenders examined during this period (24.8% of all cases;
27.8% of those judged to be abnormal). Oligophrenias accounted for about 24%
of the 100 cases of murder and attempted murder, about 17% of the cases of
manslaughter and 18.9% of the total number of violent crimes (including
infanticide and physical maltreatment). In Werner's view the relatively high
rate of serious aggression reflected a selective factor, since less serious
acts of violence by persons showing a considerable degree of mental defect
may in country districts (and Münsingen has an almost exclusively rural catchment area) be dealt with on the basis of retaliatory or disciplinary and
educational measures, or simply accepted, without being brought before a judge.
Werner's findings also show the different risks attached to different grades
of mental deficiency: it was the high-grade defectives as a rule who committed
murder or homicide. Only one case of manslaughter in his total material was
committed by a low-grade defective. As Werner summed it up: 'the old legend of
the highly dangerous low-grade defective is thus not confirmed'.

Bochnik *et al.* (Hamburg) found 15 violent offenders among 45 medium-
to high-grade defectives (out of a total of 329 male offenders), and 27 violent
offenders among 146 'intellectually subnormal offenders' (18.4% of all the
mentally subnormal). In their view a marked degree of defect, like slight mental
subnormality, was associated more with crimes of violence and theft, rarely
with fraud.

When considering all these studies, however, it is necessary to bear
in mind what we have already said about the way in which uncontrollable
selective factors affect the populations studied. It may also well be that
tolerance of aggressive behaviour on the part of the mentally defective depends
on culture and class and that, as postulated by Werner, there are differences
between urban and rural areas.

H.W. Müller & Hadamik, who examined mental defectives committed
under Section 42b of the Penal Code in the Rhineland, found a considerably
smaller proportion of violent offenders among them than did, for example,
Werner. Out of 311 mental defectives (46% of the 675 abnormal delinquents
studied) only 10 had committed acts of violence (3.2% of all oligophrenics;

12.5% of the 80 violent offenders of all diagnostic groups). So far as violence within the institutions was concerned, the mental defectives were involved to a marked degree, being responsible for 100 incidents.

This review of the available data on violent crime in the mentally deficient certainly does not give the impression that the relevant crime rate is high for this diagnostic category. The more closely the methodology conforms to epidemiological standards, the more clearly do the studies point to a criminal rate which is not very different from that of the general population. It is further clear that severely defective individuals are hardly ever involved in crimes of violence, while the risk of criminality seems to rise markedly as the degree of defect becomes less severe.

There is much to support the view that lack of intelligence or immaturity of personality as such do not provide an adequate explanation for crimes of violence by mentally defective offenders (Shapiro, 1968). It would seem much more likely that environmental factors play an essential part, and this is borne out by consideration of the less severe grades of mental defect. These views will form the basis of our hypotheses, which will be tested (as far as this proves possible) by analysis of our data.

3   QUESTIONS POSED, POPULATION STUDIED, METHODOLOGY

3.1   Questions posed and aim of the investigation

In order to have some criteria for evaluating earlier studies of
violent crimes committed by the mentally ill, we have in the introductory
chapters already had to develop a large part of our methodology. These two
chapters should therefore be regarded as providing a basis for the methodological considerations which apply to our own survey, particularly in regard
to the special problem of ensuring that the mentally abnormal offenders
studied form a representative population. We must, however, say at the outset
that we have by no means succeeded in meeting all the important methodological requirements to an equal extent and in a fully satisfactory manner.
We have tried to keep methodological needs clearly in sight and to base our
practical procedures on them whenever circumstances permitted. We have also
tried to indicate clearly the considerable number of defects and difficulties
which we have not been able to overcome in our survey and so to make clear
the limits of reliability and validity that apply to our results.

In the present study we have tried to examine the complex question
of the 'dangerousness' of the mentally ill. In doing so we aimed at compiling
relatively reliable quantitative data on the offender-incidence rates for
dangerous crimes committed by the mentally ill, so that these could be compared with the corresponding criminal rates for the general population. A
supplementary aim was to formulate the requirements of effective prevention
and treatment. We were therefore interested, on the one hand, in demographic
data on the offenders, such as age, sex and family status, so that these could
be compared with similar data on 'normal' offenders and on abnormal non-
offenders, and on the other hand in specific risk factors affecting the incidence of the crimes in question.

We began by studying factors concerned with illness, since these
affect the different quantitative and qualitative risks associated with different groups of illnesses, including mental subnormality. At the same time we
enquired into the duration of illness, including details of any treatment given

or care and control exercised up to the date of the crime. In addition we tried to obtain information which might throw light on the possible influence of hereditary characteristics, familial and other environmental factors, and finally premorbid personality, particularly earlier social and aggressive behaviour, and on the risk of criminality in mentally abnormal offenders as a whole as well as in the different groups of illnesses.

A further important aim was to investigate the motivation for the crime and its relationship to the illness, particularly the question of motives that might be specific to the illness, such as delusion or imperative sensory hallucinations; this was done within the limits of quantitative analysis that our material permitted. Because of their practical importance, we also looked for preliminary warning signs that might be present in the history of the illness, in stresses and crimes having nothing to do with the illness, or in the shape of certain patterns of reaction, and that might alert one to the risk of impending violence.

The same hope of finding a basis for preventive measures prompted us finally to examine the risk that certain individuals might become the victims of violent attacks by the mentally abnormal. We therefore studied the relationship between the victim and the offender (relative, acquaintance, etc.), as well as the quality of that relationship, in so far as this was possible (conflict, quarrels, etc.), to see if these would throw light on the cause and motivation of the crime.

Finally we were interested in the crime itself: its planned nature or lack of premeditation, the circumstances surrounding it, and the behaviour of the offender in regard to the crime, up to the point of suicide, again in relation to the groups of illness, the sex of the offender, and other variables.

3.2 Criteria for inclusion in the study

The population included in any survey is governed not only by the hypotheses to be studied but also of necessity by methodological requirements and by the practical possibilities of their fulfilment. In order to test the working hypotheses outlined above, we had to have a sufficiently large number of subjects. Only in this way could we hope to have adequate representation of the main diagnostic categories, that is to say of the most frequent groups of illness, thus permitting analysis on demographic lines and correlation of the main variables. As regards the relationship to criminal violence of the less common disorders (e.g. epileptic dementia), or of the commoner disturbances which are expected to carry a small risk of violence (e.g. senile dementia), we would in any case expect to obtain only pointers, because of the small numbers involved. It therefore seemed best to attempt a comprehensive survey covering 'mentally abnormal offenders'. Pilot studies carried out with the co-operation of some of the necessary authorities (Federal Statistical Office, Federal and Regional Criminal Bureaus, Public Prosecutors' Offices and Courts, psychiatric hospitals, regional units, ministries, etc.) showed that this could probably be done. It also had the advantage of providing the best practical solution to the difficult problem of obtaining a representative population.

After looking at the expected annual numbers of mentally ill and mentally defective offenders, taken from Federal Statistics of Convicted Offenders and from the incomplete records of the Federal and some Regional Criminal Bureaus, we decided to make our survey cover ten years. In terms of the criteria we had selected, we considered we would then be able to count on a total of 500 to 700 offenders. In fact we found 533 mentally ill or mentally defective violent offenders whose crimes were committed within the decade from 1 January 1955 to 31 December 1964. This formed the material for our investigation.

Criteria for inclusion of the crime

General considerations

In order to minimise the influence of uncontrollable factors of selection, our first consideration was given to two requirements: (1) the chance of the crime being detected, and (2) the chance of an existing mental illness being detected. Both had to be as high as possible. The first requirement called for high rates of solved crime for the offences in question, the second for high rates of psychiatric assessment for all categories of offender. From the point of view of legal practice, these requirements are most easily met in cases of serious crimes involving danger to life. The solution rates for such crimes - murder, manslaughter, bodily harm resulting in death - stood at more than 90% in the GFR in the decade 1955-1964, if we except infanticide for which the rate averaged just over 70%.[1] These were precisely the violent crimes which were central to our limited enquiry, including finally the question of prevention.

There can be no doubt that the overall criminality of the mentally ill is of the utmost practical interest. It covers less serious crimes, such as crimes against property and the so-called 'impulsive crimes' or sexual offences. Many of these offences are certainly related to psychopathology, particularly to neurotic disturbances and personality disorders. The assumption that all deviations of sexual behaviour are an expression of mental illness

is, however, a generalisation as meaningless as the idea that all acts of
violence are symptoms of mental illness in those who commit them. The fact
that social norms show particularly marked variations in this area leads to
considerable shifts in socially acceptable behaviour, in the tolerance shown
towards deviant behaviour, and thus in the readiness of the victims and of
witnesses to report such acts. Between the recorded and the 'real' rates of
crime there is therefore a considerable gap, the extent of which is veiled
in darkness. Epidemiological investigation thus becomes very difficult, if
not impossible. In regard to the relationship between 'impulsive acts' and
mental illness, moreover, the establishment of a reliable dividing line between
situational minor offences by the mentally healthy and abnormal behaviour
dependent upon mental illness is especially difficult, particularly in border-
line conditions.

As the example of petty sexual or impulsive offences shows, the
chief arguments against including less severe crimes in our study were methodological. In addition to the dark area between reported and actual rates, which
varies according to the offence, the rate of detection of known crimes is
usually relatively low for this type of offence. We had therefore to accept the
possibility, for example, that the chances of detection were lowest for offenders with higher intelligence, better social adjustment and a lesser degree of
mental handicap. This again would lead to over-representation of the mentally
ill and mentally defective in the recorded offenders who formed the population
of our survey. In addition, the chances of any mental illness being recorded
in those committing petty crimes is also less: our pilot studies showed that
the proportion of individuals referred for psychiatric assessment was relatively
low for these categories of offender.

We must again emphasise, therefore, that we did not examine the
total criminality of all the mentally abnormal, but surveyed only crimes of
violence committed by mentally ill and mentally defective persons in the decade
1955 to 1964 in the GFR. The end of the decade (31 December 1964) had to be
set relatively far back in time because of the need to ensure that our records
were complete and that they included final details of legal procedures and
court decisions.

As we were able to take as a starting point the crime and its
committal on a clearly defined date, it was easy to base the investigation on
the incidence of mentally ill violent offenders. Fixing the time of onset of
a mental illness is, however, always much more difficult and the cases examined
by us were no exception. This is one of the main reasons why exact data on the
true incidence of mental illness are in general so extraordinarily difficult
to obtain.[2]

In order to arrive at a reasonably clear and practical definition of a 'crime of violence', which we required as a starting point for our case-finding, we took first all attacks by mentally abnormal persons which led to the death of the victim. Accidental offences such as accidental homicide were of course excluded. The 'successful' execution of the act, i.e. the killing, seemed, however, too narrow a criterion, since it often depends on circumstances which are outside the offender's control: for example on interruption due to unforeseen circumstances, on speedy medical aid for a severely injured victim, or finally on inadequate preparations for the crime or lack of knowledge of the means and tools being used in its execution.

With reference to the last example quoted, we had to consider the possibility that mentally ill or mentally defective individuals might have less chance of carrying out a successful crime as compared with 'normal' violent offenders, if death of the victim is the criterion used. As it turned out, diagnostic variables in successful acts were related also to the victim: when the victims were the offender's own children, and these were the most common victims of depressed violent women, the chances of the deed being successfully executed were above average, provided that other factors, such as the decreased chance of the crime being reported if it was attempted murder of one's own children, do not explain this association.

If we included attempted murder, therefore, we should have to accept a much less sharp delineation of the population surveyed. If we held firmly to the unambiguous criterion of 'accomplished killing', we should have a clearly defined population but so far as hypotheses were concerned we would introduce an equal degree of ambiguity. The issue was decided on practical grounds: the inclusion of bodily injury endangering life corresponds to the realistic concept and to the criminological problem of violence, and in addition prevents the number of offenders from falling too low. In order to exclude the numerous and ill-defined cases of minor or trivial bodily harm, we included in our definition of crime of violence only attacks[3] which would have led to the death of the victim if circumstances outside the control of the offender had not intervened.

This can be clarified by means of two examples. Extended suicide by a depressed mother, who poisoned herself and her children by means of sleeping pills, was included even if prompt medical intervention saved all the intended victims. A patient suffering from delusional jealousy, who beat his wife, would not be included even if she suffered some minor injuries. However difficult this operational definition and dividing line may seem, it proved in practice to be simpler than we anticipated. It also ensured that all the available records of the violent crimes by mentally ill and mentally defective individuals which had led to serious or major harm to the victim and which ought to be covered by our survey, were in fact included.

Within the framework of our investigation the definition of a crime of violence was therefore as follows: an attack on a human being which either led to the death of the victim or would have done so if circumstances outside the control of the person committing the attack had not intervened.

Legal classification of the offenders

The simplest way of collecting material for our study seemed to be to abstract from the Federal Statistics of Convicted Offenders all those cases in which the mitigating circumstances of mental illness or mental deficiency, in terms of Section 51, para. 1 or 2, of the Penal Code, had been deemed to apply. But apart from the fact that this would have excluded a large proportion of offenders, namely those who did not appear before the courts, the Federal Statistics did not provide a sufficiently detailed analysis. In addition there were difficulties in adapting the penal descriptions of the crimes to our own operational criteria. (German criminal law is normative law. Classification of offenders and penal measures are mostly detailed very fully in the Penal Code. The judge has to give his verdict in accordance with this Code, so that the verdict carries with it a classification of the offenders in terms of defined standards.)

Violent crimes endangering life are covered in the German Penal Code by Sections 211 (murder),[4] 212 (manslaughter),[5] 213 (manslaughter in extenuating circumstances),[6] and 226 (bodily harm resulting in death).[7] The relevant law distinguishes between murder and manslaughter according to: very different criteria of motivation (particularly motives such as a pathological urge to murder, gratification of sexual drives, greed or other 'base motives'), the means used (means that constitute a public danger), mode of killing (insidious or ferocious) and the purpose of the deed (homicide aimed at furthering or concealing another crime is murder under Section 211 of the Penal Code). It is clear that from the point of view of empirical psychological research these are very heterogeneous criteria, some of which, such as 'base motives', make objective assessment difficult. For studies of mentally ill violent offenders such distinctions are of little practical use, especially since criteria which would betoken murder, such as 'base motives' or 'ferocious execution of the crime', are not as a rule evaluated when the motivations or impulses which lead to the crime are of a morbid nature.

Steigleder (1968) has shown in his detailed analysis of this problem that the criteria which differentiate murder from manslaughter are not precise. In his view, therefore, we still do not know where the boundary lies between these two crimes. Looked at from the psychological point of view, the legal definition of murder is highly complex: 'The diversity of the overt act, and even more the manifold and closely interwoven psychological and psycho-pathological processes in those who commit it, would seem to make an unambiguous classification almost impossible from this point of view' (*op. cit.*, p. 7). For these reasons Steigleder rightly takes the view that for medical specialists the distinction between murder and manslaughter is fundamentally of little importance. We share Steigleder's opinion, though not for the reasons which he advances. In our view, the categories in the Penal Code are most inadequate, and the various unsatisfactory divisions of the crime and the criminal are insufficient to form a basis for differentiating murder from manslaughter.

Similarly Rasch (1964), in attempting to describe certain murder-victim syndromes, had to abandon the distinction between murder and manslaughter, because 'such a demarcation and classification has to be mostly elaborated *de lege lata* according to highly abstract and quasi-psychological criteria and yet is essentially a question of the evaluation and significance of the case concerned' (*op. cit.*, p.1).

Even a cohort composed of cases of criminal homicide (according to Sections 211, 212 and 213), attempted homicide[8] and bodily harm resulting in death (Section 226) would not have included all the offenders covered by our definition. The two further very special homicidal crimes which the Penal Code cites - killing on request (Section 216)[9] and infanticide (Section 217)[10] - are of no particular importance so far as violent crimes by the mentally abnormal are concerned: killing on request represents a very rare motivation and infanti-cide a very restricted category of offender (unmarried women immediately after childbirth). To anticipate our findings, the former crime did not feature at all in our survey, and only one of our 533 cases was confirmed as infanticide.

The 'intentional' homicidal crimes mentioned above and defined in the Penal Code, even if they are not subdivided, form a general category which could be fitted in to the framework of our operational definition of a violent crime. This category is not complete, however, since the German Penal Code contains a series of further definitions such as Sections 177 (rape followed by death), 227 (brawling), 307 (very serious cases of arson), 311 (causing an explosion), 312 (deliberate flooding endangering human life), 324 (poisoning of water supply) and 330a (crimes committed in drunken frenzy), which in special circumstances comprise or include criminal homicide. We will discuss

the problems arising from this when we come to compare our results with the
Federal Statistics of Convicted Offenders.

The greatest difficulties encountered in adapting legal criteria of
crime to our operational definitions were those presented by 'bodily injuries'.
We had already formulated reasons why we considered it necessary to include
serious attacks which did not end in the death of the victim and we could therefore not be satisfied with the category of 'bodily harm resulting in death'
defined by Section 226. The remaining provisions of the Penal Code which cover
bodily harm other than that caused accidentally (Sections 223, 223a, 223b, 224,
225[11]) range so widely that they go beyond any definition of violent crime
that would make epidemiological sense. They are defined partly according to
criteria that may be grounded in legal history and legal politics, but that
could not be considered adequate in relation to psychiatry. The less serious
offences covered by these Sections are, moreover, greatly affected by the dark
area of low rates of reporting and clearing up such crimes.

So far as bodily harm not ending in death was concerned, therefore,
and in contrast to the homicidal crimes, we did not have even an incomplete
core group of offences to draw upon which was defined in terms of a valid
criterion that conformed both to the Penal Code and to our requirements.
Regardless of the criminal side of the case, we could record instances of
bodily harm only if they corresponded to the criteria of our 'operational'
definition of a violent crime, as detailed above. Strictly interpreted, this
meant that bodily harm in the sense of Sections 223, 223b, 224 and 225 were
excluded from our definition of a violent crime, since one of their most
important common criteria is that there should be no intention to kill on the
part of the offender. The same applies also to Section 226 (bodily harm
resulting in death), since this likewise excludes any intention to kill in
the strict sense.

In a psychological study of offenders the main difficulty encountered in using legal categories based on court verdicts is that psychological
examination may reveal intentions which the offender has the basic right to
deny in court. The verdict of the court, in accordance with which the offender
is placed in a certain category, is based on legal arguments with all their
procedural rules and limitations and not on the rules of objective empirical
examination of psychological content. This is the reason why an unknown number
of normal offenders, who according to our criteria would be considered to have
committed crimes of violence, were found guilty only of causing bodily harm or
of neglect in rendering aid, and not of attempted homicide, murder or manslaughter. In addition there are many different reasons for acquittal, none

of which shows up in the Federal Statistics of Convicted Offenders.

Apart from this discrepancy at the level of case identification, there is also a limited discrepancy in the criteria of classifications: intention to kill, as defined by us, includes the legal concept of intent to kill, but it covers much else besides. An act of violence by an epileptic, for example, who in a state of blind agitation inflicts grievous bodily harm, would clearly fall within our definition, though in the legal sense it would hardly be possible to prove that there was any intent to kill. In other words, even emotional excitement which discharges itself in a life-endangering attack is covered by our rather widely stretched definition of intent to kill. In this way we endeavoured to record practically all the offences that led to grievous bodily harm. This means, of course, that we had to sacrifice some points of differentiation that are made in the rough psychological divisions of the Penal Code, but we are sure that this is advantageous to our study.

From what has been said it will be clear that we hoped at all events to cover with some degree of reliability all possible cases of intent to kill. As mentioned, we encountered fewer difficulties than we had feared: in so far as it does not mean a lack of critical insight on our part, this may be due to the fact that we were able to begin with basic psychiatric and psychological studies of the offenders that had nothing whatsoever to do with the courtroom. We formed the impression, however, that the most important reason lay in the fact that, contrary to a widely held view, mentally ill offenders are more transparent in their intentions, particularly when these are of morbid origin, and more frank in their statements about such intentions than are the mentally 'normal'. This may be because, amongst other things, the mentally ill offender who is being investigated psychologically sees that his chances of a lower sentence lie less in denying the crime and its motivation than in complying with a defence on grounds of diminished responsibility or unfitness to plead.

The incomplete concordance between the legal criteria and our operational definition of a violent crime reduces the comparability of our material with the categories of offender listed in the Federal Statistics of Convicted Offenders and partly also with the Police Criminal Statistics. It is true that mentally abnormal violent offenders who have caused the death of their victim, can, if they are brought together in one category, be compared with the analogous group of mentally normal offenders. The category of mentally abnormal offenders who would have killed if circumstances outside their control had not prevented the death of their victim, are classified in the Penal Code under various paragraphs relating to attempted homicide. As we have tried to show, however, these paragraphs probably cover only a proportion of those mentally healthy culprits who are analogous to the mentally abnormal violent offenders, according to our criteria.

Although we think that a relatively small proportion of the offenders in our survey whose victims were only injured should be matched against controls drawn from 'mentally normal' offenders found guilty of bodily harm, it would not make sense to compare these groups on the basis of Criminal Statistics and Statistics of Convicted Offenders. This view is further supported if we compare the small number of offenders found guilty of criminal homicide in the narrower sense with the relatively high numbers of mentally abnormal offenders found guilty of causing bodily harm, as shown by the Statistics of Convicted Offenders and the Police Criminal Statistics Report (cf. Table 14).

Criteria used to identify mental illness or mental defect
in offenders

The legal criterion of diminished responsibility or unfitness to plead, which is based partly on medico-psychological assumptions,[12] naturally provided an important basis for case-finding: every accessible case of violence which was judged under Section 51, para 1 or 2, because of mental illness or mental defect, was included in our survey.

We could not, however, restrict ourselves to this criterion, firstly because there are, as has been said, many mentally ill or mentally defective violent offenders who do not come to judgement (for example those who commit suicide after the crime); secondly, the medico-psychological hypotheses underlying in particular Section 51, para 2 of the Penal Code extend beyond the diagnostic categories of 'mentally ill' and 'mentally deficient' which form the framework of our criteria.

It is, for example, possible for pleas of diminished responsibility or absence of responsibility to be granted to otherwise mentally healthy individuals whose consciousness is disturbed owing to alcoholic or other drug intoxication. As we were concerned solely with all violent crimes on the part of the mentally abnormal, and not just with violent crimes committed in a state of diminished responsibility or absence of responsibility (we did not want to follow the dogmatic assumption of K. Schneider, Gruhle and Haddenbrock that basically no mentally abnormal person is responsible for his crime), we could use neither a legal nor a purely psychological definition of responsibility as our criterion. A plea granted under Section 51, para 1 or 2, of the Penal Code could thus be used only as a pointer in our case-finding.[13]

As we have already pointed out, the psychiatric identification of cases had to be based on two provisos: a high probability of confirming the presence of mental illness or mental handicap in the course of the criminal enquiry or legal proceedings; and adequate validitý and reliability of diagnosis within the categories used. Both these provisos are adequately met in cases of severe mental illness and in those showing a high degree of mental defect.[14] Diagnoses such as neurosis or personality disorder (or psychopathy as it used to be called) are not only less reliable but are to some extent also of inadequate validity when it comes to differentiating them from crisis situations or abnormal modes of behaviour in the mentally healthy. Moreover the large number of these forms of mental disturbance would have added inordinately to the difficulties of conducting an epidemiological study of their relationship to crimes of violence.

In collecting our material, therefore, we included, in addition to mental deficiency, all 'psychoses', or 'genuine' mental illnesses, and all syndromes of mental deterioration and defect. The material then comprised the following groups: (1) schizophrenias; (2) affective psychoses (endogenous depressions, manic-depressive illness); (3) exogenous psychoses (acute and chronic mental disorders based on disturbances of cerebral functioning or on cerebral diseases); and (4) syndromes of defect and deterioration in the narrower sense (psychological and mental defects due to injury of various origins, dementia based on cerebral atrophies, arteriosclerosis, etc.). Although it is debatable whether the psychoses should be kept separate from other mental illnesses, with some subdivisions, for example, in the case of the depressive disorders, this division into the psychoses and the non-psychotic illnesses, together with the use of the above groupings, provided sufficiently high reliability.[15]

So far as the recorded diagnosis of depression was concerned, within the framework of our enquiry the depressive syndromes mostly belonged unambiguously to the group of psychotic depressions, since the depressed violent offenders with whom we were dealing clearly represented a selection of severe depressions. It could, of course, happen that the behaviour of less severely depressed offenders might convey the impression of acknowledged guilt and remorse, so that to the jurists they would not seem at all sick, a fact which must greatly lessen their chances of being referred for psychiatric assessment and diagnosis.

The delineation of mental deficiency also presents problems. This diagnosis is based on intelligence quotients in which the transition from subnormal to normal is on a continuum. On grounds of IQ alone, we could have decided to equate the diagnosis of mental deficiency with an IQ of below 70;

this would, however, have introduced a precision into our criteria which was not matched by similar precision in our research material. In practice an offender was regarded as mentally defective if one of the following authorities had serious doubts about his intelligence: the parties who instituted proceedings (the police and the prosecutors), the defence, or the judge. Only then was it the rule to arrange for a psychiatric examination on grounds of mental deficiency. The second condition was that the examiner should actually find a substantial degree of defect and that the offender should then be granted diminished responsibility or held to be not responsible for his actions, or committed for this reason to an institution.

Legal practices had thus some effect on case-finding in one of the subgroups of our research population. In order to give some idea of the effect of these uncontrollable variables, we can only point out once more that in severe cases the effect tends to be nil, while in the less severe forms it increases, and in the transitional area that borders upon the normal it makes the findings difficult to assess. In other words, we have probably arrived at a fairly accurate estimate of violent criminality in severe and middle degrees of mental defect, but on the basis of our enquiry we are not in a position to predict the risk of such criminality in the 'subnormal' or less severely handicapped.

Main diagnosis (combined diagnoses) and multiple classification

In cases of multiple diagnosis, where the second or third illness was one which lay outside our psychiatric criteria, we entered the case under the diagnosis which came within our criteria and recorded the other illnesses as concurrent diagnoses. A schizophrenic with concurrent chronic alcoholism would, for example, be put under schizophrenia, and a mentally defective offender with personality disturbances would be entered in the category of mental defect. If more than one diagnosis came within our criteria, we arranged to enter the case under a main diagnosis, in accordance with the following criteria: the more severe mental disturbance and that which was demonstrably related to the crime would take precedence over the less severe and that which was not related to the crime. In fact this multiple classification was called for only in the combination of brain damage or mental defect with psychosis, chiefly in cases of *Pfropfschizophrenie* (schizophrenia combined with mental retardation). In such cases schizophrenia was always entered as the main diagnosis and mental defect as the secondary diagnosis. In some of our comparative analyses, however, we were able to start not with the number of offenders but with the diagnosis, which permitted us to take both diagnoses into consideration. Where this has been done it is always clearly indicated in the text.

The subdivision of our diagnostic groups presented certain further
difficulties in that when we recorded our cases there were several classification schemes in use in German psychiatry which differed in some respects one
from another. We had therefore to choose a classification which, apart from
the diagnoses that were common to all schemes, would provide common categories
for those classes which showed a conceptual but not a material difference. This
was relatively simple, in so far as the classification schemes in question were
to a relatively large extent technically the same for the diagnostic areas with
which we were concerned, and we could also make extensive use of diagnostic
groups which had the same validity in all the classification schemes involved.

When it came to recording details of the illnesses, especially the
symptoms shown, we tried to use features which had been recorded by the examining psychiatrists on the basis of fairly uniform concepts and relationships.
This was easy, for example, in the case of the symptoms of the main psychoses,
but difficult when it was a question of assessing personality traits.

3.3 Case-finding

The simplest approach to a study of violent offenders would have
been to use official statistics. Unfortunately, however, the Federal Statistics
of Convicted Offenders give no precise data on the proportion of convicted
offenders who are mentally disturbed. As already mentioned, the offenders
recorded in the Federal Statistics do not cover all those who are mentally ill.
Some are committed immediately to a psychiatric institution, in accordance
with the Regional laws governing compulsory admission (*Landesunterbringungs-
gesetz*), without criminal proceedings being invoked; such cases may include
not only those who attempt suicide but also those who are obviously mentally
ill or mentally defective. So far as our investigation was concerned, therefore,
the chief drawback in using Federal Statistics of Convicted Offenders lay in
their completely inadequate documentation of data which would enable conclusions
to be drawn as to the presence of mental illness or mental defect in the
offender.[16]

The authorities - police and prosecutors - who actually deal with
all identified violent offenders, are regional (*Landesbehörden*) or district
authorities. The Federal Criminal Bureau handles only a small proportion of
the documentation on offenders, namely those cases in which it has been involved
on special grounds. Even though the records of the individual Regions (*Länder*)
and of the 93 prosecuting offices in the GFR varied in quality - some regional
authorities provided excellent documentation - their lists of offenders formed
an important source for our case-finding, coming closer than anything else to

comprehensive information. Moreover the co-operation we received from all
these authorities was exemplary.

Since no single source of material was uniformly available, we
decided on three parallel methods of case-finding. We hoped in this way to
cover the relevant offenders as comprehensively as possible:

1. The records of the Federal and Regional Criminal Bureaus,
   irrespective of whether it was a question of opening an
   indictment or of sentencing an offender.

2. The records of the 93 prosecuting offices in the GFR. (These
   keep the records of identified and arrested offenders, both in
   regard to proceedings leading to a court verdict and in regard
   to proceedings instituted by the prosecuting office or the
   judiciary including files on offenders who had died after the
   crime, usually by suicide.)

These two sources supplied us with files on the cases and on offenders. The
only documents which we examined *in situ* were those of the Federal Criminal
Bureau (at Wiesbaden).

3. All regional psychiatric hospitals in the GFR to which
   violent offenders were committed. (In this way we obtained
   access in particular to those offenders who had been
   committed after a crime as constituting a danger to the
   public and/or for purposes of treatment.)

Double registration can be discounted, since surname, Christian
name and date of birth were fully documented.

3.4   Representative nature of the material

The total number of mentally ill and mentally defective offenders
whom we recorded by these three methods was 533. This may be broken down into
ten yearly rates and compared with some similar categories of violent offenders
that appear in the criminal statistics published by the police authorities
(Table 2).

When we compare our figures for mentally abnormal violent offenders
with police figures for those convicted of murder or manslaughter, including
attempted murder or manslaughter, the following points emerge: With the rise
in the general rate for violent crime, calculated for two-yearly periods, the
number of mentally abnormal violent offenders also rises slowly. If we assume
that the rate of violent crime in the mentally abnormal between 1955 and 1964
has developed on the same lines as the corresponding rate for the population
as a whole, then the parallel tendency (it cannot be called more than that on
the basis of this rather imprecise comparison) argues against the view that

Table 2. *Comparison of mentally abnormal violent offenders in the research sample with trends in general criminality (murder and manslaughter, including attempted murder and attempted homicide) 1955-1964*

	Our data on mentally abnormal violent offenders		Police statistics of recorded offenders (murder and manslaughter, incl. attempts)		
Year of crime	No. of offenders	Decrease in no. of offenders 1964-55[a]	No. of offenders	% of crimes cleared up	Decrease in no. of offenders 1964-55[a]
1955	45	} 62%	904	(92.4)	} 67%
1956	44		906	(92.3)	
1957	36	} 56%	914	(91.7)	} 69%
1958	45		950	(94.4)	
1959	55	} 70%	1003	(92.5)	} 77%
1960	46		1071	(91.4)	
1961	57	} 82%	1065	(92.7)	} 84%
1962	61		1201	(93.1)	
1963	68	} 100%	1261	(92.0)	} 100%
1964	76		1426	(93.6)	

[a] Calculated in two-yearly rates: 1963 and 1964 = 100%.

Notes on Table 2

1. Up to 1960 the yearly percentages given in the police statistics included the GFR except for West Berlin and Saarland; in 1961 Saarland was included, and from 1962 both West Berlin and Saarland.

2. We have abstracted from the police statistics only those offenders who were recorded in the statistics because of murder, manslaughter, attempted murder or attempted manslaughter (Sections 211, 212, 213 of the Penal Code). As discussed above in more detail, these categories correspond fairly well to our operational definition of a violent crime. They by no means cover, of course, the whole of violent crime. Apart from the small number of special homicidal acts such as 'killing a new-born child', we omitted all cases of 'grievous bodily harm' (average yearly rate of around 28 700) and bodily harm ending fatally (yearly rate between 260 and 910). The reason for this was mainly that when the police statistics were reorganised, from 1 January 1963, traffic offences, which till then had been included with bodily harm, were for the first time removed from this category. This led to a sharp fall in the annual rate from 1963. If these offences were included, comparison between these categories would be possible only to a very limited degree. We also excluded from our comparison of annual rates those female offenders whose crime was the killing of new-born children, since police statistics for the years 1955/6/7/8 contained an error (till then male offenders were also included in this category although under the Penal Code it is an offence which can be committed only by the mother).

our case-finding might have become much less comprehensive with the passage of time.

Admittedly our material is comprehensive only to a certain degree. Our methods of case-finding nevertheless represent the optimal possibilities available at present in the GFR for obtaining a sample of mentally abnormal violent offenders which is both representative and of adequate size.

It would seem, however, that the representative nature of our material is limited in two categories of offender, namely, the mentally defectives and the depressives. Referral of mentally defective offenders for psychiatric examination depends on the assessment of the responsible judges and prosecuting authorities. In the border area of subnormality, which we have already mentioned, there are uncontrollable selective factors at work. For this reason it is unlikely that the subgroup of mentally defective offenders is as representative as our material as a whole. So far as depressed offenders are concerned, we have to consider two factors which may increase the dark figure:

1. They more frequently commit suicide. If the offender is no longer alive, and if his illness was in its initial phase, the chance of its being identified are less.

2. Most depressed offenders were married mothers, who committed an extended suicide. If the act is not completed, but leads for example only to injury or to reversible damage (poisoning, etc.) of the offender's own young children, then there is a chance that it will be concealed from the authorities. The family doctor or the hospital psychiatrist often fall in with the understandable inclination of the family to hush up the offence. Their motives range from a desire to improve the prospects of rehabilitation to a very understandable underestimate of the dangerousness of depressed female offenders. Since the official figures for such crimes is therefore certainly not comprehensive, and since most psychiatric hospitals at the time of our study had no documentation beyond the history of the illness that would give details of the offence, we were hardly in a position to achieve comprehensive cover of depressed offenders who had attempted homicide. Where actual homicide is concerned, the register of depressed offenders is more nearly complete. [17]

To conclude this section we would add that the chance of an offender being included in our register was higher, the more authorities were concerned with his crime. If the offender survives after a serious crime of violence, ending in the death of the victim, the case usually involves the police, the

prosecuting authorities and the mental hospital, so that, as we have often
mentioned, the chance of his being included in our material may be assumed
to be maximal.

3.5 Conduct of the enquiry; validity of the data obtained

After exploring possible methods of case-finding and after a pilot
study which one of us (Häfner) carried out on a small sample of cases and case
histories in order to develop working hypotheses and categories to be used, we
drew up data sheets, in close collaboration with our statistical advisers
(G. Wagner and C. Köhler). These were designed for transfer to IBM cards and
contained 79 items. After a trial run by A. Schmitt, again carried out on a
small number of cases, and a further revision of the schema, work was begun in
1966 on the first part of the enquiry. (The data sheets are reproduced on
pp. 336-49).

Two medical members of the team (W. Böker and A. Schmitt) visited
those regional psychiatric hospitals in the GFR which receive mentally abnormal
offenders within the categories described above. At the same time details were
requested from the relevant authorities (Federal Criminal Bureau, Regional
Criminal Bureaus, state prosecuting officers) about the same categories of
offender and - at our request - files were supplied covering committal or
court proceedings.

The two sources of information, hospital records and judicial files,
showed a high degree of concordance in regard to most of the items in question.
Thus, for example, we usually received copies of the same psychiatric assessment,
which was our most important source of information about the mental state of the
offender at the time of the crime. So far as the various sections of the
schedule were concerned, demographic and social data about the offender and
about the victim were usually very reliably documented in the files of
committal and of court proceedings, and particularly in documents of sentencing,
if sentence was passed. Family data and details of the previous history and
behaviour of the offender before the crime were provided by both sources with
varying degrees of accuracy. They were used to supplement our records.

Our data were thus based not on our own examination of the
offenders but on the findings of a relatively large number of other investigators. This is admittedly a doubtful procedure. But in a retrospective study
there is hardly an alternative. Our own psychiatric examination of the
offenders, carried out on average five to six, or even twelve, years after
the crime, would have contributed much less to an assessment of these long
distance facts than an evaluation of findings recorded at the time. Moreover

we could count on a degree of accuracy in the psychiatric documentation that was relatively above the average. Forensic psychiatric assessments, particularly when a crime of violence is involved, are as a rule very thorough and are supplemented by a considerable number of facts from the previous history and from the evidence. The objection that with soft data, particularly those which depend to a fairly large extent on judgement, there is bound to be an uncontrollable amount of unreliability, cannot, however, be refuted. In order to counter the objection that our documentation of the different items varied in its comprehensiveness, we have drawn express attention to those instances in which the proportion of 'not knowns' was fairly high, and where it was more than 30% we refrained from giving any results at all.

On the other hand it should be pointed out that our research population offered one particular methodological advantage: if we include the incomplete cases in our data, the success rate was 100%, which is hardly ever attained in comparable epidemiological or social science enquiries.[18]

In spite of the above considerations, we set out initially with a plan to interview personally a sample of around 100 offenders and to compare the findings with those obtained from secondary sources. With this in mind A. Schmitt conducted 99 and W. Böker six interviews. However fruitful this was in terms of psychiatric experience, it proved unproductive so far as the intended evaluation was concerned. The information and insight obtained personally in this way did in many cases make an inescapable impression of authenticity and supplemented, if they did not alter, earlier interpretations; but just as frequently we encountered descriptions of the crime or of its motives which could only be distortions of realities, false memories answering the need to cleanse oneself of guilt or at least to give a much more positive account of one's role in the crime. How could one make such a distinction objective? Taking into account the normal gaps in memory for long distance events, the effects of an illness that had often lasted for several years and the equally important effects of hospitalisation under very artificial living conditions, we were in the end unable to regard these interviews as of sufficient scientific relevance. We therefore did not evaluate them quantitatively in any way and used them solely to supplement our data (in the case of hard data only) and as a source of experience which might help us to interpret our findings.

Since our material was assembled by two investigators (W. Böker 190 cases, A. Schmitt 343 cases) we had to allow for differences in judgement, especially where certain assessments were concerned. Before evaluating our results we therefore carried out a test of concordance. Those items in which

the two assessors differed significantly, within a probability of error of
α = 0.05, were dropped from our evaluation as unreliable.[19]

The reliability of the data recorded naturally varies: data
about family relationships between the offender and the victim can be expected
to reach a high standard of completeness and validity, while data about
motivation for the crime depend heavily on value judgements and therefore do
not attain the same degree of completeness in their documentation. We took
account of this when we prepared our data sheets and in evaluating the results
we shall try where possible to use the valid data in order to make indirect
checks of our hypotheses - for example, checking hypotheses about motivation
by using offender-victim relationships. The predictive value of the findings
nevertheless still varies, depending as it does on the quality of the data
underlying them. This predictive value is comparatively high for demographic
items and for items such as the diagnosis, duration and symptoms of the illness,
but comparatively low for psychological items which depend on value judgements,
such as personality factors and motivation for the crime.

3.6   Control populations and comparative groups

In order to test individual hypotheses, we contrasted the mentally
abnormal violent offenders in our sample with various control populations and
comparative groups.

Comparison with the general population of the GFR (i.e. those
who had reached the age of 'legal responsibility')

Our results were analysed on demographic lines and compared for
age and sex with the general population of the GFR who had reached the age of
legal responsibility (all inhabitants of the GFR aged 14 and over). We took
for this purpose the arithmetical mean and the total figures for the years
1955 to 1964 covering the age groups relevant to our study. For the years
1955 to 1958 the figures were taken from the Federal Statistics of Convicted
Offenders (then called the Penal Research Statistics) and for 1959 to 1964 from
the Statistical Report (*Population and Culture, Series 9: Administration of
Justice* issued by the Federal Statistical Bureau in Wiesbaden (continuation
of the Federal Statistics of Convicted Offenders)).

Comparison with all convicted violent offenders

When we looked for a representative control population of violent
offenders we were faced with a choice between Police Criminal Statistics and
Federal Statistics of Convictions. Since only the statistics of convictions

provided detailed and reliable demographic data on the offenders, we had to
rely on them, in spite of their variations in classification and their attend-
ant imperfections. We therefore compared our cohort of offenders with convicted
violent offenders of the relevant decade,[20] which presumably gave us, at
least according to judicial principles, only 'mentally normal' offenders.
Apart from the demographic data, the comparison had to be limited to individual items connected with the crime, since the other data and statistical
records were not sufficiently reliable. The basis of comparison covered all
convicted offenders whose crime of violence was classified under Sections 211,
212, 213, 216, 217, 225 and 226 of the Penal Code.

Comparison with mentally abnormal persons in the general population
The important problem of the risk of violent crimes being committed
by mentally abnormal persons in general or by those belonging to specific
diagnostic groups presented great difficulties. There are no epidemiological
data about the frequency, age of onset of first attack, age distribution, etc.,
of mental illnesses in the general population of the GFR. In order to obtain
at least some orientation in regard to such risks in the absence of such data,
we took our findings on the comparative frequency of illness in the total population of violent offenders convicted during the decade in question and related
them to mean global figures for the prevalence of mental illness and mental
defect in other countries. In calculating the risk of violence in individual
diagnostic groups we used for purposes of comparison the only adequate data
available in Germany at the time, namely, the results of a study of 'consultation rates' for mental illness in Mannheim (Häfner et al., 1969; Häfner, 1970;
Reimann & Häfner, 1972). The problems raised by this procedure and the limits
of its reliability are discussed in more detail elsewhere.

Group comparison with a sample of mentally abnormal 'non-
offenders'
Since the comparison with 'mentally healthy' violent offenders was
possible only within narrow limits, comparison with groups of mentally ill and
mentally defective 'non-offenders' became particularly important so far as the
testing of our working hypotheses was concerned - especially in regard to the
calculation of special risk factors. Again the ideal group for comparison
would have been a representative sample of all mentally abnormal persons living
in the GFR, including the true proportion of untreated cases. But, as already
pointed out, the necessary epidemiological data are lacking. It would therefore
have been impossible for us to obtain such a representative sample, even if we

had been able to cope with the enormous expense. We had instead to look for a
sample of the mentally abnormal that would be manageable and would meet at
least to some extent the requirements of a control group. It proved opportune
to select the admissions to a large regional psychiatric hospital, taking
admission to hospital as an 'index event' that was analogous to the crime.

The disadvantage of using hospital admissions - or first admissions - is that they represent only to a limited extent the real incidence of
mental illness. The demand for admission to a mental hospital is influenced by
a profusion of factors, such as the readiness of the patient and his family to
seek help and the decisions taken about admission by doctors and functionaries
concerned, which in turn depend on attitudes, on the availability of alternative forms of treatment and on social factors. This leads to different
patterns of admission, particularly in regard to the range of diagnoses and
the age distribution of the patients admitted. In the case of severe, acute
disturbances, such as schizophrenic attacks, the effect is probably slight,
but social factors play a decisive role in determining, for example, whether
senile patients and mental defectives are admitted to hospital or not. For
this reason our control group of mental defectives, who are more often admitted
to hospital because of secondary symptoms such as socially disturbing behaviour
than because of the mental defect alone, can hardly be regarded as representative, while the group of endogenous psychoses, especially the schizophrenics,
should come close to being a representative sample.

To obtain our sample of non-violent mentally abnormal persons we
took the admissions to a large mental hospital in the Region (Land) of
Rheinland-Pfalz. The 'Pfälzische Nervenklinik Landeck' is responsible for the
catchment area of Pfalz, with a population of over 1.3 million, and includes
the large industrial town of Ludwigshafen on the Rhine, as well as country
areas.[21] The clinic is a little larger than the average regional clinic (in
1959 it dealt with an average of 1692 occupied beds, representing an
average of 830 men and 962 women).

Taking the admission registers for the years 1955 to 1964, we
selected every fifth admission to this hospital - regardless of whether it was
a first admission or a readmission - and recorded details of age, sex and
diagnosis. Cases admitted for forensic psychiatric assessment were not
included. From this sample (n = 3496) we calculated the total number of
patients admitted during the decade (including children and adolescents) as
being 17 480. In order to make the sample match the research cohort of abnormal
offenders and the other control groups from the general population who had
reached the age of responsibility, we eliminated all patients under the age of
14. The final sample from Landeck consisted of 3392 cases.

Inter-group comparison

Our next group came from admissions between 1955 and 1964 to the Regional Mental Hospital of Wiesloch, which is near Heidelberg and is responsible chiefly for the cities of Mannheim/Heidelberg and for the administrative area of Nordbaden, with a total population of 1.75 million: on the basis of the 1959 figures this meant an average bed occupancy of 1676. From these admissions we formed a matched sample of 533 mentally abnormal non-offenders, each case selected corresponding in sex, age and diagnosis to one of our 533 violent patients. Concordance between the groups in regard to these items was statistically valid (see Chapter 7). Each case in this control group was subjected to the same recording procedure - except for the data about the crime - as the abnormal offenders.

Sub-group comparison

Finally, it seemed promising and reasonable, so far as testing our hypotheses was concerned, to divide the research cohort of abnormal offenders into subgroups, for example according to diagnostic categories, and to compare these in respect of different variables.

Any quantifying or scaling of the items was to a large extent abandoned on methodological grounds: in a secondary investigation scaled assessments of items which have possibly been classified or estimated by the original examiner on a different basis can hardly be justified.

Differences were submitted to chi-square testing. In Chapter 5 the most important data are given in several dimensions (sex, age, diagnosis) and subjected to cross-comparisons. In order to be able to test these factors and their interactions, we calculated multiple chi-square values, using Lancaster's method (1969). For inter-group comparisons (Chapter 7) we used chi-square values calculated according to Irvin & Snedecor for $2 \times n$-tables. At a level of maximal $\alpha = 0.05$ we regarded the correlation as significant. Our aim was not only to look for significant differences or correlations but also to assess the weight to be attached to those variables which seemed to be important and to include this in our interpretation.

Unfortunately, in spite of the breadth of our categories, the numbers in most diagnostic classes proved to be small. A fairly complete group comparison with the 'statistical twins' drawn from the control group of hospital admissions was therefore possible only for the group of schizophrenics. Although the numbers of cases of mental deficiency were generally adequate, the comparison was of limited predictive value, because the control population was open to the influence of unverifiable selective factors. For the affective psychoses

our comparison had to be limited to a few items only. So far as those illnesses
were concerned which occurred less frequently in the research cohort of
violent offenders, such as exogenous psychoses, or epilepsy, or heterogeneous
groups such as the broad category of organic cerebral damage, we could not
carry out a statistical comparison of any kind, since the numbers of cases
were so small. Predictions about violent offenders in these groups can therefore be presented only on the basis of a quantitative analysis which is of low
general applicability, and at times only on the basis of case histories. From
findings such as these, based on small numbers, the trends which can be discerned
vary in the degree of certainty which attaches to them.

The results of our quantitative evaluations are set out in the
following chapters.

4.   RESULTS I : GENERAL DATA

4.1 Number of offenders and their sex distribution

We begin this quantitative and qualitative analysis of our findings with a brief summary of the general data: in later chapters these will be broken down into separate items which will be subjected to group comparisons.

In the decade from 1 January 1955 to 31 December 1964 we found that in the GFR, including Saarland and West Berlin, 533 mentally ill or mentally defective individuals committed a crime of violence against the life of another person. Of these offenders 410 (77%) were men and 123 (23%) women.

4.2 Location of the crime by Federal region *(Land)*

Table 3. *Distribution of mentally abnormal violent offenders by federal region 1955-64*

	No. of offenders	
Federal region *(Land)*	*n*	%
Baden-Württemberg	105	19.7
Bayern	55	10.3
West Berlin	23	4.3
Hamburg and Bremen	39	7.3
Hessen	49	9.2
Niedersachsen	68	12.8
Nordrhein-Westfalen	149	28.0
Rheinland-Pfalz	21	3.9
Saarland	1	0.2
Schleswig-Holstein	23	4.3
Total	533	100.0

Table 3 shows clear differences in the regional rates; for example for Saarland (only 1 case) and West Berlin (23 cases), the ratio between the rates in the two populations is approximately 0.4 : 1. The numbers are so small, however, that we would not be justified in drawing any conclusions about the prevalence of violence among the mentally abnormal in these two geographical areas. Moreover such discrepancies lie within the range of random statistical distribution. Different methods of selection and documentation probably also play a part.[1]

4.3 Date of crime

The number of cases per calendar year has already been given in Table 2 (p. 61).

4.4 Nature of crime

In accordance with our definition of a violent crime, it was to be expected that not all the offenders would actually have killed or seriously injured their victim or victims. In some cases the crime, or series of crimes, was interrupted; in others its accomplishment was prevented by favourable circumstances such as a gun that misfired, or speedy recovery and prompt medical attention in a case of poisoning, so that the victim was not seriously harmed. We included such cases in our survey only if, in the terms of our definition, it was highly probable that without the intervention of these special circumstances, the victim would have died.

Altogether 19 offenders (3.6%; 14 men and 5 women) had initiated such an attack which did not lead to serious or permanent injury to the victim. These

Table 4. *Distribution of 533 mentally abnormal offenders by sex and by outcome (fatal or non-fatal) of crime*

Nature of crime	Men		Women		Total	
	n	%	n	%	n	%
Not resulting in death	234	57.1	45	36.6	279	52.3
Resulting in death	176	42.9	78	63.4	254	47.7
Total	410	100.0	123	100.0	533	100.0

Significance test: $\chi^2 = 15.9209$ df = 1 $\alpha = 0.001$

cases will be analysed further in Chapter 8. In the preliminary legal and
medical reports 17 of these 19 crimes were classed as 'attempted homicide'.
This concept implies that the offender intended or desired to cause death –
an assumption that was made, or not made, by those responsible for the
preliminary examination of the offender after the crime (such examination,
if it takes place, being usually carried out at the time of the first police
interrogation). Since such a classification seems of doubtful value where the
mentally abnormal are concerned, and since our operational definition of a
violent crime did not completely coincide with the judicial concepts of murder,
manslaughter, attempted homicide, bodily harm resulting in death, etc., we
did not apply this categorisation to the remaining offenders whose crime led
to death or injury.

    The number of offenders who killed one or more victims was 254,
or 47.7%. In the remaining 279 cases, or 52.3%, the violence did not result in
death. Two hundred and eighty-six offenders, or 53.7%, injured one or more
victims. In 26 cases (4.9%) the crime caused the death of one victim and the
injury of others. Dividing the cases according to whether or not they resulted
in death, we arrived at the distribution between the sexes shown in Table 4.
The proportion of crimes ending in death was thus very much higher for female
than for male offenders. This finding is at first sight surprising and its
interpretation is discussed in Chapter 8, where we consider the correlations
between specific diagnoses and the characteristics of the offenders.

4.5 Number of victims

	No. killed			*No. injured*	
279	cases not resulting in death	–	247	cases not injured	–
232	cases with 1 death	232	249	cases with 1 person injured	249
13	cases with 2 deaths	26	27	cases with 2 persons injured	54
7	cases with 3 deaths	21	5	cases with 3 persons injured	15
1	case with 4 deaths	4	3	cases with 4 persons injured	12
1	case with 10 deaths	10 [a]	1	case with 10 persons injured	10 [b]
			1	case with 22 persons injured	22 [a]
533	Total no. of deaths	293	533	Total no. of persons injured	362

Notes:

[a] This was the attack by the Volkhoven flamethrower in June 1964 on a school
in Cologne, carried out by a man who in all probability was a chronic paranoid schizophrenic. (The case, which caused a great sensation and was the
subject of a criminological report by Kiehne, published in 1965, led to a
parliamentary question in the federal parliament.)

Notes (contd.)

(b) A 22-year old schizophrenic, who hit unknown passers-by on the head with a hammer because his imperative voices commanded him to do so.

Neither of these offenders - at least in so far as the number of victims is concerned - can be regarded as typical of the mentally abnormal violent offender.

In all, therefore, 655 persons were killed or injured by 533 offenders. Violent crimes directed against one individual are by far the most frequent. Only in a small fraction of the cases (19 out of 533, or 3.6%) were three or more victims attacked. Violent crimes in which three or more persons were killed were committed by nine offenders (1.7%) in our study. Multiple murders by the mentally disturbed are thus very rare in our material.

Analysis of the victims by age (adults or children) and sex, the relationship between characteristics of the victim and the sex and diagnosis of the offender, etc., will be discussed in Chapter 8, when the victims are considered.

5. RESULTS II : OVERALL COMPARISONS OF SEX, AGE AND
   DIAGNOSIS

In this chapter we shall compare the mentally disturbed violent
offenders with our control groups in regard to their sex, age and diagnosis.
Sex and age were the only items for which a comparison could be made between
the abnormal offenders, the normal offenders, the non-violent patients of the
Regional Psychiatric Hospital of Rheinland-Pfalz (Landeck), and the general
adult population. The marital status of the 'normal' offenders could not be
ascertained from the Federal Statistics of Convicted Offenders. Any indication of the relationship between marital status and the risk of violence in
the mentally abnormal had therefore to be based solely on a comparison between
groups of mentally abnormal patients (533 violent and 533 non-violent: see
Chapter 7), who were matched for age, sex and diagnosis. The diagnostic
classification of the abnormal offenders and of the group of non-violent in-
patients was tested on a sample of 3392 patients admitted to the Regional
Psychiatric Hospital of Rheinland-Pfalz.

5.1 Sex

Criminal statistics and other reports on mentally normal violent
offenders from different federal regions (Bromberg, Brückner, von Hentig,
Rangol, Steigleder, Wolfgang and others) have shown that men are significantly
more often involved in murder and other serious crimes of aggression than
their numbers in the general population would suggest. The first question
that interested us, therefore, was whether the male sex was also over-
represented in our group of abnormal offenders.

As Fig. 1 and Table 5 show, there are marked differences in sex
distribution between the groups of offenders and non-offenders: this is
confirmed by further statistical analysis. In the non-violent group of
patients the distribution is much the same as in the general population: in
both groups there are significantly more women than men. The sex distribution of the violent patients, on the other hand, is very different: more
than three-quarters of this group consist of men. These mentally abnormal

violent offenders have, however, practically the same sex distribution as the
'normal' violent offenders taken from the Federal Statistics of Convicted
Offenders, who show the same high proportion of men.

When we applied Lancaster's multiple chi-square test to the absolute
figures given in Table 5, and looked for significant differences in the sex

Fig. 1. Sex distribution of (1) mentally abnormal violent offenders
(n = 533), (2) normal (convicted) violent offenders (n = 3808),
(3) mentally abnormal non-offenders (n = 3392) and (4) the general
population of responsible age (n = 42 647 000).

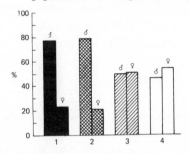

Table 5. *Sex distribution in absolute and relative figures of mentally
abnormal violent offenders, normal violent offenders, mentally abnormal
non-offenders, and the general adult population*

Sex	Mentally abnormal violent offenders		Normal violent offenders		Mentally abnormal non-offenders		General population of legally responsible age	
	n	%	n	%	n	%	n	%
Male	410	76.9	2996	78.7	1685	49.7	19 546 640	45.8
Female	123	23.1	812	21.3	1707	50.3	23 100 360	54.2
Total	533	100.0	3808	100.0	3392	100.0	42 647 000[a]	100.0

[a] The figures for the general population and for the Federal Statistics of
Convicted Offenders cover all federal regions except Saarland and West
Berlin from 1955 to 1960; from 1961 they cover all federal regions.

distribution of the first three groups as compared with that of the general
population of responsible age, we confirmed that both the abnormal and the
normal violent offenders did indeed show a highly significant difference in
distribution:

$$\chi^2 \text{ (abnormal offenders)} = 207.5187, \quad df = 1, \; \alpha = 0.001$$

$$\chi^2 \text{ (normal offenders)} \quad = 1654.5038, \; df = 1, \; \alpha = 0.001$$

Although the sex distribution of the third group (psychiatric in-
patient admissions) is not at first sight very different from that of the
general adult population, there was in fact a significant difference here too:

$$\chi^2 \text{ (abnormal non-offenders)} = 20.1675, \quad df = 1, \; \alpha = 0.001$$

The difference can be accounted for by the fact that the number of men admitted
to the Landeck hospital was higher than expected.

Finally, if we compare the sex distribution of the mentally
abnormal offenders with that of the Landeck sample, the difference is again
highly significant:

$$\chi^2 = 158.2788, \quad df = 1, \; \alpha = 0.001$$

The most important finding is undoubtedly that men are over-
represented to much the same extent among the mentally abnormal violent
offenders as among the normal convicted violent offenders, the ratio of men
to women being between 3 : 1 and 4 : 1. On the other hand, the sex distribution of the mentally abnormal non-offenders (patient admissions sample) and of
the general population was, in spite of the highly significant difference
between the two groups, approximately 1 : 1. The preponderance of men among
the mentally abnormal violent offenders is in keeping with the assumptions and
findings of other authors whom we have already mentioned, although there is
some variation in the ratios reported. For example, Lanzkron in the USA found
a ratio of 4 men to 1 woman in mentally abnormal murderers, a figure which
comes very close to our own, while Varma and Iha in India reported a considerably different ratio of 10 : 1. This unusually high preponderance of men is
probably affected by cultural aspects of crime and punishment. West, in his
1965 study of murder and suicide in London, reported some national figures of
sex distribution in murderers who committed suicide after the crime (in his

view a high proportion of them were mentally ill, suffering particularly from depression).

Although the findings in the literature are not strictly comparable, we reproduce some of them here. In the USA (Wolfgang, 1958) the ratio of men to women was around 11 : 1; in Australia (McKenzie, cited in West, 1965) around 3 : 1; in Denmark (Siciliano, 1961) around 1 : 1; in England (West, 1965) around 1.7 : 1. The considerable differences in these findings would suggest that they are affected not only by socio-cultural influences but also by the different methodological assumptions on which the various surveys were based: for example, differences in the definition of a crime of violence, or in the reliability of case-finding.

To recapitulate our findings in regard to sex distribution: the statistics for mentally abnormal violent offenders were more closely related to those for normal violent offenders than to those for mentally abnormal non-offenders or for the general population. This is seen in the striking similarity in sex distribution found (a) between the general population and non-violent psychiatric patients on the one hand and (b) between 'normal' and mentally abnormal violent offenders on the other. It is also seen in the significant difference found between groups (a) and (b).

5.2   Age

General experience suggests that crimes of violence are more common in the younger age groups, particularly in men between the ages of 20 and 40. Federal German statistics show a peak in violent crimes between 18 and 40. We therefore examined the age distribution of the mentally abnormal offenders, to see whether it followed the same trend.

Looking first at the group of non-violent patients (Table 6), we see that their age distribution, like their sex distribution, is to a large extent the same as that of the general population,[1] though the patients admitted to Landeck hospital contained a higher proportion of the older age groups.

One explanation for this age bias in admissions is probably the growing pressure on psychiatric hospitals to admit elderly patients in need of care, for whom society provides too few alternative possibilities. Another reason is that patients with endogenous psychoses and other mental illnesses requiring in-patient care often relapse and have to be readmitted, thus raising the average age of the hospital population; in other words, there is an illness-dependent factor which, together with the pressure for in-patient care, limits for our purposes the comparability of the admission group.[2]

(It is only when we come to inter-group comparisons with the patient group, which is matched for age as for other items, that comparability is restored.)

The mentally abnormal violent offenders differ considerably from the non-violent patients and, as we had anticipated, their age distribution resembled that of the mentally normal convicted offenders; in other words, the younger and middle age groups (21-40) featured more prominently than in the

Fig. 2. Age distribution of (1) mentally abnormal violent offenders (*n* = 533), (2) normal (convicted) violent offenders (*n* = 3808), (3) mentally abnormal non-offenders (*n* = 3392) and (4) the general population of responsible age (*n* = 42 647 000).

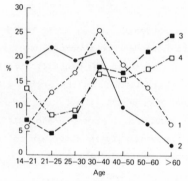

Table 6. *Age distribution in absolute and relative figures for mentally abnormal violent offenders, normal (convicted) violent offenders, mentally abnormal non-offenders, and the general adult population*

Age	Mentally abnormal violent offenders		Normal (convicted) offenders		Mentally abnormal non-offenders		General population of legally responsible age	
	n	%	*n*	%	*n*	%	*n*	%
14 - 21	31	5.8	717	18.8	250	7.4	5 847 890	13.7
21 - 25	69	12.9	838	22.0	158	4.6	3 384 630	7.9
25 - 30	88	16.5	746	19.6	271	8.0	3 798 770	8.9
30 - 40	138	25.9	805	21.2	603	17.8	7 014 540	16.5
40 - 50	99	18.6	374	9.8	566	16.7	6 734 660	15.8
50 - 60	74	13.9	251	6.6	716	21.1	7 351 660	17.2
60 and over	34	6.4	77	2.0	828	24.4	8 514 850	20.0
Total	533	100.0	3808	100.0	3392	100.0	42 647 000	100.0

general population. There are, however, clear differences between the two
groups of offenders.

Crime begins at a later age in the abnormal offenders than in the
normal offenders. As compared with the general population, the convicted
offenders are already over-represented in the 14-21 age group (the mean age
of the normal offenders was around 26.4 years); the abnormal offenders (mean
age 34.7 years) do not reach this stage of over-representation until the age
of 21-25. From the age of 30 to 40, the proportion of abnormal offenders
exceeds that of normal offenders (calculated as percentages of the relevant
total figures). Between the ages of 40 and 50 the normal offenders begin to be
under-represented, but this does not happen in the case of the abnormal
offenders until between the ages of 50 and 60. The results of multiple chi-
square tests are:

$$\chi^2 \text{ (abnormal offenders)} = 159.9066, \quad df = 6, \ \alpha = 0.001$$

$$\chi^2 \text{ (normal offenders)} = 2511.8160, \quad df = 6, \ \alpha = 0.001$$

Here again the in-patient control group, in spite of its being closer
to the general population than to the two groups of offenders, shows an age
distribution that differs significantly from that of the general population
of responsible age:

$$\chi^2 \text{ (abnormal non-offenders)} = 217.0385, \quad df = 6, \ \alpha = 0.001$$

The admissions group contains fewer young and more elderly individuals than
might be expected judging from the age distribution of the general population.

When the mentally abnormal violent offenders are compared with
the in-patient control group, significant differences again emerge:

$$\chi^2 = 23.7510, \quad df = 6, \ \alpha = 0.001$$

The difference in the age curves for the mentally abnormal and the 'normal'
violent offenders is an interesting finding which has also been described in
the literature. East, for example, compared the ages of normal convicted
murderers and mentally abnormal murderers in Broadmoor Institution, England:

Convicted murderers			Mentally abnormal murderers		
Age*(a)*	Men (%)	Women (%)	Age*(b)*	Men (%)	Women (%)
16-21	8	19	16-21	4.6	1.5
21-30	38	56	21-30	24.8	28.7
30-40	25	17	30-40	34.4	46.0
40-50	16	5	40-50	16.0	16.3
50-60	10	1	50-60	11.2	5.0
Over 60	3	1	Over 60	9.0	2.5

From von Hentig (1948).

(a) Age at time of murder; England and Wales 1904-28.
(b) Age at time of admission to Broadmoor; 1922-43.

Mowat (1966) also reported the age distribution for 110 morbidly jealous murderers detained in Broadmoor, as follows:

	Average age	Standard deviation
63 men (murder)	47.5	$\pm$ 9.7
38 men (attempted murder)	46.0	$\pm$ 13.3
8 women (murder)	44.2	
1 woman (attempted murder)	(48)	

Mowat concluded that mentally abnormal murderers are older than 'normal' murderers and that morbidly jealous murderers are older than the average mentally abnormal violent offender. He suggested that the cause might be the development of delusions, which do not usually occur before middle age and which lead only years later to violent tendencies. On the other hand the delusional theme of 'jealousy' points to a selective factor based on marital status, which influenced Mowat's findings: most of his offenders were married, and killed or injured their wives.

The question therefore arises whether the different age distribution of our 533 violent offenders, who were on average 8.5 years older than the 'normal' offenders, is directly due to the illness, or whether factors correlated with the illness, e.g. marriage, marital conflict, professional problems, etc., play an essential role. We shall return to these points later.

Finally we cannot exclude the possibility of an interaction between the variables of sex and age in the populations compared. Such an

interaction would mean that the distribution of one characteristic might be
different at different values of the other.

If we look first at the interaction between sex and age in the
two groups of offenders as compared with the general population of responsible
age, then complex and significant differences do emerge:

$$\chi^2 \text{ (normal offenders)} \quad = 32.4641, \quad df = 6, \quad \alpha = 0.001$$

$$\chi^2 \text{ (abnormal offenders)} = 26.0872, \quad df = 6, \quad \alpha = 0.001$$

In the normal offenders, with the exception of the age group 21-25, there were
fewer women than expected, the difference becoming more marked in the older
age groups. Up to the age of 50, but particularly in the younger age groups,
the overall numbers of men are greater than expected. In mentally abnormal
violent offenders the differences are not so marked as in 'normal' offenders,
but here too there are more men than might be expected in the lower age groups.
The figures for women are throughout lower than might be expected, especially
in the older age groups.

The sample group of patient admissions, on the other hand, shows
no significant interactions as compared with the general population. But if
we compare this group with the abnormal offenders, there is a significant
difference:

$$\chi^2 = 32.4641, \quad df = 6, \quad \alpha = 0.001$$

It is probably accounted for by the fact that the mentally abnormal offenders
include more men in the lower age groups (up to the age of 30) than do the in-
patients admitted to hospital, the difference being more marked than that
between the abnormal offenders and the general population; the in-patient group,
on the other hand, contains more persons of both sexes over the age of 60. With
the exception of the group aged between 25 and 30, there are proportionately
fewer women among the mentally abnormal violent offenders than in the general
population.

It is therefore clear that the age and the sex distributions of the
mentally abnormal violent offenders, as compared with those of the normal
offenders and the general population, are influenced to some extent by intervening variables. We hope that the findings to be presented later will throw
light on these 'variables, especially on diagnosis-dependent factors which
affect age and sex.

5.3 Diagnosis

The question we asked was: Are there any differences in the distribution of diagnoses between the mentally abnormal violent offenders and a random selection of patients admitted for in-patient treatment in psychiatric hospitals? Or, to be more precise: Are there diagnoses which occur with particular frequency in cases of violent crime? For purposes of comparison we again used the sample of patients admitted to the Regional Psychiatric Hospital of Rheinland-Pfalz (Landeck).

As has already been discussed in Chapter 3, we found ourselves at the time of our enquiry faced with the problem that several different and to some extent discordant diagnostic schedules were being used in German mental hospitals. (At that time the one most commonly used was the so-called Würzburg Schema.) In arranging our diagnostic codes we therefore tried to form operationally feasible categories into which the heterogeneous records of different mental hospitals and different assessors could be clearly and consistently fitted and which would cover the diagnostic groups that were essential to our enquiry. In making our comparison we used the following eight diagnostic groups:

1. *Unclassified endogenous psychoses,* in which we included all psychoses that could not be classified as schizophrenia or affective psychosis and which were not associated with organic processes such as cerebral degeneration, cerebral trauma, inflammation, etc. For example, cases diagnosed in the Landeck hospital as 'endogenous psychosis', 'adolescent psychosis', 'climacteric' and 'puerperal' psychoses, or 'involutional psychoses', were entered in this category.

2. *Schizophrenic illness* (the group of schizophrenias).

3. *Affective psychoses* (manic-depressive illness), in which we included, in addition to mania and cyclothymia, those depressive psychoses of endogenous and reactive onset, such as climacteric depression or depression associated with pregnancy.

4. *Mental deficiency* (mental retardation).

5. *Cerebral organic degenerative processes* (cerebral atrophies), in particular senile and presenile dementia, which covered the majority of mental disorders occurring in the older age groups in our research sample.

6. *Late acquired brain damage*[3] through trauma, inflammation, intoxication, and all exogenous psychoses and defect syndromes except epileptic psychoses. Cases in the Landeck admission

group under the age of 50 diagnosed as psychopathological
syndromes associated with endocrine disorders and cerebral
vascular processes were included in this category.

7. *Convulsive disorders* (epilepsies).

8. *Other disorders*, which included in particular neurotic-
psychopathic syndromes, alcoholism and other addictions
(recorded in the violent group only as a secondary diagnosis)
and, for the Landeck admissions, abnormal crises and developments, as well as vague concepts such as 'vegetative dystonia',
'dystrophy of puberty', and other similar diagnoses.

The individual categories in this classification scheme cover
some very heterogeneous diagnoses and comparisons are therefore possible only
on the basis of groups of illnesses.

Fig. 3 shows the relative frequencies of the diagnoses used by us
in the two groups of patients, and illustrates the clear differences between
the main diagnostic groups. Among the non-violent patients the more frequent

Fig 3

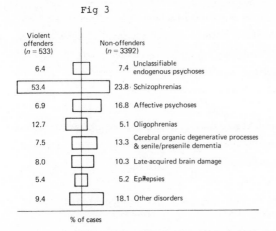

Violent offenders (n = 533)		Non-offenders (n = 3392)	
6.4		7.4	Unclassifiable endogenous psychoses
53.4		23.8	Schizophrenias
6.9		16.8	Affective psychoses
12.7		5.1	Oligophrenias
7.5		13.3	Cerebral organic degenerative processes & senile/presenile dementia
8.0		10.3	Late-acquired brain damage
5.4		5.2	Epilepsies
9.4		18.1	Other disorders

% of cases

diagnoses are those which come within the groups of affective psychoses, organic
cerebral degenerative processes and, particularly, the group embracing 'other
disturbances', while among the violent offenders diagnoses of schizophrenia and
mental deficiency are by far the most common. But because of the various intervening factors which affect the composition of the hospital admissions group,
and which we have discussed above, these differences in diagnostic distribution
are of limited significance and the comparison can be used only to provide some
points of orientation.

There is a further methodological problem which complicates the

interpretation of these varying rates: the question arises whether the differences in diagnosis may not be related also to the factor of 'sex', which was
different for the two groups (see Fig. 1). It is known that the morbidity rate
of certain mental illnesses is related to sex: for example, more women than men
suffer from affective psychoses, and more men from alcoholism (Weitbrecht; Wyss
in *Psychiatrie der Gegenwart*, vol. 2).[4]

The influence of the sex factor must therefore be 'partialled out',
i.e. eliminated statistically. In preparing our complicated frequency tables
(frequency of different diagnoses in men and women in two patient groups) we
have limited ourselves, as an approximate solution, to testing the distribution
of diagnoses separately for men and for women. As both test tables yielded highly
significant results, we may still conclude that the different diagnostic composition of the two groups is not caused solely by differences in sex.

The following sections give an interpretation of the frequency rates
found in the main diagnostic groups.

Schizophrenias

We begin our discussion with the schizophrenics, since they form by
far the largest group among the violent offenders and since this category is
relatively clear-cut, as compared with the mentally deficient and the epileptics.
As with the other diagnoses the question to be answered is: Does the fact that
a patient is suffering from a schizophrenic psychosis imply a higher risk of
violence?

When the frequency of schizophrenia in the two populations, (Table 7),
is statistically compared (chi-square test) with all other forms of illness,
then the difference is highly significant:

Table 7. *Distribution of the diagnosis of 'schizophrenia'
in the violent and non-violent mentally abnormal*

Mentally abnormal violent offenders (n = 533)				Mentally abnormal non-offenders (n = 3392)			
m	f	Total	%	m	f	Total	%
232	52	284	53.4	347	460	807	23.8

$\chi^2 = 199.6348,\quad df = 6,\ \alpha = 0.001$

       The marked predominance of male over female violent schizophrenic
offenders gives the impression, which is in line with traditional ideas, that
schizophrenic men represent a high proportion of all mentally abnormal violent
offenders (see the review of the literature on this subject in Chapter 2). At
the same time the suspicion is strengthened that a schizophrenic illness actually
increases substantially the risk of committing a violent crime. We must
remember, however, that the above differences in frequency represent raw
figures which may be influenced by other variables (sex and age are of
particular relevance here). Therefore the fact that the control group consists
of hospital admissions is important. Since we cannot refute the objection
that the admission policy of the mental hospital in question might be affected
by various uncontrollable factors which would cause the diagnostic composition
of the control population of hospital admissions to be unrepresentative, we
can at this stage do no more than formulate a suspicion. In order to increase
the reliability of our predictions about the risk of violence attached to
specific diagnoses, we shall at a later point undertake a comparison with a
population of psychiatric patients which is not based solely on hospital
admissions.

Other endogenous psychoses
       This section covers briefly the group of affective psychoses taken
together with the general group of unclassifiable endogenous psychoses.
       In contrast to the schizophrenic groups, the hospital admission

Table 8. *Distribution of non-schizophrenic endogenous
psychoses (affective and other) in the violent and
non-violent mentally abnormal*

Mentally abnormal violent offenders ($n = 533$)				Mentally abnormal non-offenders ($n = 3392$)			
m	f	Total	%	m	f	Total	%
25	46	71	13.3	206	615	821	24.2

sample here contains almost twice as many patients with 'other endogenous
psychoses' as the sample of mentally abnormal violent offenders (Table 8).
If we compare the rate for this group of non-schizophrenic endogenous psychoses with all other forms of illness in the two populations, we find again a
highly significant difference in favour of the hospital admissions group:

$$\chi^2 = 31.0667, \quad df = 1, \quad \alpha = 0.001$$

If we take only those patients with manic-depressive illness,
then the hospital admissions group has more than double its share (16.8%
compared with 6.9%). Again, however, these differences do not permit us to
draw any firm conclusions (in this instance even less than in the other cases
mentioned) about the risk of violence in such forms of psychosis: they are
nevertheless worth noting.

In the control group of non-violent patients the diagnoses sub-
sumed under 'affective psychoses' or 'depression' were probably used in a
broader sense than in the case of the mentally abnormal violent offenders.
But the comparison still provides a pointer which has to be checked against
a control group drawn not only from mental hospital admissions.

The proportion of women in the non-violent group is very high.
This is associated with the higher rates of hospital admission and the higher
morbidity for manic-depressive psychoses and other depressions in women, and
we shall deal with this topic in detail later.

Mental deficiency

Since the comparability of the hospital admissions group and the
violent offender group seems particularly dubious for this diagnostic category,
the findings here should be viewed with great caution. Mental defectives are
proportionately much more frequent among the abnormal violent offenders of all
diagnoses than in the non-violent admissions group (Table 9), which would at
first sight suggest that mental deficiency carries a clear and increased risk
of violence. (In the two populations together, the proportion of mental
defectives is significantly high as compared with all other diagnoses:
$\chi^2 = 47.9477$, $df = 1$, $\alpha = 0.001$)

This finding can hardly be accepted without further consideration,
even if we formulate it only as a tendency. As already explained, it is highly
probable that mental defectives are under-represented among admissions to
mental hospitals. For one thing, special provisions exist for the mentally
deficient which cover a considerable proportion of those requiring hospital

Table 9. *Distribution of the diagnosis of 'mental deficiency' in the violent and non-violent mentally abnormal*

Mentally defective violent offenders					Mentally defective non-offenders			
m	f	Total	%		m	f	Total	%
59	9	68 [a]	12.7		460	66	171	5.1

[a] This figure does not include the mentally defective violent offenders who were also diagnosed as schizophrenic (*Pfropfschizophrenie*). These numbered 15 cases, which were entered by us as schizophrenia, because according to our criteria this seemed to be the main diagnosis.

care. For another, many mentally retarded individuals live with their families without ever having to be admitted to hospital. The reasons for which mental defectives are admitted to psychiatric hospitals may therefore be assumed to include an undue proportion of additional disturbances such as other mental illnesses, antisocial disturbing behaviour, etc. It is possible, too, that aggressive and other socially disturbing behaviour, which is less well tolerated in men than in women, plays a considerable part and influences the sex distribution of hospital admissions in favour of men.

For these reasons we refrained from regarding this comparison as providing even a pointer towards an increased risk of violence in the mentally deficient, though we considered that the high disproportion of men, which exists also in comparison with the sex distribution of the mentally defective in the hospital admissions group, was a reliable finding and indicated a genuine trend.

Organic cerebral degenerative disorders (dementia), late acquired brain damage, epilepsies, and other disorders

While no disproportion between violent and non-violent patients was found in late-acquired brain damage (due to trauma, inflammation, poisoning) or in the epilepsies, the violent offenders included proportionately about half as many patients with cerebral degenerative disorders. (When

compared statistically with all other diagnoses, the difference was highly
significant: $\chi^2 = 14.2331$, df = 1, $\alpha = 0.001$.) As this category was over-
represented rather than under-represented in relation to the other diagnostic
groups in terms of the true morbidity rates, the finding may be regarded as
of some significance. It is also in line with the experience of other authors
quoted in the review of the literature in Chapter 2 (e.g. Bürger-Prinz &
Lewerenz, Roth, and others).

The great difference in the rates for the 'other disorders' can
be explained by the large proportion of severe personality disorders (psychopathies, alcoholism and other addictions) and the abnormal reactions (e.g.
associated with suicidal attempts) found in the group of patients admitted to
hospital. Such cases occurred among the mentally disturbed violent offenders
only in association with genuine mental illnesses, defect, or severe brain
damage, the personality disturbance, neurosis, etc. being recorded as a
secondary diagnosis.

Table 10. *Distribution of organic psychosyndromes, epilepsies and other
disorders in the violent and non-violent mentally disordered*

	Mentally disordered violent offenders				Mentally disordered non-offenders			
	m	f	Total	%	m	f	Total	%
Organic cerebral degenerative disorders	35	5	40	7.5	213	239	452	13.3
Late-acquired brain damage	40	3	43	8.0	254	96	350	10.3
Epilepsies	27	2	29	5.4	111	66	177	5.2
Other disorders	40	10	50	9.4	449	165	614	18.1

5.4   Age and sex in the main diagnostic categories

In the sections on schizophrenias and other endogenous psychoses above
we said that a special risk of violence was associated significantly with the
'male sex' and with the 'younger and middle age groups'. This finding applied
to the group of mentally abnormal violent offenders as a whole. We therefore
wished to see whether it applied also to the diagnostic subgroups.

We limited our test to the diagnoses of schizophrenia, affective
psychoses and mental deficiency, since it was important to compare relatively
homogeneous diagnostic groups. (The less common, heterogeneous groups were
therefore excluded, as were the 'unclassifiable endogenous psychoses', though
this made the group of affective psychoses - 37 cases - very small for
purposes of experimental testing.)

Answers were sought to the following questions:

1. How do the schizophrenic, depressive and mentally defective
violent offenders differ in sex and age distribution from the
group of convicted violent offenders who were held to be
responsible for their actions?

2. Are there differences in these distributions within a
diagnostic category between violent offenders and our control
group of non-violent patients admitted to Landeck?

Sex (see Table 11)

Schizophrenia

The group of schizophrenic violent offenders contains almost five
times as many men as women, while not even half of the schizophrenics in the
Landeck sample are of the male sex. (This difference is highly significant:
χ^2 = 126.2702, df = 1, α_2 = 0.001.) On the other hand, the sex ratio for the
schizophrenic violent offenders is very similar to that of the mentally normal
violent offenders, among whom there were about three and a half times as many
men as women. (Statistically the null hypothesis could not be refuted here.)

This clear finding of a marked preponderance of men among the
schizophrenic violent offenders is in line with the observations of other
authors (e.g. H.W. Maier, Wanner). It is of vital importance here that the
sex ratio for schizophrenic offenders was much the same as that of the mentally
normal violent offenders.

Mental deficiency

Sex distribution in the mentally defective showed the same pattern.
Here too it tended to resemble that of mentally normal convicted offenders

Table 11. *Sex distribution of three diagnostic groups of mentally abnormal violent offenders and non-offenders compared with that of mentally normal (convicted) violent offenders*

	Mentally normal (convicted) offenders		Mentally abnormal										
			Schizophrenias				Affective psychoses				Mental deficiency			
			Violent offenders		Non-offenders		Violent offenders		Non-offenders		Violent offenders		Non-offenders	
Sex	n	%	n	%	n	%	n	%	n	%	n	%	n	%
Male	2996	78.7	232	81.7	347	43.0	8	22.0	143	25.0	59	87.0	105	61.4
Female	812	21.3	52	18.3	460	57.0	29	78.0	428	75.0	9	13.0	66	38.6
Total	3808	100.0	284	100.0	807	100.0	37	100.0	571	100.0	68	100.0	171	100.0

Table 12. *Age distribution of three diagnostic groups of mentally abnormal violent offenders and non-offenders compared with that of mentally normal (convicted) offenders*

	Mentally normal (convicted) offenders		Mentally abnormal										
			Schizophrenias				Affective psychoses				Mental deficiency			
			Violent offenders		Non-offenders		Violent offenders		Non-offenders		Violent offenders		Non-offenders	
Age	n	%	n	%	n	%	n	%	n	%	n	%	n	%
14-21	717	18.8	8	2.8	51	6.3	0	-	4	0.7	13	19.0	52	30.4
21-25	838	22.0	40	14.1	54	6.7	1	3.0	17	3.0	17	25.0	23	13.6
25-30	746	19.6	49	17.3	95	11.8	7	19.0	27	4.7	16	23.0	20	11.7
30-40	805	21.2	87	30.6	221	27.4	15	41.0	80	14.0	14	21.0	27	15.9
40-50'	374	9.8	59	20.8	182	22.5	7	19.0	106	18.6	6	9.0	18	10.5
50-60	251	6.6	34	12.0	142	17.6	5	13.0	178	31.2	2	3.0	24	14.0
60 and over	77	2.0	7	2.4	62	7.7	2	5.0	159	27.8	0	-	7	4.1
Total	3808	100.0	284	100.0	807	100.0	37	100.0	571	100.0	68	100.0	171	100.0

(for the mentally defective offenders the ratio of men to women was about 6 : 1, for convicted offenders about 4 : 1). The non-violent defectives from the admissions sample showed, on the other hand, a ratio of men to women of about 1.5 : 1, though we must remember that there may be a selective factor that makes for an over-representation of men among mental defectives admitted to a psychiatric hospital. Werner described 29 men and 8 women among his mentally defective group who had committed offences against life and limb; that is to say he also found a preponderance of men.

It would therefore seem that both in schizophrenia and in mental deficiency around 4 to 6 times as many men as women commit crimes of violence. This corresponds closely to a ratio of 4 men to 1 woman among mentally normal violent offenders and suggests that in both diagnostic categories there is a closer relationship between sex and the risk of violence than between diagnosis and this risk.

Affective psychoses

In this group of illnesses the sex ratio for the violent offenders is a direct reversal of that found in all the other categories of illness. Here alone women predominate (n = 29) over men (n = 8) in a ratio of about 3.5 : 1.

(The 34 'unclassifiable endogenous psychoses' consisted of 17 women and 17 men and so far as sex ratio is concerned came between the group of schizophrenias and that of manic depressive illness.)

The sex ratio of depressed violent offenders corresponds to that of the same diagnostic category in the control group of hospital admissions. In the mentally abnormal violent group the proportion of men is so small and insignificant that the difference can be ignored. (We have already discussed in detail in Chapter 3 the possibility that the number of depressed offenders is low because of a high dark figure for extended suicide.)

We assumed that some married depressed women who attempted to kill their children and to commit suicide did not come before the courts and/or into in-patient psychiatric care and thus remained outside the scope of our survey. It is unlikely, however, that this factor would reverse the sex ratio found by us, since the proportion of female offenders would be increased rather than decreased thereby.

All in all, so far as violent offenders with affective psychoses are concerned, the illness does seem clearly to influence the sex distribution of the abnormal offenders. In addition to the higher morbidity for women in depression, there is also a stronger inclination in women than in men to involve their children in their own suicide. The close symbiosis between mother and child, which is particularly marked in depressive personalities, plays a part here. Depressed men seem to behave differently in this respect.

Since in the published suicide rates for the GFR men are slightly over-represented as compared with women, we must assume - in spite of our limited sample numbers - that they prefer single suicide and that extended suicide is extraordinarily rare in men as compared with women. Psychiatric literature confirms this assumption on the basis of clinical experience and various collections of case studies (Langelüddeke, Spangenberg, Popella). In the rare cases in which fathers involve their children in their suicide, the wife is usually also included (Popella, Greger and Hoffmeyer) and it becomes a 'family murder' (Jacobi, 1928).

Age (see Table 12)

Schizophrenia

It is evident that in the schizophrenic violent offenders the age group between 25 and 30 features prominently and that the violence declines after the age of 60. This delayed criminality, which by comparison with the convicted offenders occurs about 10 to 15 years later in the middle and higher age groups, seems to be attributable to the psychosis. (The difference is significant at the 0.001 level: $\chi^2 = 98.8565$, df = 6.)

This allows us to formulate two hypotheses: (1) the psychosis schizophrenia has a direct delaying effect on violence; (2) there are indirect factors involved, which are intricately associated with the illness and with the tendency to violence, such as social or family constellations, and which are affected by the timing of the illness. We shall try to decide between these alternatives in later chapters.

The non-violent schizophrenics in the hospital control group show an even more marked shift into the higher age groups. (As compared with the violent schizophrenics the difference here is highly significant: $\chi^2 = 37.1231$, df = 6, $\alpha = 0.001$.) We have already discussed possible explanations of this finding, in section 5.2. Basically it is because the hospital sample contains an excess proportion of readmissions in all diagnostic categories, and of first admissions of elderly patients.[5]

Affective psychoses

In this diagnostic category we found in our survey not a single case of serious violence in the age group under 21, and only one case in the age group up to 25. For the reasons already discussed, the preponderance of offenders aged between 30 and 40 may be attributed to the over-representation within this age group of chronically sick women who are often married and subject to relapses. If we regard extended suicide, involving the patient's own children, as the typical crime in this illness, the shift to middle age, as compared with the normal offenders, is also to be expected.

The non-violent control group of patients in this diagnostic category are distinctly older (peak between 50 and 60) than the violent abnormal offenders. Probably the same explanation applies here as in the case of the non-violent schizophrenics.

Mental deficiency

The age distribution of the mental defectives is not very different from that of the convicted violent offenders. This finding may be seen as an indication that in this diagnostic category the mental disturbance (deficiency) exercises no modifying influence on the risk of criminality in regard to age (or sex) - unless later statistical findings suggest a different explanation. The non-violent mental defectives are again older, though not to the same extent as the patients suffering from affective psychoses.

These age, sex and diagnostic distributions are based on very different comparisons, and conclusions can be drawn from them only within very different limits. Thus the differences in diagnostic composition between the group of abnormal violent offenders and the abnormal non-offenders is, according to our interpretation of the results, hardly capable of generalisation. Any answers to questions about the risk of violence attached to specific illness must at this stage be formulated only as 'trends', because the control group cannot be guaranteed to show a representative distribution of diagnoses. The high proportion of schizophrenics among the violent offenders could correspond to a high risk and the low proportion of affective psychoses (depressions) to a low risk of violence. The large number of mental defectives among the abnormal offenders, however, cannot be taken as indicating a trend. This diagnostic category is, unlike schizophrenia and affective psychoses, probably considerably under-represented in the control population of mental hospital admissions.

The findings on age and sex distribution have greater predictive value. The groups of mentally abnormal and normal violent offenders show a very similar composition: the male sex and the younger age groups predominate to a considerable extent. On the other hand the age and sex distribution of mentally abnormal non-offenders, in the sample drawn from admissions to a mental hospital, are to a large extent the same as those of the general

population. Since violent offenders, both abnormal and normal, differ considerably and highly significantly from the general population and from the abnormal
control group, we may conclude that age and sex are more important factors
than mental illness in influencing the risk of violence.

We can also place this finding within a familiar theoretical framework: age and sex act as facilitating or inhibiting factors and limit the
influence of other risk factors, including the possible influence of mental
illness or mental defect. In other words, violence is more likely to occur
when the facilitating factors are maximal - male sex, age between 18 and 40 -
and less likely when these factors are less in evidence - female sex, lower
or higher age group.

This interpretative model supports the hypothesis that mental illness does in fact influence the risk of violence. The upward shift, averaging
8.3 years, in the age maximum of mentally abnormal offenders as compared with
normal offenders is an important finding which argues in its favour. It cannot,
however, be immediately assumed that mental disorders frequently act as
facilitating or inhibiting factors or that they chiefly only contribute to a
postponement in the manifestation of violence, without diminishing quantitatively the risk of its occurring. As we have said, it is quite possible that
other as yet unknown factors, which are associated with mental disorders, raise
the age of manifestation of violence in the mentally abnormal. This will be
discussed further at a later point. [6]

These comments on age and sex distribution treat 'mental illness'
to some extent as a quasi-unitary factor and naturally apply only to predictions of global associations. The example of the affective psychoses, with
their reverse sex ratio of 1 : 3.5, proves that the global factor of 'mental
illness' is the product of different and sometimes opposing factors which
still have to be identified and assessed. The same group of illnesses also
shows that this product, while deviating from the formulated rule, was able
substantially to affect the sex-specific disposition to violence. If we
formulate the finding as an impression we may say that the risk of violence
appears to be increased in women by a depressive psychosis, but to be
decreased in men.

6.   RESULTS III : COMPARATIVE RISKS OF VIOLENCE IN THE
MENTALLY ABNORMAL AND IN THE GENERAL POPULATION

6.1   Comparison with 'recorded' violent offenders
          One of the most important aims of our study, namely to compare the
risks of violence in the mentally abnormal and in the general population,

Table 13. *Comparison between mentally abnormal violent offenders, and
'recorded' violent offenders from the Police Criminal Statistics of the GFR*

Source: Police Criminal Statistics		Our survey
Population: Recorded offenders 1955-64		Mentally abnormal offenders 1955-64
Murder and manslaughter (including attempts) [a]	10 701	Crimes resulting in death 251
Infanticide	798	Attempted homicide, incl. grievous bodily harm, not resulting in death 282
Grievous bodily harm resulting in death (Sections 226, 227, 229)	6 431	
	n = 17 930	n = 533
		Percentage of mentally abnormal offenders = 2.97%
Dangerous and serious bodily harm, incl. maltreatment of dependants (Sections 223a, 223b, 224)	362 134	
	n = 380 064	n = 533
		Percentage of mentally abnormal offenders = 0.14%

[a] This category includes recorded offenders whose crime came under Penal Code
Sections 211 (murder), 212 (manslaughter), 213 (manslaughter in extenuating
circumstances) or 216 (killing on request).

encountered particular difficulties because of the unreliability of the statistics available for this purpose. In order to obtain at least approximate figures, we carried out the comparisons shown in Table 13.

Taking the first category of offences listed in the criminal statistics - murder and manslaughter, infanticide and bodily harm resulting in death - which includes in particular criminal homicide and attempted homicide and therefore is fully covered by our definition of crimes of violence, the percentage of mentally abnormal offenders is 2.97%. If we add recorded cases of dangerous and serious bodily harm, then the percentage of mentally abnormal offenders falls to 0.14%. This latter estimate is based, however, on doubtful assumptions: the category of dangerous and serious bodily harm, which is governed by heterogeneous criteria such as the use of dangerous weapons, deceitful attack, life-endangering attack, etc., certainly extends far beyond our definition of violent crime. Nevertheless it does presumably contain an unknown number of violent offenders analogous to the mentally abnormal offenders defined by our criteria.

6.2 Comparison with convicted violent offenders

The Federal Statistics of Convicted Offenders certainly cover the 'proved' offenders as well as those sentenced. But the judicial procedures of obtaining evidence are not the same as empirical-scientific procedures. They also lead to a classification of violent crimes under a great many heterogeneous categories, many of which include in one paragraph both minor offences and serious crimes resulting in death.[1] The Federal Statistics of Convicted Offenders also sometimes include in one rubric crimes resulting in death and less serious crimes: for example, Section 177 (sexual assault) and Section 178 (sexual assault ending in death). The proportion of offenders convicted of fatal acts of violence or of otherwise defined serious violent crimes cannot therefore be reliably ascertained from the rubrics of the Federal Statistics of Convicted Offenders.

Table 14 shows how difficult it is to obtain adequate categories of offenders which can be properly compared. Most cases of dangerous and serious bodily harm cover what has been reported in this category in the Police Criminal Statistics. To include them in the comparison with the mentally abnormal offenders would serve no purpose.

Nevertheless, in spite of all the imprecision, the percentage of mentally abnormal violent offenders as opposed to convicted offenders in the population of the GFR is still of the same order of about 3%. The Police Criminal Statistics probably give more reliable reference figures than those

Table 14. *Comparison between mentally abnormal violent offenders, and convicted violent offenders from the Federal Statistics of Convicted Offenders*

Source: Federal Statistics of Convicted Offenders		Our survey	
Population: Convicted offenders 1956-65 [a]		Mentally abnormal offenders 1955-64	
Murder and manslaughter (Sections 211, 212, 213) including attempts and related fatal crimes [b]	3 808	Crimes resulting in death	251
Other crimes of violence in which there is a possibility of death: poisoning, brawling and other crimes endangering the public [c]	2 955	Attempted homicide, including grievous bodily harm, not resulting in death	282
Rape, sexual offence or sexual assault resulting in death (Sections 177, 178) [d]	10 846		
	$n = 17\ 609$		$n = 533$
Convicted and mentally abnormal offenders	$n = 18\ 142$ [e]	Percentage of mentally abnormal offenders = 2.93%	
Dangerous and serious bodily harm, incl. mal-treatment of dependants (Sections 223a, 223b, 224)	114 067		

[a] The data from the Federal Statistics of Convicted Offenders were moved forward one year to the decade 1956 to 1965 because as a rule conviction follows from several months to well over a year after the crime. This shift served to improve the comparability of the data with our own research population which was based on the year in which the crime was committed.

[b] This includes Penal Code Sections 216 (killing on request) = 21 offenders; 217 (infanticide) = 352 female offenders; 225 and 226 (deliberate grievous bodily harm and bodily harm resulting in death) = 721 offenders.

[c] This category covers the most important paragraphs of the Penal Code and of the Federal Statistics of Convicted Offenders, namely, crimes of violence, excluding the above-named homicidal crimes in the narrower sense, in which the death of the victim is expressly indicated and/or which often result in death: Sections 221 (abandonment of a child), 227 (brawling), 229 (poisoning), 251 (robbery with violence, grievous bodily harm or death of the victim), 307 (arson of a particularly serious nature), 311 (causing an explosion) and 312 (deliberate flooding endangering human life).

Continued at bottom of p.98.

taken from the Federal Statistics of Convictions, which are affected by the very special judicial classification used, with its many ambiguities and sources of error.

A further possibility would be to compare the number of victims killed by mentally abnormal offenders with the number of cases of death from similar crimes registered in the same period of time.

6.3 Comparison with the statistics of causes of death [2]

The Federal Statistics of Causes of Death for the decade in question recorded 5288 deaths under the rubric murder, manslaughter and deliberate injury by another person (ICD No. E 964-985, DAS 981-986)(Table 15).

Calculated on this basis, the percentage of persons killed by mentally abnormal violent offenders is 5.6%. The number of victims of violent crime included in the Federal Statistics of Causes of Death is nevertheless certainly too low, presumably because registration presupposes a court verdict. The police statistics for the same period show 7229 cases alone of bodily harm

Table 15. *Comparison of victims killed by mentally abnormal offenders with deaths from murder and manslaughter, 1955-64*

Source: Federal Statistics of Causes of Death		Our survey	
Deaths from murder, manslaughter, etc. 1955-64	5288	Victims killed by mentally abnormal offenders 1955-64	293
Average annual incidence	529	Average annual incidence	29

Percentage of deaths caused by violent crimes of mentally abnormal offenders : 5.6%.

Notes to Table 14 (contd.)

[d] Rape (Section 177) and sexual offence or sexual assault resulting in death (Section 178) are unfortunately included in the same rubric in the Federal Statistics of Convicted Offenders, so that the proportion of crimes resulting in death in this category, which is probably not very high, remains unknown. For this reason, and because the number of offenders is relatively high, we have treated it separately.

[e] In calculating the percentage of mentally abnormal offenders we first added these to the convicted offenders, which we did not do when comparing them with the offenders recorded in the Police Criminal Statistics. We did this because the convicted offenders are, or at least should be, fully responsible individuals who are not mentally ill or mentally defective.

resulting in death and infanticide, both crimes which by definition ended in death. Considering that there were also 10 701 cases of murder and man-slaughter, admittedly including attempted murder and homicide, the figure of 5288 cases shown in the Federal Statistics of Causes of Death must be much too low. According to our estimate, these statistics record about half the cases of death by violence. On this assumption the percentage of victims killed by mentally abnormal offenders would again be just under 3%.

6.4   Comparison with prevalence data

As no previous studies of the prevalence of mental illness had been carried out in the GFR we could use as our basis only average figures drawn from the prevalence rates published in the Scandinavian countries, Great Britain and the USA. For the diagnostic groups covered by our survey, namely endogenous and exogenous psychoses, epilepsies, degenerative processes and mental deficiency of low and middle grades, the average prevalence would seem to be between 3 and 5% of the population over the age of 14. This would put the proportion of mentally ill and mentally defective offenders at approxi-mately the same level as the proportion of mentally ill and mentally defective individuals in the adult population (over the age of 14).[3] This would allow us to predict - with all the reservations implied in the underlying methodo-logical assumptions - that mentally ill and mentally defective individuals are not on the whole more or less likely to become violent offenders than the so-called mentally healthy.

6.5   Comparison with incidence data

Since our survey has the advantage of being planned as a study of incidence, it is clear that we should compare our findings with those obtained in studies of the incidence of mental illness. Comparison of the incidence of particular groups of illnesses in the general population and the incidence of violence in the same groups offers in the main two predictive possibilities. On the one hand it enables us to test the degree of correspondence between the diagnostic distribution of the mentally abnormal violent offenders and that of the mentally abnormal in the relevant general population somewhat more reliably than can be done using the age and marital status of a sample of mental hospital admissions. On the other hand it allows us to calculate the risk of violence on the basis of 'first attacks' of mental illness and mental deficiency, as a whole as well as for those groups of illnesses for which adequate data are available.

Unfortunately, so far as the GFR is concerned, there is only one

investigation available which gives even approximate information about the
incidence of mental illnesses, namely that carried out by Häfner, Reimann and
their co-workers in Mannheim (1969, 1970). This covered all the inhabitants of
the city of Mannheim who sought psychiatric help for the first time in the
year 1965 from the out-patient and in-patient psychiatric and psychological
services (specialists, hospitals, etc.) or from other hospitals, or from the
social and advisory services. So far as mental deficiency is concerned, the
resultant 'administrative' rates come close to the 'true' incidence rates,
because of the general obligation to attend school and the investigations which
this entails. For the other groups of illnesses they are to a greater or
lesser degree below the true figures because in all diagnostic categories
there is a varying proportion of patients who have never consulted a medical
or social agency. This proportion is probably lower for the serious illnesses
such as schizophrenia and higher for the less serious such as minor affective
psychoses. Moreover the inhabitants of Mannheim, a city which is predominantly
industrial with a small share of village communities, are not necessarily
representative of the population of the GFR. These reservations must be borne
in mind when we use the Mannheim findings as the basis on which to calculate
the risks of violence. We may, however, formulate the following tendency: the
first-consultation rates reported by Häfner, Reimann *et al.* tend to be lower,
to a varying extent, than the true incidence rates, which means that the
calculated risks of violence may be higher rather than lower than the true risks.

The rank comparison (Table 16) can be interpreted only with many
reservations. The diagnosis of schizophrenia heads the list for the
abnormal violent offenders, with 53% of all cases. Among the mentally ill with
comparable diagnoses in the Mannheim population, schizophrenia comes only fifth,
with 7%. This implies a disproportionate risk of violence in schizophrenia.
Another clear feature, but in the opposite direction, is the difference shown
in the senile degenerative processes - 7.5%, fourth in the rank list for
violent offenders, against 21%, first in the rank list in the Mannheim consultation group - but this probably can be explained by the general decline in the
risk of violence with old age.

In fact the risk of violence in the general population of responsible
age reaches its peak between 18 and 40 years, falling sharply before and after
(cf. p.78). From this one would expect illnesses whose maximal manifestation
comes within this age group to show a correspondingly high rate of violence: so
far as the numerically important groups of illnesses are concerned, this
applies first and foremost to schizophrenia, and secondly, because of a slight
shift towards higher age groups, to the affective psychoses. Conversely one

Table 16. *Rank comparison of groups of illnesses (first consultations 1965) in mentally abnormal violent offenders and in the Mannheim population*

	Mentally abnormal violent offenders		Inhabitants of Mannheim (incidence of consultation 1965) [a]		
	No. (n)	% in the main diagnostic categories		No. (n)	% in the main diagnostic categories	Rate per 1000 of Mannheim's inhabitants 1965
		(round)				
Schizophrenia	284	53	Senile degeneration	508	21	1.55
Mental deficiency	68	13	Mental deficiency	498	20	1.52
Cerebral disorders and trauma (lues etc.)	43	8	Cerebral disorders and trauma	352	15	1.07
Senile degeneration (arteriosclerosis, presenile and senile dementia, etc.)	40	7.5	Affective psychoses	243	10	0.74
Affective psychoses (manic-depressive illness)	37	7	Schizophrenia	166	7	0.51
Epilepsy	29	5	Epilepsy	138	6	0.42
Other psychoses and organic syndromes	34	6	Other psychoses and organic syndromes	532	22	1.63
Total	533			2437 [b]		

[a] From Häfner & Reimann's study.

[b] Only psychoses, mental deficiency and organic syndromes.

Table 17. *Age-group comparison of mentally abnormal and normal violent offenders*

Age	Mentally abnormal offenders		Convicted offenders (Federal Statistics of Convicted Offenders)	
	n	%	*n*	%
14-20 (adolescence)	31	5.8	717	18.8
21-49 (adulthood)	394	73.9	2763	72.6
50 and over (old age)	108	20.3	328	8.6
Total	533	100.0	3808	100.0

would expect that illnesses whose maximal manifestation comes after the age of 60, for example degenerative psychoses such as arteriosclerotic and senile dementia, etc., would show a very low incidence of violence, while disorders for which the age distribution more closely resembles that of the general population should lie in between. Only where the actual rates of violence found in particular groups of illnesses differ significantly from the age-corrected expected rates, is it possible to calculate precisely a positive or negative influence of these illnesses upon the average risk of violence. The control data which would be required for such a calculation, such as the age distribution of the incidence of mental disorders and of their main diagnostic groups in the population, are not available. It is hardly to be expected that they will be available in the near future, since they could not be obtained without methodologically difficult and at the same time very wide-ranging investigations. For this reason it seemed to us justifiable to make estimates on the basis of such data as were available, even though they are less reliable.

6.6   Risks of violence (probabilities) for some groups of illnesses

In the end we used the Mannheim consultation incidence rates, adjusted to cover ten years, for three diagnostic categories which were present in adequate numbers in our material, namely schizophrenia, affective psychoses and mental deficiency, and calculated the probability that an individual who had once been mentally ill would become also a violent offender. The risk of violence for individual groups of illnesses was calculated as a conditional probability according to the multiplication theorem of probabilities (Hoel, 1962):

$$p(Gew/K) = \frac{p(Gew + K)}{p(K)}$$

where *Gew* is the ten-year incidence rate of mentally abnormal offenders
corrected for duration of illness, and *K* is the ten-year incidence of mentally
ill patients in the same diagnostic group, based on the population of the GFR.

It was necessary to correct for duration of illness of the violent
offenders in our decade because, if we use as a basis the number of violent
offenders recorded in a particular diagnostic group during that period, the
high average duration of illness leads to an appreciable increase in the
incidence rates for violent offenders within that group. Thus, for example,
in the group of 96 schizophrenics, who had on average had their first attack
7.5 years before the crime, 75% were eliminated on the assumption that their
illness had begun before the ten-year period.

Schizophrenia

Calculated as above on the ten-year incidence, the risk of violence
in schizophrenics was found to be 0.05%. This corresponds to five violent
offenders per 10 000 suffering from schizophrenia. The calculation is based
on the following data:

Correction for duration of illness:

Duration of illness (years)	Cases	% who were ill before the decade studied	Corrected no. of cases
0-1	55		55
1-5	96	25	72
5-10	68	75	17

The ten-year incidence of violent offenders diagnosed as schizophrenic,
corrected for duration of illness, is 134.

Calculation:

$$p(Gew/K) = \frac{134/\text{Pop GFR} (= 44\ 477\ 399)}{163 \times 10/S\ (266\ 610)} = \frac{1}{611\ 379 + 10^{-5}}$$

$$= 0.49232 \times 10^{-3} = c.\ 0.05\%$$

where Pop. GFR is the mean figure for the population of the GFR aged 14 and
above for the decade 1955-64 and *S* is the number of first consultations for
schizophrenics aged 14 and above, taken from the raised rates for the
Mannheim study and multiplied again to match the population of the GFR.

Affective psychoses

We carried out an analogous procedure with the affective psychoses:

$$p(Gew/K) = \frac{23/\text{Pop. GFR}}{242 \times 10/266\ 610} = \frac{0.052 \times 10^{-5}}{907\ 693 \times 10^{-5}}$$

$$= 0.005729 \times 10^{-2} = c.\ 0.006\%$$

Mental deficiency

Since mental deficiency is practically always a lifelong condition, and since the average expectation of life is considerably different from that of the general population, we had to make an estimation of prevalence on the basis of our incidence data. The prevalence of mental deficiency was calculated as follows:

Incidence (average age minus age of responsibility)
The probability of becoming a violent offender is then:

$$p(Gew/K) = \frac{68/\text{Pop. GFR}}{498 \times 14/266\ 610} = \frac{0.153 \times 10^{-5}}{0.0261505}$$

$$= 0.00585 \times 10^{-2} = c.\ 0.006\%$$

The figure for average age was obtained by using the mentally deficient population in Landeck hospital, whose average age proved to be 28 years. We realise that this may not be a reliable figure, but better data were not available.

The finding of 0.006%, or 6 per 100 000, gives the same risk of violence as in the affective psychoses.

In spite of the limited reliability of the control data (denominators) these calculations of the risk of violence in three main groups of illness confirm the tendency we have already seen in the rank comparison and, for schizophrenia and the affective psychoses, in the comparison of diagnostic distribution in these groups and their control groups of hospital admissions. The risk of violence is about ten times higher in schizophrenia than in the other two categories of illness. The figures as a whole are surprisingly low. In schizophrenia and the affective psychoses they are moreover probably higher than the true figures, because the control figures in the denominator were obtained from a secondary source and, as mentioned, are certainly lower than the true incidence rates.

7. RESULTS IV : PERSONALITY, ILLNESS AND BACKGROUND OF
    THE CRIME - PATIENT COMPARISONS

Inter-group comparisons of violent and non-violent
patients

In what follows we shall examine the previous histories of violent
and non-violent psychiatric patients to determine whether and in what way they
differ. We shall at the same time look for further factors which affect the
risk of violence in the mentally abnormal and try to obtain at least pointers
towards increased risks which might be helpful in the prevention of such
violence.

Since we wished to break the problem down into separate testable
hypotheses, we compared the group of abnormal violent offenders with a group
of non-violent mentally ill and mentally defective patients, matched for size,
sex, age and diagnosis.

As has already been explained in Chapter 3 (p.68), the control
group used in the following investigations consisted of patients admitted
between 1955 and 1964 to the Regional Mental Hospital of Wiesloch. We used
as our population base a random sample of all admissions, n = 4144.

It was not possible to obtain an equally good match for all three
items of sex, age and diagnosis. So far as sex was concerned, the groups as a
whole[1] matched exactly, each consisting of 410 men and 123 women. As regards
age, we used as our basis a scale divided into ten-yearly periods. It was not
possible to reach complete concordance between the two groups and at times
we had to make adjustments between two neighbouring classes. In diagnoses,
too, we were unable to eliminate small deviations. The largest was the
difference between the groups of 'unclassifiable endogenous psychoses', since
this description does not appear in the diagnostic classification (Würzburg
Schema) used on the control group of Wiesloch admissions, so that no criterion
of selection was possible. All we could do was admit into the control group
additional cases of schizophrenia and depression (14 of which were then, after
study of their case histories, entered as 'unclassifiable psychoses' in
accordance with the diagnostic code which had been used for the mentally

abnormal violent offenders).

The comparisons we made covered the following areas which seemed likely to affect the risk of violence:

1. Social and genetic heredity (family milieu and hereditary factors)
2. Previous history
3. Factors concerned with the illness (symptoms and course)
4. Previous treatment
5. Social factors and indicators covering the six months preceding the crime or the admission to hospital (contacts, home situation, stressful events, signs of aggressiveness, etc.)

It may with some justification be claimed that so far as comparison of the two groups of 533 as a whole is concerned, the factors of sex, age and diagnosis have been kept constant. Nevertheless, when it comes to evaluating the above items, further difficulties arise which limit the concordance achieved, to a degree which varies from item to item.

For one thing, neither in the judicial files and assessments of the group of violent offenders, nor in the case histories of the control group recorded by the Regional Mental Hospital of Wiesloch for its own purposes, was documentation complete. 'Information not available' was an unavoidable entry under various headings. These entries are, of course, included in the tables of frequency, but have been excluded from test procedures and from the calculation of percentages (100% = n minus the 'not knowns'). As a result the test groups could not always be matched for size and the condition 'same sex, same age, same diagnosis' is often only approximately met. Fortunately, in spite of the different sources of information, the differences between the two groups in respect of the number of 'not knowns' remained within narrow limits.

Another difficulty was that the groups, particularly the diagnostic groups, were in many cases very small. For this reason it was necessary to combine some groups in order to carry out particular tests of significance.

For some items we also carried out subgroup comparisons within the group of mentally abnormal violent offenders (e.g. between the diagnostic groups of schizophrenia, affective psychoses and mental deficiency on the one hand and the groups analysed by sex on the other). We shall give first the results of the inter-group comparison. We shall then return to the other investigations of differences within the group of mentally abnormal

offenders in the section on 'Subgroup comparisons in violent patients'. Finally
in Chapter 8 we shall deal with the items referring to the crime and the
victim.

7.1 Heredity

Broadening its usual and earlier definition, we have included in
this concept not only the influence of hereditary factors but also - as
social heredity - the influence of the family milieu as mediated by learning
processes and affective interaction. We had to abandon any idea of testing
genetic and milieu factors separately, because they were to a large extent
indistinguishable in our survey data. 'Family' was defined as Grade 1 relationships (in Roman law), which gave the data a more reliable foundation: thus
the survey included only parents and siblings, that is to say, the members of
the so-called primary family or family of origin. We also enquired into the
occurrence in that family circle of serious mental disorders, aggressive or
auto-aggressive and addictive (alcoholism) forms of behaviour, as well as into
the external and internal family structure (family cohesion).

We are aware that a retrospective survey based on case records and
official files must lead in this area to considerable gaps.

Family loading of serious mental disorders

First we tested the hypothesis that mentally abnormal violent
offenders may show a higher family loading of serious mental disorders than
mentally abnormal non-offenders (Table 18). We recorded information about the
occurrence of endogenous psychoses, mental deficiency, epilepsy and other
organic cerebral disorders. Since we knew from experience that precise diagnostic details are apt to be lacking in routine case histories, we included
in the category 'disorders present' such items as 'died in an institution,
diagnosis uncertain' and 'diagnosis uncertain'.

Since it soon became apparent that the number of individual
diagnoses in the control groups would be very small and the number of
'uncertain diagnoses' very large, we had to limit ourselves to entering
simply the presence or absence of recorded mental disorder.

For the violent offenders the primary family loading for mental
disorders is 30%, for the non-violent patients around 23%. Remembering that
the complex question of heredity was probably more carefully documented in
the violent group - the fact that the control group contains twice as many
'not knowns' points in this direction - we cannot assume that there is a real
difference between them and the control group. At the most it would seem that

family loading may play a part in offenders with affective psychoses or mental
deficiency. On the whole, however, the percentages are only of small predictive
value. In spite of the significant difference, the hypothesis that violent
patients show a greater family loading of severe mental disorders cannot be
reliably confirmed.

Family loading of aggressive and/or auto-aggressive behaviour
Under this rubric we recorded, again in parents and siblings, conspicuous forms of behaviour expressing aggression or auto-aggression, i.e. suicide
and attempted suicide, criminal records (including all felonies and offences
apart from traffic and driving offences, even if the offender was not prosecuted
or convicted) and chronic alcoholism. As we could not hope to obtain
detailed information about different patterns of family behaviour, such as
style of upbringing, forms of communication, etc., we limited ourselves to

Table 18. *Serious mental disorders in the primary families of violent and
non-violent patients*

	Whole group		Schizo-phrenia		Affective psychoses		Mental deficiency	
	n	%	n	%	n	%	n	%
Violent patients								
No disorders	350	70.0	186	69.4	21	60	35	58
Disorders present	150	30.0	82	30.6	14	40	25	42
Subtotal	500	100.0	268	100.0	35	100	60	100
Not known	33		16		2		8	
Total	533		284		37		68	
Non-violent patients								
No disorders	360	77.2	200	74.5	33	77	42	72
Disorders present	106	22.8	68	25.5	10	23	16	28
Subtotal	466	100.0	268	100.0	43	100	58	100
Not known	67		25		6		12	
Total	533		293		49		70	

Significance test:
Whole group χ^2 = 6.511   df = 1 α = 0.05

these admittedly very heterogeneous categories, which nevertheless covered modes of behaviour that were from our point of view important. Chronic alcoholism, for example, was included on the assumption that it may represent a masked form of auto-aggressive or aggressive behaviour (Menninger, 1938) and that alcohol at least decreases in a secondary way the individual's control over aggressive and destructive impulses.

We followed the assumption that just such forms of behaviour in the primary family of mentally abnormal individuals who later become violent offenders might have provided learning models for violent reactions, on the lines described by Brückner (1961) in mentally normal violent offenders.

It will be seen from Table 19 that family loading of behaviour

Table 19. *Family loading of conspicuous aggressive and auto-aggressive behaviour in violent and non-violent patients*

	Whole group		Schizo- phrenia		Affective psychoses		Mental deficiency	
	n	%	n	%	n	%	n	%
Violent patients								
No conspicuous behaviour	375	77.2	216	82.4	26	74	27	49
Conspicuous behaviour	111	22.8	46	17.6	9	26	28	51
Subtotal	486	100.0	262	100.0	35	100	55	100
Not known	47		22		2		13	
Total	533		284		37		68	
Non-violent patients								
No conspicuous behaviour	421	90.5	251	93.7	38	88	41	72
Conspicuous behaviour	44	9.5	17	6.3	5	12	16	28
Subtotal	465	100.0	268	100.0	43	100	57	100
Not known	68		25		6		13	
Total	533		293		49		70	

Significance test:

Whole group $\chi^2 = 31.1737$ df = 1 $\alpha = 0.001$

(No attempt was made to give separate figures for forms of disturbed behaviour, which were often multiple.)

disorders such as suicide, crime and alcoholism was recorded in about 23% of
the violent offenders but only in about 9% of the non-violent control group.
This difference is highly significant (α = 0.001), while the almost equal
number of 'not knowns' in the two groups strengthens the result. This is
clearly a more reliable finding, which, unlike the hereditary loading, cannot
be explained by differences in documentation.[2] A comparable finding resulted
from a criminological study by Duncan *et al.* (1958), who described a high incidence
of violent behaviour in the primary families of mentally normal murderers. The
psychiatrist Macdonald (1963) and the psychoanalyst Tanay (1969) both speak of
the unfavourable prognostic significance in the life history of murderers of an
upbringing characterised by cruelty and brutal aggressiveness.

Guze *et al.* (1962, 1969), in the studies of male capital offenders
which we have already mentioned, describe not only a high prevalence rate of
sociopathy and alcoholism in the offenders themselves but also a somewhat lower
but clearly above-average rate of antisocial and addictive modes of behaviour
in their immediate (Grade 1) relatives. This is either the expression of a
genetically based disposition to uncontrollable or aggressive behaviour, or
such families, characterised by considerable aggressive tensions and an antisocial way of life, provide both normal and abnormal violent offenders with a
behaviour pattern that tends to make them react, like other members of their
family, aggressively or with alcoholism. In the latter case we may speak of a
social heredity, which probably varies in strength in individual diagnostic
groups of violent offenders.

Socially deviant behaviour as defined by us was clearly more
frequent in the primary families of the violent schizophrenics than in the
families of non-violent schizophrenics (17.6% and 6.3% respectively). From this
it may be surmised that such patterns of family behaviour constitute a real
risk factor in the violence of schizophrenic patients. This prediction does not
apply to depressives, since here there is no such clear distinction between the
violent and non-violent groups. In mental deficiency, where both groups show a
very high loading, no statistical comparison can be made because of the assumed
effect of conspicuous antisocial behaviour on the chances of admission to a
mental hospital (see p. 87).

Turning now to individual forms of conspicuous behaviour in the
family, we find that the diagnostic groups sometimes show a preferred combination of such forms of behaviour: in the primary families of the depressives
suicide was the most common event recorded; in schizophrenics suicide and
alcoholism predominated; in the mental defectives, however, it was almost
exclusively crime or crime associated with alcoholism.

This finding seems to indicate that aggressive and auto-aggressive impulses in the families of depressed and schizophrenic patients more often took a self-destructive form (suicide, alcoholism), while in the mentally defective they showed themselves more often in openly antisocial (criminal) behaviour. This diagnosis-specific pattern of conspicuous behaviour - the common kernel of which may be assumed to be on the one hand a decreased control of impulses in mental deficiency, and on the other hand a strong tendency on the part of depressives and schizophrenics to act in a self-destructive manner - would appear to apply equally to the primary families of violent and non-violent patients.

The assumption that a family loading of mental illness, epilepsy or mental deficiency has a more significant effect on the risk of violence than a loading of aggressive or antisocial modes of behaviour in the primary families, is not borne out by these findings. Here again we may refer to Guze *et al*. who found that neither the offenders they investigated nor their relatives suffered more frequently from mental illnesses such as schizophrenia, affective psychoses, cerebral organic syndromes or neuroses, including homosexuality, than did the general population.

Intactness of the primary family

It is not only alcoholism, criminality and other aggressive modes of behaviour in the primary family which affect the development of the young, but also the composition of the family: whether the close relatives have been able to form a co-operative family group or whether divorce, death or desertion have led to the loss of one or both parents.

S. & E. Glueck, who carried out extensive studies, attached great importance to the complex concept of family cohesiveness (1950), amongst other things, in assessing the risk of criminality in adolescent boys. They understood by this concept a climate of belonging, of common interests and 'we-feeling' in general, the lack of which distinguished very clearly between the families of the 500 delinquents studied and those of the 500 non-criminals in the control group (24.7% and 0.8% respectively). It was not possible for us to include communicative qualities of this kind in our study of the primary families of the abnormal violent offenders, since our method of obtaining data did not permit it. Instead we limited ourselves to the external but easily ascertained characteristic of family intactness and compared the frequency of broken home milieus in both groups of patients (Table 20). [3]

These findings are almost the same for the violent and the non-violent patients, about a quarter of each group having lost one or both parents. It would thus seem that violence is not one of the specific accompaniments of this kind of disturbed primary family. This is in line with Haffter's finding (1948) when he examined the children of 100 broken marriages: he was not able to confirm that criminal behaviour on the part of the children was a consequence of the parents' divorce.

Broken homes were most frequently found (in more than half of the cases) in the group of mentally defective violent offenders, a finding which suggests that the lack of consistent upbringing is of particular significance in this group in increasing the risk of later violent crime. This is presumably associated with inadequate control of impulses, which seems to be an important factor in the violent crimes of the mentally deficient. Schizophrenics and depressed offenders, on the other hand, come mainly from outwardly intact

Table 20. *Frequency of broken homes in the primary families of violent and non-violent patients*

	Whole group		Schizo- phrenia		Affective psychoses		Mental deficiency	
	n	%	n	%	n	%	n	%
Violent patients								
Intact family	359	73.2	210	79.3	26	81	30	46
Broken home	131	26.8	55	20.7	6	19	35	54
Subtotal	490	100.0	265	100.0	32	100	65	100
Not known	43		19		5		3	
Total	533		284		37		68	
Non-violent patients								
Intact family	371	78.0	221	80.6	36	82	35	56
Broken home	105	22.0	53	19.4	8	18	28	44
Subtotal	476	100.0	274	100.0	44	100	63	100
Not known	57		19		5		7	
Total	533		293		49		70	

Significance test:
Whole group $\chi^2 = 2.8595$ df = 1   Null hypothesis not refutable

families. In the control groups of schizophrenic and depressed patients the
proportions were much the same.

Summary

Tests of some broad features of the heredity of violent and non-
violent patients showed that family loading with severe mental disorders such
as mental illness, epilepsy or mental deficiency, was recorded in both groups
to almost the same extent (about 25%). On the other hand, loading with
aggressive or auto-aggressive modes of behaviour and with alcoholism played
an important part in the previous history of the abnormal violent offenders,
who showed a significantly higher loading (23% as against 9%) than the control
group. So far as individual diagnostic groups were concerned, the families of
the mental defectives showed a particularly high loading with antisocial modes
of behaviour and this was more marked in the violent defectives than in the
control group (51% as against 28%). In addition they showed a higher rate of
broken homes (54% as against 44%). Both these findings suggest that for mental
defectives, who are particularly at risk because of inadequate control of
impulses, defects in socialisation also play an important part in increasing
the risk of violent crime. Broken families are rare in patients with affective
psychoses. The schizophrenics occupy a middle position. In both these groups
of illnesses there is no difference in the frequency of broken homes between
the violent and non-violent patients, so that family intactness clearly does
not affect the risks of violence in these diagnostic categories.

7.2   Previous history

Premorbid personality

An important problem in any study of mentally abnormal offenders
is that of determining whether their violence is linked more closely to premorbid personality and related modes of behaviour than to risk factors associated with their illness. In other words, is there perhaps an innate 'inclination' or disposition to violence?

Important basic features, such as social integration, instinctual
behaviour and emotional characteristics, were very unevenly documented in our
source material and very different concepts and dimensions of judgement were
used in assessing them. In order to record the premorbid personality of the
offender, we applied a simple rating procedure to the complex pieces of information available, though in doing so we were fully aware of the difficulties
involved. The category of 'social style of behaviour' was rated in terms of
contact activity as 'inhibited', 'normally active', 'over-active'; emotional

style as 'cold', 'sensitive', 'over-sensitive', 'aggressive'. These insub-
stantial, unreliable qualities could not be expected to provide more than an
orientation.

Violent crimes often exemplify vividly the modes of behaviour of
those who commit them and contain many indications as to their personality.
But the more flexible the descriptions supplied, the more difficult it was to
codify them and the less reliable they were for use in statistical analysis.
There were also considerable differences in the ratings made by the two medical
examiners (W. Böker and A. Schmitt). We therefore abandoned the idea of
analysing these data statistically.

For control purposes we had included in our data sheets a rough
estimate of personal history, rather along the lines of the usual clinical
comments found in psychiatric assessments (e.g. 'nothing of note in the
previous history', 'previous history of neurotic symptoms', 'antisocial and
psychopathic traits'). The original medical examiners had also used similar
terms to indicate different categories of previous history. As there were no
significant differences here between the examiners, we used in our analysis
only these crude items, which makes our prediction applicable only in a very
generalised way.

Antisocial/psychopathic and neurotic features
We started with the hypothesis that forms of behaviour regarded
as disturbing would be found more frequently in the previous history of the
violent patients than in that of the non-violent controls. An analogous hypothesis was formulated for neurotic symptoms, and we hoped that analysis of
these symptoms would also reveal further characteristics of the premorbid
personality of the violent offenders.

'Previous history' was defined for psychoses as covering the
period up to the onset of the illness, and for mental deficiency as covering
the period up to the crime or up to admission to the regional mental hospital.

The assumption that the previous histories of the abnormal
offenders would show antisocial forms of behaviour more frequently than those
of their non-violent controls, was confirmed (Table 21). The items in question
were found in about 20% of all violent offenders, but only in 7.5% of the control
group. The difference is highly significant. Mention is also found in the psychiatric literature of sociopathic behaviour in the primary personality as a
factor that increases the risk of later violent crime (Macdonald, 1963, 1967).

If we consider the diagnostic groups separately we find that the
premorbid personality structure of the depressed offenders is not strikingly

Table 21. *Frequency of antisocial/psychopathic features in the previous history of violent and non-violent patients*

	Whole group		Schizo-phrenia		Affective psychoses		Mental deficiency	
	n	%	n	%	n	%	n	%
Violent patients								
Nothing of note in previous history	348	69.1	210	78.7	28	80	10	15
Antisocial/psycho-pathic traits [a]	100	19.8	22	8.2	1	3	48	74
Neurotic symptoms [b]	56	11.1	35	13.1	6	17	7	11
Subtotal	504	100.0	267	100.0	35	100	65	100
Not known	29		17		2		3	
Total	533		284		37		68	
Non-violent patients								
Nothing of note in previous history	402	81.5	248	91.2	43	90	19	28
Antisocial/psycho-pathic traits	37	7.5	8	2.9	0	–	24	36
Neurotic symptoms	54	11.0	16	5.9	5	10	24	36
Subtotal	493	100.0	272	100.0	48	100	67	100
Not known	40		21		1		3	
Total	533		293		49		70	

Significance test: $\chi^2 =$ df $= 2$ $\alpha =$

Whole group	32.77	0.001
Schizophrenia	16.72	0.001
Affective psychoses [c]	1.13	Null hypothesis not refutable
Mental deficiency	20.09	0.001

[a] 'Antisocial/psychopathic' was defined as covering social maladjustment in the sense of lying, fraudulent, irritable/aggressive and querulant forms of behaviour.

[b] The category of 'neurotic symptoms' covered all forms of behaviour belonging to the clinical concept of neurosis, and in addition sexual perversions, excluding homosexuality.

[c] Because of the small numbers no separate tests were carried out for antisocial/psychopathic traits and neurotic symptoms, but a test was carried out for the sum of the two together.

different from that of the non-violent depressed patients. As already mentioned
in Chapter 5, the illness itself may here be regarded as an influencing factor
that obviously has a more important effect on the crime than the premorbid
personality traits which are influential in the other diagnostic groups. In
the schizophrenic violent offenders antisocial traits and neurotic symptoms
were not very frequent, though they were still found more often here than in
the corresponding control group. The mentally deficient violent offenders
included a high number who showed antisocial traits (74% of the cases),
significantly more than the non-violent control group where 'neurotic
symptoms' were more common. Such behavioural anomalies may have been the
reason why the non-violent defectives were admitted to hospital.

These findings are well in line with the data already obtained on
family loading and family structure in mentally defective offenders. It is
clear that in this group of abnormal violent offenders defects of socialisation, socially deviant behaviour and aggressiveness run like a red thread
through family, childhood and premorbid personality right up to the criminal
violence. Together they constitute the most important group of risk factors
in mental deficiency.

Alcoholism

In addition to the primary personality features just described,
we were also interested to discover how often the records examined mentioned
chronic alcoholism as featuring in the previous history (Table 22). At the
same time we looked for mention of drug dependence and perversions: they
appeared so seldom, however, that they could not be subjected to any statistical test. As there has since been a massive rise in the use of drugs, this
would possibly no longer be the case today.

The chi-square test showed in the group as a whole a slightly
significant preponderance of alcoholics among the violent offenders
($\alpha = 0.01$). About 15% of the violent offenders were alcoholics, as against
only about 8% of the non-violent patients. The finding is, however, of
dubious significance, as the violent patients were drawn from the whole of
the GFR, the control group from North Baden. It is likely that drinking
patterns differ in different regions of the GFR. If we compare the violent
offenders from Baden-Württemberg with the control patients from the same
region, we find that the violent patients show no more cases of alcoholism
than the non-violent patients (Table 23).[4]

It would nevertheless be wrong to discount any connection between
chronic alcoholism and violence. An organic cerebral decline which often

occurs after decades of excessive drinking is known to lead not only to dementia but also usually to increased irritability and to decreased affective control. In patients with brain damage due to other noxae, alcohol can lead to explosive frenzy and violence. (We will examine the immediate connection between

Table 22. *Frequency of chronic alcoholism in the previous history of violent and non-violent patients*

	Whole group		Schizo- phrenia		Affective psychoses		Mental deficiency	
	n	%	n	%	n	%	n	%
Violent patients								
Alcoholism not present	454	85.2	262	92.2	34	92	54	79
Alcoholism present	79	14.8	22	7.8	3	8	14	21
Total	533	100.0	284	100.0	37	100	68	100
Non-violent patients								
Alcoholism not present	488	91.6	284	97.0	49	100	64	91
Alcoholism present	45	8.4	9	3.0	0	–	6	9
Total	533	100.0	293	100.0	49	100	70	100

Table 23. *Comparison of the frequency of chronic alcoholism in the previous history of violent and non-violent patients from the region of Baden-Württemberg*

	Violent offenders		Control group		Total
	n	%	n	%	
Alcoholism not present	95	90.5	488	91.6	583
Alcoholism present	10	9.5	45	8.4	55
Total	105	100.0	533	100.0	638

Significance test: $\chi^2 = 0.1306$ df = 1   Null hypothesis not refutable

alcohol and crime when we come to discuss crime-victim relationships in Chapter 8.)

The lack of statistical evidence of these associations in our study may be due to the fact that brain-damaged patients and epileptics who do not drink or become violent or constitute serious social problems are as a rule not admitted to mental hospitals and for this reason are not adequately represented in the control group. It is therefore conceivable that there is a slight over-representation of alcoholics in the control group.

According to Alström's studies (1950), for example, the risk of violence is particularly high in those brain-damaged epileptics who are inclined to abuse alcohol (see review of the literature in Chapter 2). The following case history illustrates the complex associations that can exist between brain injury, traumatic epilepsy, additional cerebral damage due to chronic alcoholism, and drinking before the crime:

Case No. 480

A tradesman fell from some scaffolding in 1940 and suffered a broken skull with cerebral contusion. After a year during which he was unable to work, he had to be retrained as a merchant clerk.

In the years that followed he had to be admitted several times as an in-patient to a hospital for nervous disorders (first admission in the summer of 1942), as he suffered from traumatic epileptic attacks which were frequently associated with drinking bouts. In the state of excitement that ensued he sometimes destroyed furniture and also on one occasion attacked someone by the throat. For the first few years the picture was mainly one of tonic-clonic attacks, but this changed later to epileptic twilight states with marked aggressive features.

In addition to the epileptic disorder he developed chronic alcoholism: over several years he drank four to eight bottles of beer a day. In 1956 he was convicted of drunken driving. In 1958 he had a serious accident while driving home from an evening of beer-drinking. In 1960 he had a second car accident because of an epileptic attack and his licence was withdrawn.

He married in 1944 and had four children, the marriage being described by outsiders as a good one. The couple lived with relatives of his wife and had ideas of building their own house. Mr F. was considered by his colleagues to be 'quiet, friendly, helpful' and to be a man who apparently could accept criticism. He himself had for a long time felt uncomfortable at his place of work and felt himself becoming increasingly

irritable and sensitive to the point of tears. Because he made one or
two errors in calculation, he asked for easier work.

In the middle of March 1962 a cash box went missing from
an unlocked cupboard at his place of work and the patient was suspected
of the theft. The files record that F. was innocent. He was upset by the
insinuation and could not sleep at night. The fact that his wife took the
affair lightly hurt him very much and led to tensions between the couple.
In the following few days he suffered from a feverish cold and headache
and on 29 March 1962 went off sick because of this. On the morning of
31 March 1962, the day of the crime, he drank a few cups of tea with an
unknown quantity of rum added, in order to fight off his cold. The
general practitioner who saw him prescribed Saridon and Acedicon tablets
to relieve his aches and cough.

After the midday meal F. suddenly emitted a piercing cry,
seized a knife that was lying in the kitchen and in a blind frenzy stabbed
his wife and their 11-year-old son who had had their meal with him. He
later maintained that he remembered nothing from the moment he felt the
knife in his hand. In his state of frenzy he also slashed the furniture
and the curtains. His wife and child were killed.

The neighbours who rushed in had difficulty in overpowering
him. Even after he had been tied to a stretcher he broke loose again and
still held the knife in an iron grip.

After admission to the regional mental hospital he remained
for several days in a state of clouded consciousness and restless delirium.
He also had grand mal attacks. His blood alcohol content was 1.13 $^o/oo$.
Clearly he had committed the crime in an excited epileptic twilight state,
exacerbated by alcohol.

The patient was considered to be not responsible for his
actions and was admitted under Section 42b. During his further stay in
hospital he was regarded as a dangerous, enigmatic man, who would try
to obtain alcohol secretly and who sometimes bothered women in an un-
pleasant erotic manner.

Intelligence

A comparative assessment of intelligence would have been easier if
we had been able to start with IQ values based on uniform standardised procedures. Unfortunately it turned out that the case histories of the non-violent
patients contained hardly any intelligence test data (one could hardly expect
to find them in routine admissions, of which they are not an essential part)

Table 24. *Distribution of different grades of intelligence in violent and non-violent patients*

	Whole group		Schizo- phrenia		Affective psychoses		Mental deficiency	
	n	%	n	%	n	%	n	%
Violent patients								
Considerable degree of defect	25	4.8	2	0.7	0	–	21	31
Middle-grade defect	49	9.3	14 }	5.0	0	–	30	44
Subnormality	121	23.0	52	18.7	6	16	17	25
Normal and above- average intelligence	330	62.9	211	75.6	31	84	0	–
Subtotal	525	100.0	279	100.0	37	100	68	100
Not known	8		5		0		0	
Total	533		284		37		68	
Non-violent patients								
Considerable degree of defect	26	5.2	0	–	0	–	22	31
Middle-grade defect	46	9.2	9 }	3.3	1	2	29	42
Subnormality	63	12.5	21	7.7	1	2	19	27
Normal and above- average intelligence	367	73.1	243	89.0	45	96	0	–
Subtotal	502	100.0	273	100.0	47	100	70	100
Not known	31		20		2		0	
Total	533		293		49		70	

Significance test:	χ^2 =	df =	α =
Whole group	19.85	3	0.001
Schizophrenia	17.32	2	0.001
Mental deficiency	0.12	2	Null hypothesis not refutable

(The brackets in the frequency table show which classes were put together in the significance test: the test was not applied to the affective psychoses because the expected values were so low.)

and the same applied frequently to the files of the violent offenders. In most cases, therefore, our only resource was a crude estimate of intelligence based on scholastic and professional attainments and on any observations that might have been recorded by the physicians who examined or treated the patients.

So far as could be ascertained, marked degrees of mental defect were of significance only in 14% of all violent offenders: 23% were of slightly less than average, and 63% of average or above-average intelligence (Table 24).

In contrast to their educational level (see below) there was a significant difference in the estimated or measured intelligence of the offenders as compared with the control group. While the gradings of 'consider-

Table 25. *Educational level of violent and non-violent patients*

	Whole group		Schizo- phrenia		Affective psychoses		Mental deficiency	
	n	%	n	%	n	%	n	%
Violent patients								
Primary school not completed	154	29.6	60	21.5	0	–	61	90
Primary school completed	301	57.7	174	62.0	25	74	7	10
Advanced schooling	66	12.7	46	16.5	9	26	0	–
Subtotal	521	100.0	280	100.0	34	100	68	100
Not known	12		4		3		0	
Total	533		284		37		68	
Non-violent patients								
Primary school not completed	144	29.2	51	18.3	3	6	60	91
Primary school completed	303	61.5	194	69.5	39	83	6	9
Advanced schooling	46	9.3	34	12.2	5	11	0	–
Subtotal	493	100.0	279	100.0	47	100	66	100
Not known	40		14		2		4	
Total	533		293		49		70	

able degree of defect' and 'middle grade defect' showed much the same distribution, the category of 'subnormal' was significantly more often applied to the
violent offenders. This finding reflects perhaps the variations in the standard of assessment in the two groups: the offenders were subjected to a more
thorough examination of their intellectual capacity than the patients who were
routinely admitted to the regional mental hospital. The less marked intellectual

Table 26. *Marital status of violent and non-violent patients*

	Whole group		Schizo- phrenia		Affective psychoses		Mental deficiency	
	n	%	*n*	%	*n*	%	*n*	%
Violent patients								
Single	239	44.9	144	50.7	1	3	57	84
Married	238	44.6	112	39.4	34	92	9 }	13
Divorced, widowed	56	10.5	28	9.9	2	5	2	3
Total	533	100.0	284	100.0	37	100	68	100
Non-violent patients								
Single	284	53.3	183	62.5	6	12	62	88
Married	191	35.8	83	28.3	37	76	4 }	6
Divorced, widowed	58	10.9	27	9.2	6	12	4	6
Total	533	100.0	293	100.0	49	100	70	100

Significance test: χ^2 =   df = α =

Whole group   9.05   2   0.025

Schizophrenia   8.84   2   0.025

Mental deficiency   0.316   1   Null hypothesis not refutable

(The brackets in the frequency table show which classes were put together
in the significance test: the test was not applied to the affective psychoses because the expected values were so low.)

defects were therefore more frequently picked up. It was in order to control this artefact that we included the question about schooling in our questionnaire.

No test of significance is required to show that violent and non-violent patients had more or less the same education (in most cases primary school)(Table 25). The large number of schizophrenics who did not complete their primary schooling can probably be explained by the fact that in accordance with our criteria for main and secondary diagnoses we counted cases of *Pfropfschizophrenie* as schizophrenia.

Marital status

It seemed of interest to find out whether the majority of the abnormal offenders were unmarried or married, and whether perhaps divorced and widowed patients tended to be more violent than those still living within an unbroken marriage.

Table 26 shows that with the age and sex distribution kept constant, there were more married persons among the violent offenders than in the control group (about 45% and 36% respectively). For the schizophrenics the difference between the two groups would seem to be accounted for by this diagnosis. Depressed patients - who were mostly women - were nearly all married, whether violent or not. The mentally deficient were nearly all single.

The unmarried state cannot therefore be regarded as constituting a risk factor, and indeed would appear to lessen the risk. The factor of 'marriage' seems to carry most risk in the affective psychoses. At all events for the married patients there are typical risks concerned with conflict and motivation: this is borne out, for example, in the case of depressives and schizophrenics by the high number of family members found among the victims (see Chapter 8).

In general the higher proportion of married persons in the violent group indicates a greater degree of vitality and social initiative, whereas the patients in the control group are more inclined to passivity and to autistic withdrawal (see also p.199).

Occupation at the time of the crime or at the time of admission

In view of our finding that a history of sociopathic-aggressive behaviour disorders was more common in the abnormal offenders than in the control group, it seemed possible that such personality traits would also affect occupational level and that low-status jobs, or lack of a job, would likewise be more common among the offenders than in the control group.

The occupational ratings given in Table 27 represent a somewhat

Table 27. *Distribution of occupational groups in violent and non-violent patients*

	Whole group		Schizo-phrenia		Affective psychoses		Mental deficiency	
	n	%	n	%	n	%	n	%
Violent patients								
Unemployed	144	27.2	76	27.0	1	3	17	25
Being educated	15	2.8	6	2.1	0	-	2	3
Temporary worker	165	31.1	87	30.8	1	3	44	66
Skilled worker, employee	106	20.0	71	25.2	10	27	1	2
Higher grade employee, self-employed	10	1.9	7	2.5	1	3	0	-
Housewife	90	17.0	35	12.4	24	64	3	4
Subtotal	530	100.0	282	100.0	37	100	67	100
Not known	3		2		0		1	
Total	533		284		37		68	
Non-violent patients								
Unemployed	164	30.9	86	29.5	5	10	28	40
Being educated	14	2.6	11	3.8	0	-	3	4
Temporary worker	173	32.6	87	29.9	13	27	38	54
Skilled worker, employee	110	20.7	74	25.4	9	18	1	2
Higher grade employee, self-employed	14	2.6	7	2.4	2	4	0	-
Housewife	56	10.6	26	9.0	20	41	0	-
Subtotal	531	100.0	291	100.0	49	100	70	100
Not known	2		2		0		0	
Total	533		293		49		70	

Significance test:

Whole group $\chi^2 = 10.18$ df = 5 Null hypothesis not confirmed

simplified version of those used in the questionnaire. We had originally
distinguished, for example, between 'unemployed' and 'incapable of work, or
invalided'. But as it was not always possible to make such a distinction on
the basis of the documents available, we combined the two categories under the
heading 'unemployed'.

As can be seen from the table, there were more unemployed patients
in the control group than among the offenders, while the proportion of housewives was somewhat smaller in the control group. This finding supports the
assumption formulated above, namely that the offenders as a group were somewhat more active and had more social contacts than the control patients.
(This is a trend which became apparent in our preliminary test data and which
later analyses strongly confirmed.)

The high number of housewives among the offenders is explained by, .
amongst other things, the high marriage figures for depressed offenders, in
whom there seemed to be close associations between the crime, the clinical
picture and a closely knit conjugal family. Apart from this, however, there
are only slight deviations in the distribution of occupations; the test result
is not significant.

Delinquency (previous criminal record)

In considering the premorbid personality of the violent offenders
we were very interested to find out whether the index crime represented the
first occasion of this kind in a previously uneventful career, or whether
there was a history of previous delinquency. The psychiatrist who is
responsible for such patients, and particularly for discharging them back into
the community after a period of in-patient care, must pay very special attention to the question of a possible relapse into crime.

We classified previous delinquent episodes according to whether
they were offences against life and limb or other offences not associated
with the use of violence, including relevant incidents which had not come
before the police and excluding traffic and driving offences; we recorded
all such items occurring up to the time of the crime or the date of admission.

Crimes against life and limb

Comparison between the two groups (Table 28) shows highly
significant differences: crimes against life, dangerous sexual assault and
especially bodily harm, feature much more frequently in the previous histories
of the violent patients - more than 35% as against only 4% for the non-violent.
Most of the violent crimes consisted of bodily harm (29.2% of the violent

Table 28. *Frequency of offences against life and limb in the previous histories of violent and non-violent patients*

	Whole group		Schizo- phrenia		Affective psychoses		Mental deficiency	
	n	%	*n*	%	*n*	%	*n*	%
Violent patients								
No violent offences	342	64.4	188	66.4	34	92	28	41
Bodily harm	155	29.2	85 ⎤		0	–	28 ⎤	41
Sexual assault[a]	17	3.2	3 ⎥	33.6	0	–	9 ⎥	13
Life-endangering attacks	17	3.2	7 ⎦		3	8	3 ⎦	5
Subtotal	531	100.0	283	100.0	37	100	68	100
Not known	2		1		0		0	
Total	533		284		37		68	
Non-violent patients								
No violent offences	506	95.7	279	95.9	48	98	64	93
Bodily harm	18	3.4	11 ⎤		1	2	2 ⎤	
Sexual assault[a]	5	0.9	1 ⎥	4.1	0	–	3 ⎥	7
Life-endangering attacks	0	–	0 ⎦		0	–	0 ⎦	
Subtotal	529	100.0	291	100.0	49	100	69	100
Not known	4		2		0		1	
Total	533		293		49		70	

Significance test:	χ^2 =	df =	α =
Whole group	163.4	3	0.001
Schizophrenia	78.725	1	0.001
Mental deficiency	38.999	1	0.001

(The brackets in the frequency tables show which classes were put together in the significance test. The test was not applied to the affective psychoses because the expected values were too low.)

[a] Only those assaults which were accompanied by threats to life, e.g. rape accompanied by strangling to keep the victim quiet.

offenders); sexual assaults were rare (about 3%) and are of importance only
in the group of mentally defective offenders. Previous life-endangering crimes,
i.e. the category of violent offence in which we were most interested, were
recorded in only about 3% of all the abnormal offenders. Because of the
practical importance of this question in terms of affecting decisions about
discharge and continued detention, we give in Table 29 a summary of the 17
relevant cases, restricting our review to brief information about the diagnosis,
the crime, and the previous crime.

The figure of about 3% is remarkably low. If we consider only the
eight previous homicides we find that of the 251 offenders who were in our
cohort because of a homicidal crime, 3.1% had previously committed homicide.
In assessing this relatively low rate of relapse, it may be suggested that
perhaps a high proportion of the abnormal offenders who are at risk as regards
committing further homicides are prevented from doing so because they are sent
to institutions or detained in prison for a long period of time.

Other investigators in the USA have reported similar findings.
Genert (1966) published a study of 2568 individuals in Pennsylvania who had
been convicted of homicide (both normal and abnormal offenders), of whom only
13 (0.5%) had repeated this crime. This relapse rate is lower than that found
in our study, and makes it clear that it is the crime rather than the mental
illness that is associated with the low rate of repetition.

Macdonald (1967) examined 100 patients who had been detained in
psychiatric institutions because of murder threats. Three of them had already
killed someone before being committed to hospital. In a follow-up study five
to six years later, in which 75 patients were covered, it was found that four
of them had committed suicide and three had committed murder. In particularly
aggressive patients the risk of murder is higher if there is no previous history
of suicide attempts.

At all events our 17 patients who had repeated the crime of murder
or attempted murder included three whose previous crime was an attempt at
extended suicide. When we investigated suicide incidents within the six months
preceding the crime (see also Chapter 6) both the offenders and the non-
offenders in our study showed a rate of attempted suicide amounting to about
10% which does not exactly argue in favour of Macdonald's hypothesis. [5]

Probably the factors which determine whether aggressive tension
is discharged against the self or against another person not only lie in the
personality structure of the offender but also depend to a large extent on the
situation, for example the behaviour of the victim (see Chapter 8).

Table 29. *Summary of histories of violent patients who had committed previous life-endangering crimes*

Case no.	Sex	Diagnosis	Crime	Previous crime	Calendar year of	
					First crime	Second crime
003	m	Ment. def. (middle grade)	Killed sweetheart with an axe	Killed wife	1934	1957
022	m	Cyclothymia	Tried to kill lodger (excited mania)	Extended suicide attempt	1937	1962
070	f	Schizophrenia	Strangled her child (infant), extended suicide attempt	Strangled her child	1963	1964
091	f	Ment. def. (middle grade)	Tried to poison daughter-in-law (E 605)	Put insecticide in father's food	1955	1960
095	f	Atypical endogenous psychoses	Threw daughter (aged 1) out of train	Gave infant intentional overdose of sedatives	1963	1964
100	m	Cerebral trauma	Tried to strangle second wife	Strangled wife	1952	1962
102	m	General palsy	Killed wife and 2 sons with knife and axe	Turned on gas in family's bedroom	18 Feb 1962	26 Feb. 1962
104	m	Schizophrenia	Tried to strangle wife	Attacked wife with axe	1949	1964
131	f	Reactive depression	Two children killed by gas in extended suicide attempt	Extended suicide attempt	1960	1961
147	f	Endogenous depression	Extended suicide with son aged 3	Extended suicide attempt	1954	1958
249	m	Schizophrenia	Tried to kill wife with flat-iron	Tried to kill wife with hammer	1956	1957
264	m	Frontal lobe syndrome	Tried to shoot wife, daughter and son-in-law	Shot a fellow soldier	1945	1964
308	m	Schizophrenia	Grievous bodily harm to fellow-prisoner with razor-blade	Nearly killed friend with flat-iron	1955	1960
315	m	Schizophrenia	Strangled fellow-prisoner	Choked wife to death	1959	1964
336	m	Schizophrenia	Shot a neighbour	Killed landlady	1956	1961
338	m	Schizophrenia	Attempted robbery and murder. Knocked down old woman	Killed aunt with cudgel	7 Dec. 1956	8 Dec. 1956
534	m	Ment. def. (middle grade)	Rape and murder	Rape and murder	Jan. 1962	Apr. 1962

Other crimes

Under this heading we enquired into crimes not associated with the use of violence, namely indecent behaviour without violence, crimes against property, abusive behaviour, defamation of character, threatening behaviour and combinations of these. In Table 30 we have distinguished between crimes associa-

Table 30. *Frequency of other crimes, with or without threats but not associated with open violence, in the previous histories of violent and non-violent patients*

	Whole group		Schizo-phrenia		Affective psychoses		Mental deficiency	
	n	%	n	%	n	%	n	%
Violent patients								
None	264	49.6	144	50.7	33	89	16	24
Crimes with no threat	69	13.0	21	7.4	0	–	24	35
Crimes with threat	199	37.4	119	41.9	4	11	28	41
Subtotal	532	100.0	284	100.0	37	100	68	100
Not known	1		0		0		0	
Total	533		284		37		68	
Non-violent patients								
None	359	67.9	203	69.8	46	94	25	36
Crimes with no threat	72	13.6	31	10.7	0	–	30	44
Crimes with threat	98	18.5	57	19.5	3	6	14	20
Subtotal	529	100.0	291	100.0	49	100	69	100
Not known	4		2		0		1	
Total	533		293		49		70	

Significance test:	χ^2	df = 2	α =
Whole group	48.88		0.001
Schizophrenia	33.71		0.001
Mental deficiency	7.30		0.001

(The test was not applied to the affective psychoses because the expected values were too low.)

ted with threats and those not so accompanied, which enables us to detect
aggressive patterns of behaviour.

Previous crimes accompanied by threats are, like violent crimes,
more frequent in the group of offenders than in the control group but here
again the reason for the difference may be that in the case of the offenders
the original examiner was looking more carefully for aggressive modes of
behaviour in the previous history. Crimes not accompanied by threats were
about the same for both groups, at around 13%. The fact that these relatively
minor events were recorded as frequently in the control group as in the
offenders may perhaps be taken as an indication that the other data covering
this feature are not too unreliable.

Unlike the other diagnoses, the violent and non-violent depressed
patients (mostly women) showed no difference in respect of the frequency of
'other crimes' in their previous histories. The schizophrenic offenders, on the
other hand, had a more frequent history of crimes, mainly 'crimes with threats'
(41.9% as against 19.5% in the control group). The same was true of the oligophrenics, in whom an entirely crime-free record was much more rare than in
patients with other diagnoses.

Summary

The educational and occupational history of the violent offenders
did not differ from that of the control groups. Their social ties, from the
point of view of marital status, were no fewer than those of the comparable,
non-violent patients. The married state was in fact a little more frequent
among the violent offenders; viewed in conjunction with the findings on
occupation, this may be taken as implying to some extent that social or family
rootlessness is not one of the essential factors heightening the risk of
violence in the mentally abnormal - with the exception of the mentally defective.
But some features of the premorbid personality and some trends in behaviour
that are analogous to the relevant criminal behaviour do point to a danger of
violence that should not be underestimated; aggressive patterns of behaviour,
threats and violence, mostly on a smaller scale than the crime which brought
them into our study, were considerably more frequent in the mentally abnormal
offenders than in the non-violent patients. The group of affective psychoses
came well below the average for violent offenders in this respect (8% of cases
showed aggressive crimes including homicide and attempted homicide; 11% crimes
with threats); the schizophrenics came close to the average (34% with
aggressive crimes, etc.; 42% crimes with threats); the mental defectives, however, easily headed the list (58% aggressive crimes, etc.; 41% crimes with

threats; only 24% with no previous crimes). One has no hesitation in concluding from these data that where a tendency to aggressive behaviour is rooted in the personality - and in the mentally abnormal such a tendency has usually become manifest long before the onset of the psychosis - this has a far stronger effect than the illness itself on the risk of violence.

This prediction applies to the group as a whole, to schizophrenics, and particularly to mental defectives, with the qualification that in the latter group the mental defect has of course existed before manifestation of this behaviour pattern. It is therefore an open question whether the mental deficiency and the development of such behaviour patterns are interdependent. Since criminal violence does not appear to be more frequent among the mentally defective than chance would lead us to expect, it is at least not very likely that this interdependence, if it exists, plays a great part. What is certain is that the above items, and other antisocial personality traits, are decisive risk factors so far as mental deficiency is concerned. Or conversely: the probability that a mental defective without antisocial personality traits, without a previous history of aggressive behaviour patterns and without previous crimes containing an aggressive component or at least accompanied by threats, will commit a serious crime of violence is small: it is less than 20%.

These findings are in line with our findings on the nuclear family. They make it clear that family loading with aggressive or antisocial/ psychopathic modes of behaviour and with the analogous features of alcoholism and the like, is of more significance as a risk factor than loading with mental illness or mental defect. The latter loadings, which concern hereditary illness in the narrower sense, were in part slightly more frequent among the violent offenders, but there was no reliable difference between the violent and the non-violent groups. Again the case-rate for aggressive and auto-aggressive or antisocial/psychopathic features was highest in the members of the nuclear families of mentally defective offenders (51% of cases).

This summary of some of our findings shows clearly that the mentally abnormal patients who commit violent crimes are mostly individuals who maintain an active, if restricted and hazardous, capacity to live their own lives and are as a rule, with the exception of the mentally defective, able to be at least as well integrated, so far as occupation and personal life is concerned, as the average mentally abnormal non-offender. But they show considerable signs of maladaptation, which seemed to be associated with aggressive patterns of behaviour. The risk of their becoming violent would appear to be influenced more by these factors of family, personality and behaviour than by factors of illness in the narrower sense. Their disposition

to violent crime - to put our interpretation in more substantive terms - can
be traced back more clearly to a generation-long predisposition to aggressive
or antisocial forms of behaviour than to a predisposition to illness.
Occupational status and social class would not appear to affect the issue at
present, since in respect of the items which we studied and which are relevant
to social gradients, the mentally abnormal violent offenders were above rather
than below the control group of non-violent patients. A conclusive answer would,
however, call for a special study tailored to fit the question.

      The violent offenders with affective psychoses represent a special
case. Their previous history, like their family history, shows extraordinarily
few incidents of aggressive behaviour. In the small number of cases which did
have a previous history of aggressive crimes, the index crime followed the same
pattern as the earlier offence, the most common being attempted homicide
associated with attempted suicide (8% of the cases) and straightforward
crimes accompanied by threats; other previous crimes showed 0%. It
thus becomes increasingly clear that in this group of illnesses it is
other risk factors which are decisive. They are not based on antisocial or
openly aggressive patterns of behaviour in the offender and his family, but
are closely associated with the illness. As already mentioned, they are also
specifically associated with sex. Most of the offenders in this category are
married (92%), 65% are housewives, not in gainful employment - a group which
is also over-represented to a considerable extent among the non-violent patients
with this diagnosis in our control group (41%). Family history, premorbid
personality and social history are thus not reliable pointers to an increased
risk of violence in the affective psychoses, in which respect they differ both
from mental deficiency and from schizophrenia.

7.3 The illness

      In section 5.3 we considered how far the 533 abnormal offenders
differed in regard to diagnosis from the population (n = 3392) of non-violent
patients in a regional mental hospital: in other words, whether violent crimes
occur with particular frequency in certain groups of illness. In the sections
which now follow we shall try to see whether individual symptoms or symptom
clusters can be picked out which seem to be associated with a high or low risk
of violence.

      Earlier investigators had already developed some hypotheses bearing
on this problem (see Chapter 2). According to Brandt, Janzarik, Lanzkron, Mowat,
Stierlin, Wanner and others, it seemed plausible to assume that schizophrenics
who suffer from systematic delusions, for example of persecution, are more
likely to become violent than those who do not misinterpret reality in a

delusional way. In our pilot study of case histories we ourselves also formed
the impression that delusional perceptions of an imperative nature (in
particular the so-called imperative voices) [6] and a frequent tendency to
excited mood disorders in the course of the illness were more common among the
offenders than among the non-violent patients.

According to Wilmanns' analysis (1940), the initial phase of the
illness is particularly significant in schizophrenia so far as the occurrence
of violent crime is concerned. In the view of other authors, however, for
example Mowat (1966), violent crimes by delusional patients are usually
preceded by a build-up of symptoms over several years. It was therefore of
interest to include in our comparative study both the duration and the course
of the illness up to the time of the crime or (for the control group) the
date of admission to hospital, and in this way to test such observations and
assumptions.

Symptoms

It was not possible to cover in our data sheets the frequency and
severity of the full range of symptoms that are to be found in mental disorders. Our list therefore included only those symptoms which might be expected
to be present in quantities suitable for statistical analysis and which would
in all probability be documented if they did occur. In particular we examined
the symptoms of delusion, delusional perceptions and thought disorders that
are frequently found in schizophrenics, and the 'mood disorders' ('affectivity')
which feature prominently in the description of manic and depressive syndromes.
'Affect' or 'mood' is a complex concept, the assessment of which can depend on
the individual examiner, and in recording it we concentrated on such features
as excitement, suspicion, lability, etc., which seemed to us of particular
importance in any estimation of the risk of violence.

It was only in relation to 'affect' that we were able to compare
the violent and non-violent patients as a whole, and also to compare them for
the three diagnostic groups of schizophrenia, affective psychoses and mental
deficiency. Although we recorded the frequency of 'delusion' in the group as
a whole and in the diagnostic groups of schizophrenia, affective psychoses and
mental deficiency, we restricted our analysis of delusional symptoms to schizophrenia alone. The items 'hallucinations' and 'thought disorders' are to a
large extent specific to schizophrenia and were analysed for that group only.

In our first analysis we compared the distribution of the four
classical subgroups of schizophrenia in the abnormal offenders and their non-
violent matched controls (Table 31). A simple course was found in

Table 31. *Frequency of the psychopathological subgroups in violent and non-violent schizophrenics*

	Violent patients		Non-violent patients			
	n	%	*n*	%	Total	% difference
Simple schizophrenia	49	17.3	85	29.0	134	+ 11.8
Catatonia	27	9.5	33	11.3	60	+ 1.8
Paranoid-hallucinatory schizophrenia	164	57.7	157	53.6	321	- 4.2
Paraphrenia	44	15.5	18	6.1	62	- 9.4
Total	284	100.0	293	100.0	577	

Significance test: $\chi^2 = 21.19$ df = 3 $\alpha = 0.001$

17.3% of the schizophrenic offenders, but in 29% of the control group. There were thus almost twice as many in the control group. Paranoid-hallucinatory and catatonic courses were almost equally represented in the two groups. There was, however, a considerably higher proportion of paraphrenics among the violent offenders.

Catatonic and simple schizophrenic syndromes can with justification be classed as 'unproductive', in contrast to the 'productive', paranoid-hallucinatory and paraphrenic subgroups, in which the tendency to delusions, hallucinations, etc., is taken as a criterion of 'productivity'. It is evident that these productive, delusional subgroups are significantly more common among the violent schizophrenics than in the control group of non-violent schizophrenics.

Delusion

Since the phenomenon of delusion features prominently both in the literature and in our analysis of schizophrenic symptoms in the violent group, we shall now examine more closely the occurrence, structure and content of this symptom.

Our first aim was to see how often delusion was recorded in the two cohorts of patients studied and to find out whether, in accordance with the hypothesis formulated at the beginning of this section, delusions were more frequent among the violent patients as a whole than among their non-violent controls.

The significance test in Table 32 shows that 'delusion' does occur more often in the whole group of violent patients than in the non-violent patients, to a degree that is beyond chance expectation. If we take only the schizophrenic patients, the difference becomes more marked (ratio of delusion in violent and non-violent schizophrenics around 89% to 76%, as against 65% to 47% for the group as a whole); the level of significance is the same. Depressive offenders likewise suffered markedly more often from delusions, but no such difference was found in the mental defectives.

The second question which interested us was the structure of the

Table 32. *Occurrence of delusion in violent and non-violent patients*

	Whole group		Schizo-phrenia		Affective psychoses		Mental deficiency	
	n	%	n	%	n	%	n	%
Violent patients								
No delusion	186	35.1	32	11.3	16	44	66	97
Delusion present	344	64.9	251	88.7	20	56	2	3
Subtotal	530	100.0	283	100.0	36	100	68	100
Not known	3		1		1		0	
Total	533		284		37		68	
Non-violent patients								
No delusion	281	53.4	69	24.1	36	74	69	99
Delusion present	245	46.6	217	75.9	13	26	1	1
Subtotal	526	100.0	286	100.0	49	100	70	100
Not known	7		7		0		0	
Total	533		293		49		70	

Significance test:	$\chi^2 =$	df = 1	$\alpha =$
Whole group	34.72		0.001
Schizophrenia	16.00		0.001
Affective psychoses	6.05		0.05

delusional phenomena described in the patients. We suspected that, so far as
motivation for the violent crime was concerned, it might matter whether or not
the patient had developed a logically elaborate, closed delusional system,
usually built round a central theme, as a result of which he may, for example,
deludedly and for a long time have believed that a certain man was his enemy
or persecutor, at times to the complete exclusion of all other thoughts. In
the presence of some additional factor, or possibly just as a consequence of
the delusional development, it is conceivable that such a patient may erupt
into violence that is in keeping with the delusional motivation. On the other
hand it is conceivable that in a state of delusional confusion, for instance
in the kind of anxious and uneasy delusional mood that can often be observed
as an unstructured background to delusion, the patient may suddenly give way to
unpredictable and relatively undirected aggressive impulses. In accordance with
these assumptions we drew a distinction between 'delusional mood', with no
structural theme, and 'delusional system', in the sense of a structured delusional
complex. Our findings are given in Table 33.

Even a simple comparison of the figures shows that systematic forms
of delusion are far more frequent, both absolutely and relatively, in the group
of violent patients as a whole as well as in the schizophrenics, the difference
being significant at the 0.001 level. This finding is an important one: patients

Table 33. *Frequency distribution of structured and unstructured
forms of delusion in delusional offenders and non-offenders
(only for the whole group and for schizophrenics)*

	Whole group		Schizophrenics	
	n	%	n	%
Delusional offenders				
Delusional mood	86	25.0	57	22.7
Delusional system	258	75.0	194	77.3
Total	344	100.0	251	100.0
Delusional patients in control group				
Delusional mood	145	59.2	119	54.8
Delusional system	100	40.8	98	45.2
Total	245	100.0	217	100.0

with a diffuse anxious delusional mood do not often act aggressively, but the presence of a systematic delusion seems to increase the risk of violent crime.

A further question now arises: if we compare patients with delusional symptoms, does the offender group show specific characteristics so far as delusional content is concerned? To answer this question we looked only at those schizophrenic patients in whom, according to Table 32, delusional phenomena had been noted in the course of the illness. This gave us 251 violent and 217 non-violent delusional schizophrenics. Table 34 shows the distribution of certain delusional themes which recurred again and again in the case histories of these patients.

The category covering delusions of interpretation, reference and injury represents the general concept of core paranoid syndromes, as well as unsystematised, vague 'ideas of reference without justification' such as are

Table 34. *Distribution of typical delusional themes in delusional schizo-phrenic violent offenders and their control group of delusional schizo-phrenic non-offenders*

Delusional theme	Violent schizophrenics		Non-violent schizophrenics	
	n	%	*n*	%
Delusions of interpretation, reference and injury	170	67.5	177	81.6
Delusions of grandeur, religious delusions	24	9.7	19	8.7
Delusions of love, jealousy	28	11.2	3	1.4
Hypochondriacal delusions, delusions of guilt	11	4.4	8	3.7
Other themes	18	7.2	10	4.6
Total	251	100.0	217	100.0

Significance test:	$\chi^2 =$	df =	$\alpha =$
Whole group	21.2708	4	0.001
Delusions of interpretation, reference, injury, love, delusional jealousy	19.4835	1	0.001
Delusions of grandeur, religious delusions, hypochondriacal delusions, delusions of guilt	0.0225	1	Null hypothesis not refutable

found in the initial stages of schizophrenia (Conrad, 1958), and structured
forms of delusion with such well-defined and constantly held themes as are
not covered by other categories in the table. We shall give in a later section
a separate comparison based on the classical delusion of persecution accompanied
by a feeling of being under threat.

Table 34 shows that the group covering delusions of interpretation,
reference and injury was found more frequently in the non-violent patients than
in the violent offenders. The explanation may lie in the fact that in the non-
violent patients the predominant syndrome was one of vague delusional mood with
unsystematic delusions which as a rule contained paranoid elements (see Table 31),
while the violent schizophrenics included more paraphrenics, i.e. patients with
systematised delusions and well-defined delusional objects.

The clear preponderance of delusions of love and jealousy in the
violent offenders is worth discussing. Since a majority of the jealous offenders
came from Bavaria, it may be asked whether this might be due to a cultural factor
affecting a rural population or whether it is a significant finding which applies
to the whole group of delusional offenders. This is a suitable point at which to
discuss an important condition which clearly affects the risk of violence in
delusional patients.

There is much to support the view that when other persons are involved
in the patient's delusion, the risk of their becoming victims is greatly increased
whereas delusions which centre essentially on the patient's own person, such as
hypochondriacal delusions or delusions of grandeur, do not, at least immediately,
tend to lead to attacks upon others. Delusions of love and jealousy, however,
are forms of delusion which involve partners in a particularly intense way and
in which the patient is constantly, in his thoughts and suspicions, entangled
with another person.

It should be remembered here that very close and conflicting human
relationships, particularly where the primal emotions are concerned, represent
a cardinal problem in the pathology of schizophrenics, as family research on
these patients has shown. Unlike megalomania or delusions of guilt and sin,
delusional love and particularly delusional jealousy may represent a revival
of that ambivalent primal relationship and may result in an extremely tense
and highly charged emotional situation.

According to studies by Rutter (1966) and Hoenig & Hamilton (1967),
for example, the inclusion of children in the delusions and hallucinations of
a schizophrenic parent frequently leads to behaviour disorders and health
problems in the offspring. It also leads as a rule to disturbed relationships
between those affected. From these findings, and from the experience exemplified

by the following case, it may be assumed that such tense and often deeply
ambivalent one-to-one relationships, taken especially in association with their
delusional components, may give rise to elementary feelings not only of anxiety
but also of hate. They may therefore constitute a particularly dangerous situation so far as violence is concerned, especially in a partner who is limited
both in orientation to reality and in self-control.

Case No. 329: Paranoid schizophrenia

Karl S., born 1909, son of a master tradesman, was, like his
two brothers, apprenticed to an upholsterer after leaving school. As a
young man he was said to have been sensitive, easily upset and shy. He
was exempted from military service because of a mitral defect. He had
numerous relationships with women and in 1939 had to get married because
a child was on the way. His reputation was on the whole good. It was only
with his step-father (his father had died shortly after the First World
War as a result of a war wound) and his elder brother that he sometimes
got involved in quarrels.

His marriage was full of tension, because he soon (from 1940)
felt that his wife was deceiving him and was tormented by violent jealousy.
He accused his wife of wanting to get rid of him and also involved his
son in this steadily growing suspicion. In November 1956 he became acutely
excited and was admitted to a clinic for nervous disorders, where he
complained of symptoms of poisoning. Although no signs of poisoning could
be found, the diagnosis of paranoid schizophrenia was abandoned, since
there were no other relevant symptoms, and he was considered to be a case
of 'abnormal mental development'. On the insistence of one brother,
who threatened legal proceedings if he was not discharged, he was brought
home against the advice of the doctors.

In 1957 his marriage ended in divorce, because his wife was
afraid of serious violence. Years before he had already threatened to kill
her. In November 1958 he was committed by the court doctor to a regional
mental hospital after he had come to blows with his elder brother, with
whom he worked in an upholstery shop. He thought he was being persecuted
by his divorced wife and by this brother and several times said in front
of witnesses that he would kill himself and his wife because of this. He
said that the tuberculosis from which he had been suffering for some time
was caused by poison. The brother who had been attacked believed that the
patient owned a pistol, felt himself to be in serious danger, and asked
for him to be committed.

In the hospital he was at first friendly and grateful for the help, feeling that he had been taken into protection. Soon, however, he refused any further treatment and in this he was supported by the rest of his family. Both his son and one of his sisters believed that he had real grounds for his delusional fears and kept trying to get him out of hospital. The sister insisted that her brother 'could only get worse' in hospital; it was all the fault of his divorced wife and elder brother. The patient was finally discharged in February 1959, in an improved state; he returned to his previous environment and resumed work with his brother.

After his divorce the patient had become friendly with a 33-year-old woman but gradually came to believe that she too, like his ex-wife, was deceiving, harming and poisoning him. In the summer of 1959, in the weeks preceding the crime, he hardly went to work, brooded a lot over his jealous ideas and seemed to his relatives absent-minded. On the evening before the crime he felt he was dying. He thought his headache, buzzing ears, palpitations and bodily aches were due to poison which his lover had administered to him in order to get rid of him in favour of another. He thereupon decided to kill her.

On the night of 28 August 1959 he first had sexual inter-course with this friend, who fell asleep beside him. Shortly after he attacked her on the head with a wine bottle and pressed her face into the pillows. Finally he choked her until there was no sign of life.

After admission to the institution under Section 42b, his mental state scarcely altered. His further behaviour confirmed the diagnosis of paranoid schizophrenia.

This case illustrates the development of a delusional illness in the course of which the wife and then the lover were persecuted by the patient's jealousy. The delusion later extended into a paranoid conviction that his life was in danger and that his near relatives were also involved in this malevolence. The crime took the form of revenge for imagined unfaithfulness, as well as self-protection against a delusional threat to his own life.

The points of view presented above throw light on the frequency with which the themes of love and jealousy appear in the delusions of the abnormal offenders. The explanation presumably does not lie in any cultural selective factor. Mowat (1966) also attributes great significance to delusional jealousy and in his own study describes its influence on murderous acts.

There is another syndrome in which account must also be taken of a connection between the violence of delusional patients and the involvement of the victims in the delusion. Delusional guilt or nihilistic delusion, found mostly in depressive patients, may be assumed to conceal a special risk of violence if close relatives, above all children, are involved in the delusion. Killing them as well as oneself is seen in the delusional reasoning as sparing them shame, suffering or destruction. As Table 34 shows, these forms of delusion are found in association with hypochondriacal delusions only slightly more frequently in the group of schizophrenic offenders than in the control group of non-violent schizophrenic patients (4.4% as against 3.7%). But the very frequent occurrence of the delusional belief that the act will bring release to the victims provides a very clear pointer in the case of the depressive offenders.

Delusional threat to the patient's own life

From examples in the literature (Brandt, Gaupp, Janzarik and others) and from study of our own case histories, we repeatedly found a delusional theme closely related to that described above, in which the paranoid patient feels threatened by imaginary persecutors and in an upsurge of panic or after years of cold planning attacks his supposed enemies with the intention of destroying them. It is known that many paranoid patients deludedly feel that their lives are in danger or that important parts of their bodies or their functions, e.g. potency, are imperilled. We therefore decided to find out whether such deep-seated anxieties and feelings of danger were recorded more frequently in our abnormal offenders than in the control groups.

The following brief example shows the kind of delusional theme we had in mind:

Case no. 466: Catatonic schizophrenia

Bachelor, son of a farming family, born 1933, with a family history of 'nervous troubles'; lived up to the time of the crime with his elder sister on his parents' farm which he was expected one day to take over.

As a child he showed a certain amount of obstinacy and timidity, but his upbringing presented no serious difficulties. He was an active boy of normal intelligence, who completed his schooling with reasonable success and from then on worked at home. His life was uneventful until his twenty-seventh year.

In 1960/1 he developed a schizophrenic psychosis, expressed in fears of persecution and poisoning and in auditory hallucinations. After three weeks of in-patient treatment he was discharged home. In the autumn of 1961 there was a second, more severe episode in which the patient, believing that his father was a stranger who wanted to kill him,

became anxious and excited and attacked his father during the night with
a knife. After three months of in-patient treatment he was discharged
back to his old environment and from then on he was noticeably odd: he
became solitary, suspicious and unfriendly, began to drink, to smoke
furiously, and to be miserly. Although he continued to receive tranquilli-
sing drugs from the general practitioner, which often had to be
administered without his knowledge, he would have severe mood disturbances
every four or six weeks in which he would get into a rage over trifles and
be unable to work.

In the middle of August 1964 his mental state was again worse
and his parents advised him to have treatment in a psychiatric hospital,
which he refused to do. At the beginning of September he got into a state
of anxiety in which he thought the farm was full of foreigners and spies
who were plotting against his life. Over the next few days his anxiety
mounted and he became convinced that his enemies had poured hydrochloric
acid over his mother.

On the evening of 25 September 1964 he stayed in his room,
fully dressed, wandering to and fro in a panic-stricken state, expecting
some incomprehensible disaster. Next morning the world seemed to him
strange and threatening; the house was full of gas. He was convinced that
his mother had been killed by his father, who in fact was one of the spies
and was also trying to kill him. In excited tones he told his father to
produce his mother immediately, otherwise he would kill him. When the
mother then appeared, he thought she was a stranger. Hardly had she gone
away when he rushed at his father with a pitch-fork, injured him badly,
threw him to the ground and strangled him. Neighbours helped the mother
to pull him off but they could not overpower him. (Later he said that
during the struggle a voice had kept repeating to him 'This is not your
father'.)

Finally he ran off to the barn, which he set on fire 'in
order to smoke out the spies'. When the flames were burning high he
pulled his mother towards the fire and threatened her with a horrible
death. He was then finally brought into custody.

This example illustrates both the patient's inharmonious and
complicated relationship with his parents, which was acutely heightened by his
delusions, and the delusional motivation for his violence against his father
as the 'partner' drawn into his delusion of persecution who was, he believed,
threatening sometimes his own and sometimes his mother's life. The case also
shows in a striking way the severe, morbid misidentification of reality which

appeared first as an acute delusional mood and probably made it to a large extent impossible for him to control the impulse to kill. In this respect, however, the patient represents an exception rather than the rule among delusional offenders.

On the assumption that the delusional experience of being threatened may constitute a special risk so far as violence is concerned, we then examined the records to see whether schizophrenics had experienced threats of this kind to life and limb, irrespective of the theme of their delusion.

Such an experience was in fact encountered much more frequently in the group of violent schizophrenics: 137 out of 251 delusional schizophrenic offenders (about 55%) felt themselves threatened in this way, against only 65 out of 217 non-violent controls (about 30%). Delusions of interpretation, reference and injury, to which this experience essentially belongs, had in the group of violent offenders much more clearly assumed the character of dangerous persecution and threats to life and limb.

The chances of such threatening anxiety leading to violence can, however, be assessed only in relation to a delusional quality which we have already discussed, namely the fixation or otherwise of the delusion upon certain delusional objects, in this case 'delusional enemies'.

It seems clear that feelings of hate which are dealt with project-ively and concentrated on one supposed persecutor provoke both anxiety and fantasies of destruction directed against that person. As the delusion develops, such a patient may seek to protect his endangered life and safety by trying to get rid of the enemy who threatens him or at least by converting his anxiety and hatred into a serious act of revenge. If, on the other hand, the delusion is not concentrated on individuals, and the threat comes from vague, anonymous or supernatural powers, as often happens in an unstructured delusional mood, it is unlikely that the defence against such a danger will take the form of a planned act of violence directed at specific individuals.

The finding that systematic delusions were almost twice as frequent in violent schizophrenics (77%) as in the non-violent control group with this diagnosis (45%) clearly takes on a new significance. When a systematic delusion of persecution is accompanied by the experience of danger or threat to life, and is concentrated on a personal partner, then this apparently constitutes a real risk of violence by schizophrenic offenders.

Auditory hallucinations

From our preliminary examination of the case material we had, as mentioned, formed the impression that many violent acts by abnormal offenders

were carried out under the influence of hallucinations that were either abusive
or constituted direct orders to commit the crime. Our interest was particularly
aroused by the striking and frequently described phenomenon of auditory hallucinatory commands, or so-called 'imperative voices'. The following case may serve
as an illustration:

Case no. 369: Schizophrenia

    A farmer's son, of below-average intelligence, inclined to
depressive rumination, the youngest of three children, felt himself from
childhood overshadowed by his older, cleverer and more active brother,
who would one day inherit the farm. There was frequent tension and
quarrelling between the two. At the age of 22 the patient suffered from
delusions of guilt and persecution, accompanied by depression. After
six weeks of in-patient treatment, with the diagnosis of 'schizophrenia',
he was discharged home in a state of remission and over the following
two years developed the delusion that his hated brother was not his
father's son but the son of the pastor, who was inciting him against
the patient. Soon he heard voices commanding him to kill his brother,
these voices coming at times from the pastor, at times from his siblings.
The delusion compelled him to believe that it was quite right for him
to kill his brother, since he would in any case have to die in the next
war. Voices ordered him to stab his brother with a hay-fork; the victim
himself wanted this. These imperative hallucinations were sometimes,
though less often, directed against his sister. Finally he resolved to
kill his brother secretly. Shortly afterwards he hit him on the head
at night with a wooden pestle, causing grievous bodily harm.

    Our first step was to compare the occurrence of auditory hallucina-
tions in the two groups, as well as their content (Table 35). The preponderance of productive forms, i.e. rich in symptoms, among the violent schizophrenics is reflected also in the frequency of hallucinations. But auditory
hallucinations occurred in both groups of patients, in two-thirds of the
violent offenders (66.5%) and in more than half of the controls; the difference is barely significant. Taking all the schizophrenics with a history of
auditory hallucinations and dividing them according to the content of these,
we find a slightly higher proportion of imperative voices in the offender
group as compared with the control group, but, contrary to our expectations,
the difference is again not significant (Table 36). Their presence, therefore,
clearly cannot yet be taken as implying an increased risk of violence. The
difference might have been greater had we enquired about imperative voices
inciting to kill. We did not do this, however, because we would have had to

expect a bias in favour of the offenders.

It is interesting to note that auditory hallucinations with abusive content were more frequently recorded in the control group than among the offenders. This may conceivably represent self-reproaches disguised as hallucinations, the content of which is governed by earlier codes of conduct and social sanctions and which may be regarded as a form of reaction to unwelcome impulses.

Table 35. *Frequency of auditory hallucinations in violent and non-violent schizophrenics*

	Violent		Non-violent	
	n	%	*n*	%
No auditory hallucinations	87	33.5	115	43.9
Auditory hallucinations	172	66.5	147	56.1
Subtotal	259	100.0	262	100.0
Not known	25		31	
Total	284		293	

Significance test:

Presence of auditory hallucinations $\chi^2 = 5.397$ df = 1 $\alpha = 0.05$

Table 36. *Frequency of abusive and imperative voices in violent and non-violent schizophrenics*

	Violent		Non-violent	
	n	%	*n*	%
Abusive voices	62	36.0	72	48.9
Imperative voices	45	26.2	27	18.4
Other auditory hallucinations[a]	65	37.8	48	32.7
Total	172	100.0	147	100.0

Significance test:

Whole group $\chi^2 = 5.88$ df = 2   Null hypothesis not refutable

[a] If the hallucinations appeared in combination, we took the one that most frequently occurred. 'Other auditory hallucinations' covered voices that were neutral or were experienced positively.

The difference in frequency is therefore not without interest: it may possibly
reflect a weaker reaction formation - or a defect in socialisation - in the
violent offenders and a stronger reaction formation in the non-violent schizophrenics.

Bodily hallucinations

In investigating this symptom we proceeded on the assumption that
psychotic violent offenders might also possibly be partly induced to commit
their crime by tormenting physical sensations which in delusion are often
traced back to damaging influences, e.g. rays. The existence of haptic
hallucinations might thus be seen as a possible motivation for violence
against someone who is deludedly held to be responsible for such sensations.
At the same time we enquired about simple feelings of malaise (e.g. headaches)
which were regarded by the patient as being caused by the influence of other
persons.

Bodily hallucinations and paranoid feelings of malaise were
significantly more frequent among the violent offenders, more than half of
whom had suffered from these symptoms as against only just over a third of
the control group (Table 37). In fact the difference in this relatively
refined symptom may not be quite so great: we do not believe, however, that
it represents only a difference in documentation. It is worth noting that

Table 37. *Bodily hallucinations and feelings of malaise in violent
and non-violent schizophrenics*

	Violent		Non-violent	
	n	%	*n*	%
No bodily hallucinations	105	39.9	178	64.5
Paranoid feelings of malaise	22	8.4	7	2.5
Bodily hallucinations	136	51.7	91	33.0
Subtotal	263	100.0	276	100.0
Not known	21		17	
Total	284		293	

Significance test:

Whole group $\chi^2 = 35.21$ df = 2 $\alpha = 0.001$

the distribution is very similar to that of the delusional experience of threats to life and limb.

Thought disorders

This psychological phenomenon is one of the characteristic symptoms of severe psychoses and provides a measure of the severity of personality disintegration. We included it in our questionnaire because we wished to test the hypothesis that aggressive impulses erupt more easily when the controlling effect of the cognitive apparatus is reduced. (This implies, of course, that thought disorders are in fact a sign of decreased cognitive control, which is by no means certain.)

We established two categories: 'subjective thought disorders' were understood as thought inhibition, disconnected thought, thought diffusion, hearing one's thought spoken aloud; 'objective thought disorders' covered incoherence, fragmentation, etc. Again we applied this evaluation only to schizophrenic patients.

While subjective thought disorders show no great difference in distribution, objective thought disorders were recorded somewhat more frequently in the violent group than in the non-violent control patients, though the difference is only slightly significant (Table 38). It may be objected that this difference is due to differences in documentation, but against this it

Table 38. *Frequency of thought disorders in violent and non-violent schizophrenics*

	Violent		Non-violent	
	n	%	*n*	%
No thought disorders	90	32.5	115	40.2
Subjective thought disorders only	69	24.9	82	28.7
Objective thought disorders	118	42.6	89	31.1
Subtotal	277	100.0	286	100.0
Not known	7		7	
Total	284		293	

Significance test:
Whole group $\chi^2 = 8.08$ df = 2 $\alpha = 0.025$

can be pointed out that the much less obtrusive symptom of 'subjective thought disorders only' was recorded more frequently (by a few per cent) in the non-violent group. Incoherent, fragmented thinking reflecting fairly severe cognitive disintegration would thus in fact appear to affect the control of aggressive impulses in a proportion of the cases, though statistically this can be regarded only as a trend.

Predominant affect in the illness

We began by asking ourselves whether patients who later became violent might during their illness have already shown in their affective style of behaviour a tendency to moods which might conceivably provide an emotional background for aggressive discharge (e.g. increased moodiness, suspiciousness, or coldness of affect).

We could not, of course, use a rating scale for this item, since in a secondary enquiry such as this the available documentation was based on value judgements which varied considerably from examiner to examiner. We there-fore restricted the study to a qualitative rating according to categories which we selected, which covered a limited number of items only and which cannot be said to be free from arbitrariness. (For example we frequently came across patients described in the case records as 'anxious and perplexed', which we entered as 'suspicious' - a category that thus had to cover a spectrum ranging from general anxiety to personal mistrust.)

The recorded mood was based as far as possible not only on the opinion of the preliminary medical examiner, but also on descriptions of behaviour entered by the nursing staff, though we could not be sure that this did indeed give us the dominant mood either in respect of intensity or in respect of occurrence during the course of the illness. Table 39 must therefore be treated with caution and one cannot claim any high degree of validity for the findings.

It will be seen that forms of affect which are usually associated with violence, such as 'coldness of affect' and 'irritability', as well as 'lability of mood', were in fact recorded more frequently for the abnormal offenders than for the non-offenders. The question therefore arises whether the categories attributed to the violent patients were the result of rater bias, in other words whether they were influenced by the raters' expectations. It is a question which cannot be answered reliably. In the control group 'apathy' was seen as the most characteristic affect in almost a third of the cases: it was not infrequently found in the violent offenders too - even heading the list for the mental defectives - but it was clearly more frequent among

Table 39. *Distribution of dominant forms of affect in violent and non-violent patients*

	Whole group		Schizo-phrenia		Affective psychoses		Mental deficiency	
	n	%	n	%	n	%	n	%
Violent patients								
Cold affect	39	7.6	16	5.7	0	–	16	30
Suspicious	147	28.5	116	41.8	0	–	0	–
Irritable	61	11.8	30	10.8	0	–	9	17
Sad and depressive	98	19.0	34	12.2	29	79	0	–
Elevated mood	22	4.3	12	4.3	2	5	0	–
Apathetic	92	17.9	48	17.3	2	5	28	53
Labile	56	10.9	22	7.9	4	11	0	–
Subtotal	515	100.0	278	100.0	37	100	53	100
Not known	18		6		0		7	
Total	533		284		37		60	
Non-violent patients								
Cold affect	4	0.8	0	–	0	–	4	7
Suspicious	136	27.4	127	43.2	1	2	3	6
Irritable	35	7.1	11	3.8	0	–	4	7
Sad and depressive	100	20.1	27	9.2	44	90	4	7
Elevated mood	38	7.7	26	8.9	3	6	1	2
Apathetic	147	29.6	80	27.7	0	–	36	64
Labile	36	7.3	21	7.2	1	2	4	7
Subtotal	496	100.0	292	100.0	49	100	56	100
Not known	37		1		0		14	
Total	533		293		49		70	

Significance test:	$\chi^2 =$	df = 6	$\alpha =$
Whole group	56.91		0.001
Schizophrenia	35.05		0.001

the non-violent patients. The result as a whole seems to depend mainly on the
schizophrenic offenders, in that for individual items such as 'depressive'
and 'apathetic' the figures for the mentally defective and depressed groups
are diametrically opposed and cancel each other out.

Again our results are in keeping with earlier findings which showed
the violent offenders as being altogether more active personalities and more
inclined to be at odds with their environment than the non-violent patients.
The same kind of difference is seen in the schizophrenics, where productive
syndromes are over-represented in the offenders and non-productive syndromes
in the non-offenders. Suspicious and depressed moods are more or less equally
distributed. Affective psychoses, which were omitted from the significance
test because of the low number of cases, were again fundamentally different
from the other diagnoses. As might be expected, the depressive mood prevailed
almost exclusively.

Duration and course of illness

Impressed by cases in which the dramatic onset of a state of
excitement was followed by a violent crime (case no. 466 (p.141) is an
illustration of this), earlier psychiatrists developed the theory that this
initial phase of the illness was significantly associated with the outbreak
of violence (see Chapter 2: Birnbaum, Mikorey, Mezger, Wilmanns and others).
The crime thus ranked as an initial symptom. In order to test this assumption,
which is of great practical importance, we studied the duration of illness
(from its presumed onset, so far as this could be determined, to the date of
the crime or, for the control group, to the date of admission to hospital) and
examined also the course of the illness (e.g. whether it was episodic, phasic
or chronic/progressive; whether the patient was in an improved or deteriorated
state before the crime).

Duration

We looked at the interval of time between the first manifestation of illness and the crime, irrespective of remissions and relapses, for
the group as a whole, for the schizophrenics and for those with affective
psychoses (Table 40). We did not include the mentally defective in this test
since theirs is not an 'illness' in the narrow sense, nor can one speak of its
'duration'.

Comparison with the non-offenders here provides no more than an
orientation, since 'admission' and 'crime' are not events which take place
under analogous conditions. Differences in duration were, of course, to be

Table 40. *Duration of illness in violent and non-violent patients (excluding the mentally defective)*

	Whole group		Schizo-phrenia		Affective psychoses	
	n	%	n	%	n	%
Violent patients						
Up to 1 month	17	3.3	8	2.9	4	11
1-6 months	34	6.6	16	5.8	8	22
Up to 1 year	38	7.3	21	7.6	1	3
1-5 years	143	27.5	96	34.7	12	33
5-10 years	99	19.1	68	24.5	4	11
10 years and over	188	36.2	68	24.5	7	20
Subtotal	519	100.0	277	100.0	36	100
Not known	14		7		1	
Total	533		284		37	
Non-violent patients						
Up to 1 month	61	11.8	40	14.2	4	8
1-6 months	31	6.0	14	5.0	13	27
Up to 1 year	21	4.1	10	3.6	5	10
1-5 years	119	23.1	82	29.2	8	16
5-10 years	73	14.1	56	19.9	8	16
10 years and over	211	40.9	79	28.1	11	23
Subtotal	516	100.0	281	100.0	49	100
Not known	17		12		0	
Total	533		293		49	

Significance test:	χ^2 =	df =	α =
Whole group	37.2919	5	0.001
Schizophrenia	28.4307	5	0.001
Affective psychoses	1.0342	2	Null hypothesis not refutable

expected between the different illnesses. Nevertheless it is remarkable that
the average duration of illness in the offenders was one to five years, the
deviations varying according to the illness, while the control group more
frequently showed illnesses that were of very short duration or that had lasted
more than ten years. The simple table of duration of illness in the violent
offenders is of particular interest. The view that the prodromal stages are
particularly dangerous is not confirmed by these findings.

Wilmanns had developed the 'prodromal' theory in respect of schizophrenics, but this is precisely the group to whom it least applies: within a
ten-year period (1955-64) only eight out of 284 schizophrenics had committed
a violent crime against the life of another person in the first month of their
illness! This clearly confirms what we said in Chapter 2 in regard to
Wilmanns' findings, namely that a large proportion of the offenders described
by him as schizophrenic were in fact patients with prison psychoses who did
not become ill till after the crime, while they were in prison. From the
practical and preventive point of view, much more significance is attached to
those illnesses which have lasted for years and which we have already discussed
when dealing with the development of delusions of jealousy (see p. 80). Violent
crimes committed within four weeks of the onset of the illness are somewhat
more frequent in the affective psychoses (11%). Because of the low number of
cases, however, this rate can only be regarded as imprecise and as including
deviations in both directions.

Course

If our findings now show that there is no increased risk of violence
in the acute initial stages of illness - with the affective psychoses probably
constituting a slight exception - then the next question that arises is whether
the violence may be partly caused by an acute exacerbation of an already existing mental illness.

We drew a distinction between a phasic or periodic (*Schub*) course
and a chronic/progressive illness. 'Exacerbation' covered a clear deterioration
in the patient's state in the days preceding the crime or the admission to
hospital.

Theoretically this enabled us to distinguish between a flaring up
of subjectively experienced symptoms and an objectively perceived worsening of
behaviour or an increase in observed conflict and tension with the environment.
In our retrospective enquiry, however, it was not often possible to make such
a distinction and we therefore had to content ourselves with a more general,
aggregate concept of exacerbation. In mental defectives exacerbation does not
indicate deterioration in intellectual performance, as in this sense the illness

Table 41. *Course of illness, and in particular the occurrence of acute exacerbations, in violent and non-violent patients*

	Whole group		Schizo- phrenia		Affective psychoses		Mental deficiency	
	n	%	n	%	n	%	n	%
Violent patients								
Episodic or phasic								
No exacerbation	87	16.6	54	19.2	20	54	O	-
Exacerbation	94	17.9	70	24.9	15	40	O	-
Chronic/progressive								
No exacerbation	265	50.6	113	40.9	1	3	67	99
Exacerbation	78	14.9	44	15.6	1	3	1	1
Subtotal	524	100.0	281	100.0	37	100	68	100
Not known	9		3		O		O	
Total	533		284		37		68	
Non-violent patients								
Episodic or phasic								
No exacerbation	72	13.7	28	9.6	35	71	O	-
Chronic/progressive	139	26.5	118	40.3	11	23	O	-
No exacerbation	201	38.4	98	33.4	1	2	52	74
Exacerbation	112	21.4	49	16.7	2	4	18	26
Subtotal	524	100.0	293	100.0	49	100	70	100
Not known	9		O		O		O	
Total	533		293		49		70	

Significance test:	χ^2	df =	α =
Whole group	24.98	3	0.001
Schizophrenia	22.0	3	0.001
Affective psychoses	1.94	1	Null hypothesis not refutable
Mental deficiency	15.095	1	0.001

(Affective psychoses and mental deficiency were tested only for the occurrence of exacerbation before the crime or the admission to hospital.)

is not subject to exacerbation, but denotes the accompanying disturbances of
social behaviour.

As Table 41 shows, the frequency of an episodic or chronic course
was much the same for the violent patients as a whole, the violent schizophrenics and the violent manic-depressive patients, as for their non-violent
controls. Admittedly it was not always possible to rate the patients without
making arbitrary and uncertain distinctions, but nevertheless it must be
emphasised that in regard to the traditional concepts of course and type of
schizophrenic psychosis there is no significant difference between the violent
and the non-violent patients.

It was therefore of interest to find out whether relatives,
colleagues and other associates had noticed any exacerbation in the patient's
state before the crime or before admission. To our surprise this happened
significantly more often in the non-violent group of patients (about 48% as
against 33% of the violent offenders), even though the control group contained
more clinically quiet schizophrenics.

When one considers that after a crime has occurred the tendency
may well be for the examining psychiatrist and the relatives questioned to
over-estimate rather than to deny 'exacerbations' in the form of psychological
symptoms, anomalies of behaviour and conflict or tensions that were observed
in the offender before the event, this finding acquires particular significance.
In interpreting it we must consider several points of view.

It is possible that anxiety and inner tension may be reduced by
anticipation of a serious act of aggression, whether imagined or planned, so
that sometimes there appears to be an improvement (or at least the individual's
condition seems no worse) such as is often observed in those who have taken
the decision to commit suicide.

In this connection it is worth considering the hypothesis put forward
by the American psychoanalysts Dalmau and Podolsky (Podolsky, 1966), according
to which aggressive criminal behaviour may serve as a means of ridding the
threatened ego of its severe intrapsychic anxiety and tension. Their further
assumption that violent acts might even help to prevent a psychopathic breakdown
has, however, no empirical foundation. [7]

On the other hand the manifestation of violence has many other
determinants, for example motivating conflict situations (such as long-standing
marital tensions), the behaviour of the victim, factors such as alcohol that
decrease or remove self-control, and much else besides. The development of a
systematic delusion, such as was often found in our schizophrenic offenders, may
even be viewed in psychoanalytic theory as an ego-stabilising process, and yet

the crime may 'logically' follow from such a delusion, for example as an act
of self-defence. Its interpretation as a 'primitive measure of self-preservation
on the part of the ego apparatus' is not, to say the least of it, in this
connection enlightening.

A further possible explanation lies in the behaviour of close
associates: according to the findings of psychiatric family studies it may be
assumed that the relatives of delusional schizophrenics are often, and in
varying degree, involved in their conflicts and pathological modes of behaviour,
so that they may be ill-equipped to provide a realistic and objective assessment of the delusion and of many other phenomena. At times they are not only
passively drawn into their sick relative's delusional development, but they
also defend his delusion against the normal critical world. They often deny,
more or less consciously, the morbid phenomena that are already obvious to
the impartial observer. This tendency to denial may have the effect not only
of making the relatives less able to perceive the start of any deterioration
in the patient's state, but also of making them less ready to arrange for
treatment. In this way they may involuntarily contribute to a dangerous
intensification of the patient's aggressive tensions. This is borne out, for
example, by the fact that almost half of the schizophrenic offenders had, in
spite of their long-standing psychiatric illness, never been admitted to a
psychiatric hospital up to the time of their crime (see Table 42 below).

Our case material contained numerous examples of this kind of
denial:

Case no. 528. Paranoid-hallucinatory schizophrenia

The 22-year-old youngest son of a 64-year-old father and his
62-year-old wife, of independent means. At the age of 18 (1958), after an
unfortunate love affair, his scholastic performance declined gradually
and he showed an autistic alteration in personality, on account of which
he had to leave school.

In the autumn of the same year he spent several weeks under
observation in a psychiatric clinic, where he was diagnosed as 'process
schizophrenia' with thought disorder, bodily hallucinations and hypochondriacal ideas. His delusionally altered thoughts centred on erotic
fantasies and megalomaniac marriage plans.

Treatment was begun but before it could be completed his
mother failed to bring him back after an outing from the clinic and
insisted, against the urgent advice of the doctors, on keeping him at
home. Although from 1959 onwards he sat around the house doing
nothing and at times got excited and even boxed his mother's ears or

struck her with a broom (according to him 'because she refused to take
him to see a girl he might marry'), she did not consider him ill and
denied that he needed treatment. He was nevertheless seen on one occasion
by two doctors as an out-patient, but the parents did not give a true
account of his history, so that he did not receive any appreciable
specialist treatment.

Even after the patient struck an 11-year-old girl violently
in the face on the street in October 1961, because of delusional ideas
which were not further specified, the mother did not alter her attitude
of denial. Finally in January 1962 the patient attacked a 10-year-old
girl who was skating with her 8-year-old brother. He nearly strangled
the child and hit her brutally with his fist. He said he did it because
it angered him to see a boy and a girl skating together. His father's
interpretation was that his son had at the time 'had difficulties about
skating, and also the cold contributed to it'. When her son was thereupon committed to a psychiatric clinic, the mother complained in a
paranoid way about the doctors who 'wanted to carry out experiments on
her child in the institution'.

Case no. 351

A farmer, born in 1921, developed a schizophrenic psychosis
in 1950/1, which began insidiously but in 1954 led to grossly abnormal
behaviour with hallucinations, eccentricities and motiveless abuse of
his neighbours. In 1955 he accused his wife of poisoning him and had
vague ideas of jealousy. He thought his siblings were making a fool of
him, and that they had forced him to marry; he also complained of
numerous bodily ills. At the same time he expressed grandiose ideas,
he was 'in command' and had to concern himself with governing the world.
He thought his 9-year-old daughter was sexually experienced, because
his younger son had once slept with her in the same bed, and that she
had intercourse with boys. The girl was not really his child but had
another father. His wife would not listen to all this and was going to
get rid of him 'because of this affair'. Since he was 'Commander', he
could on no account have an illegitimate child in the family.

On 25 October 1956 he went of his own accord and without
telling his family to the nearby psychiatric hospital and asked to be
examined. After he had been under observation for a day and a half the
doctor noted his symptoms as 'grimacing, delusions, refusal of food' and
diagnosed paranoid hallucinatory schizophrenia. He suggested to the
family that the patient should be admitted for treatment.

His relatives, however, among whom his sister was particularly
lacking in insight, did not believe the urgent statements of the doctors
about his long illness and pressed for early discharge. On 27 October his
wife took the patient back to the farm, against his will. He himself tried
to resist. Before he left he lay in protest on the floor and had to be
carried to the car. In the weeks that followed his wife continued to make
light of his severely disturbed behaviour, so that no medical treatment
was given. On 8 December 1956 the patient strangled his 9-year-old daughter
in her sleep, under the influence of delusional jealous thoughts.

In the affective psychoses, unlike the other diagnoses, exacerbations
were somewhat more frequent in the violent offenders before the crime than in
the non-violent patients before admission (16 out of 37 as against 13 out of
49). This may be in line with the hypothesis already discussed in Chapter 5,
that in this group the morbid process itself is the most important determin-
ant of the crime.

Summary
Schizophrenia

The chief difference between the two groups of schizophrenics
concerned their delusions: non-violent patients did not suffer from delusions
as often as the violent. Moreover in the violent group delusions consisted
not so much of delusional mood or unsystematic delusional ideas as of systematic delusions associated with specific themes such as jealousy, injury or
persecution. This special form of delusion seemed to be accompanied by a
delusional experience of menace to life and limb, either at the hands of
particular individuals or at least at the hands of persons with a special
role in the patient's life, for example wife or girlfriend. This, like
systematic delusions, was found more frequently in the violent group. Violent
and non-violent patients with systematic delusions did not differ, however,
in the frequency with which they believed their life was in danger (about
two-thirds of the cases). Systematic delusions are clearly concerned mainly
with fixed ideas of menace and danger.

The predominance of productive forms of illness in the violent
group (i.e. delusions, hallucinations and paraphrenic symptoms) is reflected
also in the frequency of further symptoms: auditory and bodily hallucinations
(and paranoid feelings of physical malaise) were also more frequent.

The less reliable affective features, such as irritability, coldness of affect and sad, depressive moods, were also noted more frequently in
the violent schizophrenics than in the control group.

Most schizophrenic offenders had already been ill for years, while
in the control group there were many patients who had not been ill for long
(only eight, or 2.9%, of the 284 offenders with this diagnosis had committed
their crime within a month of falling ill). There was no difference between
the two groups in regard to the frequency of episodic or chronic/progressive
forms of illness, though an acute exacerbation of symptoms was more common in
the control group before admission than in the violent group before the crime.

This may in part be related to the larger number of short, acute
illnesses among the patients in the control group. An abrupt onset and acute
schizophrenic symptoms, such as heightened delusional mood, experiences of
world catastrophe, inadequate affective behaviour, disjointed motor behaviour
and disconnected thinking, are among the first signs that strike the layman
as implying sickness, and may more readily lead to admission to hospital.

We have already discussed other possible interpretations and
implications of these findings. One additional point deserves mention: the
psychopathological subgroup of paraphrenics ('paranoia patients'), which
formed a higher proportion of the offenders than of the non-violent patients,
make a less morbid impression on those around them. These patients often
strike their fellow men more as cranks, if indeed they are perceived as in
any way 'not normal'. They are considered to be suspicious, irritable, cold,
showing unusual personality attributes or unusual modes of behaviour rather
than symptoms which in lay understanding signify illness. Delusion and the
much more deep-seated disturbance in human contact which is mostly shown
towards relatives and intimate partners, are often hidden from the rest of
the world. But it is just this situation which stimulates the patient to
aggressive behaviour and to a dangerous intensity of emotion. If therapeutic
measures are neglected and the delusion is not seen as an illness, then the
opportunity is also neglected of discharging the patient's tension and avoiding the accompanying progression of the delusional process of destruction. The
paraphrenics themselves do not wish to be regarded as 'ill', since they find
it difficult to accept the passive side of the sickness role. They often force
their partners to view the delusion as at least partly justified by reality
and the abnormal behaviour as a logical consequence of that reality, that is
to say they force them to deny the illness.[8] The partner relationship is
therefore often maintained by both sides until catastrophe occurs, in spite
of mounting conflict and tension, since the absurd, 'mad' behaviour, for
example, that of a morbidly jealous partner, is seen partly as 'normal'. Even
the modest chance of improvement offered by treatment is therefore often
not utilised.

Affective psychoses

In none of the items investigated (symptoms, affect, duration and course of illness) was there a significant difference between the violent offenders and the control group. Phasic forms of illness clearly predominated over the chronic/progressive forms (in 35 out of the 37 violent offenders). Here too the crime was usually committed after a very long period of illness. The proportion of offenders who had been ill for only a short time was nevertheless slightly higher than that found in the control group (11% committed the crime within a month of onset of illness).

Mental deficiency

In mental deficiency, which is a permanent state already apparent in childhood, changes in the course of illness in the narrower sense cannot be significant so far as the occurrence of violent crime is concerned. Here it is a question of conflicts that arise from the interaction between this permanent state and the external world: these are of paramount importance, in which respect the mentally defective are like the patients with delusions. The conflicts are partly associated with personality factors and patterns of reaction and behaviour which have probably developed from the interplay of learning processes in childhood and a disposition that has been affected by heredity or by brain damage.

7.4 Treatment data (previous treatment)

We hoped that our statistical analysis would provide an answer to one question of particular importance so far as prevention is concerned, namely: Would the risk of a violent crime be lessened (1) by better psychiatric treatment; (2) by non-specialist medical treatment; (3) by some form of intensive social care? Since this complex question does not lend itself to a summary answer, we broke it down into the following testable components and hypotheses:

1. Are there differences between the violent offenders and the control group in respect of the number and duration of previous in-patient admissions?

2. In the six months preceding the crime is the proportion of abnormal offenders receiving in-patient or out-patient specialist care lower than that of the non-violent control group?

3. Is the proportion of patients who terminate such in-patient treatment against medical advice or who abscond from a

psychiatric hospital higher for the offenders than for
the non-offenders?

4. If one regards a violent crime which follows an earlier
period of psychiatric treatment as hypothetically analogous
to a relapse on the part of a non-violent patient who has
also had previous treatment, are there differences in the
time that elapses between the last discharge from a
psychiatric hospital and the crime or next admission?

We had made provision in our questionnaire for information about
social aid and general practitioner care during the six months preceding the
crime. It turned out, however, that the records contained very few details on
this point, so that we were unable to test the hypothesis that such therapeutic
measures might affect the risk of a violent crime. The lack of information may
in itself provide an answer, since it strengthens the assumption that these two
forms of care were very rarely given to those who later committed violent crimes.

Previous in-patient treatment

The lengthy illness that generally preceded the crime, especially
in the case of the psychoses, led us to expect that a large proportion of the
offenders would have received in-patient treatment at least once before the
crime. Such previous treatment not only offers an opportunity of assessing the
risk but also makes it easier for those concerned with the patient to recognise
that abnormal behaviour on his part is a sign of illness and to consider further
specialist intervention (Star, Nunnally and Cumming).

Surprisingly enough, this was not the case. As Table 42 shows, a
very large number, in fact half, of the abnormal offenders had up to the time
of the crime never been in a psychiatric hospital, while this was true of only
39% of the non-offending patients. The difference is all the more remarkable
because short illnesses were more common in the control group, so that one
would have expected to find a higher number among them who had not been admitted
previously. Taking the schizophrenics only, 41% of the offenders had no
previous admissions to hospital against only 27% of the control group.

Although the proportion of patients with productive forms of
schizophrenia, i.e. with striking symptoms such as delusions and hallucinations,
was higher for the violent than for the non-violent schizophrenics, whose illness was usually clinically quiet, the schizophrenic offenders had clearly less
often received in-patient psychiatric treatment.

In interpreting this finding we would refer to what we have already
said about the phenomenon of denial (see p.155) which is found in the families of

Table 42. *Occurrence and duration of previous in-patient treatment in violent and non-violent patients before the crime or before the current admission to hospital*

	Whole group		Schizo-phrenia		Affective psychoses		Mental deficiency	
	n	%	*n*	%	*n*	%	*n*	%
Violent patients								
No previous hospital treatment	264	49.9	116	41.1	19	51	40	59
Duration of treatment:								
less than 1 year	177	33.4	115	40.8	15	41	8	12
1-5 years	66	12.5	43	15.3	3	8	7	10
5 years and over	22	4.2	8	2.8	0	-	13	19
Subtotal	529	100.0	282	100.0	37	100	68	100
Not known	4		2		0		0	
Total	533		284		37		68	
Non-violent patients								
No previous hospital treatment	207	39.1	80	27.3	29	59	31	46
Duration of treatment:								
less than 1 year	211	39.9	138	47.1	17	35	18	26
1-5 years	68	12.9	44	15.0	3	6	12	18
5 years and over	43	8.1	31	10.6	0	-	7	10
Subtotal	529	100.0	293	100.0	49	100	68	100
Not known	4		0		0		2	
Total	533		293		49		70	

Significance test: $^{(a),(b)}$ χ^2 =   df = α =

	χ^2	df	α
Whole group	16.69	3	0.001
Schizophrenia	22.07	3	0.001
Affective psychoses	0.225	1	Null hypothesis not refutable

[a] Only two classes (previous hospital or no previous hospital admission) were tested for the affective psychoses.

[b] Comparison between the mentally defective group and the other diagnostic groups seemed particularly meaningless here. We have therefore tabulated only the frequency figures and have not carried out any significance tests.

schizophrenics and which is accompanied not only by increased tolerance of
abnormal behaviour but also by mistrust and reservations towards therapeutic
activities, sometimes carried even to the point of manoeuvres that prevent
admission to hospital (cf. cases nos. 351, 528 and 329).

Anticipating the section on inter-group comparisons, we may mention
here that amongst those schizophrenic offenders who had not received previous
in-patient treatment, the adolescent patients (hebephrenics) and the patients
with systematic delusions (paraphrenics) were more numerous than, for example,
those whose illness began with acute excitement (catatonics). This is not
surprising, since catatonia is certainly the subgroup which makes the strongest
impression on those concerned with the patient. On the other hand, when only
the hebephrenics were examined, it was found that half of the violent patients
had never been in hospital, as against about one-seventh of the non-violent
patients with the same diagnosis. This difference is interesting and suggests
that violent hebephrenics may have a specially intense involvement in their
relationships with others. So far as the risk of violence is concerned, this
involvement may tend to prevent their having treatment; or the conflicts
arising from such relationships may become intensified over the years, thus
strengthening the motivation for the crime (cf. the years of mounting sibling
rivalry in case no. 369, p.144).

Unlike the violent patients of all diagnostic groups, and unlike
the schizophrenic offenders, the violent depressive patients had been treated
in hospital somewhat more frequently than their non-violent control group. The
difference is not, however, significant. One possible explanation is that,
unlike the paraphrenics, depressed patients whose symptoms have reached a certain
stage strike their relatives as seriously ill and also are themselves more easily
persuaded to go into hospital than are the paranoid patients. Since their
aggressive tensions are principally directed inwards against their own personality, they have not such a hostile, defensive attitude towards medical intervention and offers of help from those around them.

So far as the mentally defective are concerned, the proportion of
those who had never been in hospital was somewhat higher in the violent group
than in the control patients: 40 out of 68 as against 31 out of 68. When
violent defectives had been in hospital it was usually for a long period, which
may be connected with the fact that in the previous history of those 28
offenders who had received in-patient treatment there were 17 instances of bodily
harm, sexual assault or homicide and it was presumably considered unsafe to
discharge them earlier. (Thirteen offenders had been in hospital for five
years or more before the crime.) Here again is evidence of the trend we have

already mentioned, namely that sociopathic criminal tendencies are liable to
be a permanent feature of personality and of behaviour in a considerable
proportion of mentally defective offenders. The mental hospital does not act
here as a treatment centre but rather as an institution whose object is to
keep such individuals in a form of 'safe custody'.

As a further check we also investigated the number of admissions
before the crime for the three diagnostic groups of schizophrenic, affective-
psychotic and mentally deficient violent offenders and compared the findings
with those of the control group. It emerged that the non-violent patients as
a group had also had more frequent admissions to hospital than the abnormal
violent offenders.

Psychiatric treatment in the six months preceding the crime
or the admission to hospital

In addition to studying the most intensive form of psychiatric
treatment, namely full admission to a mental hospital, we were also interested
to see whether the two groups varied in regard to out-patient specialist
treatment during the six months immediately preceding the crime or the
admission to hospital.

We chose this period because any kind of specialist treatment in
the period immediately preceding the crime is of basic importance from the
point of view of recognising the risk of violence and adopting preventive
measures. We also hoped that by narrowing the period to some extent we would
be able to obtain adequate information about visits by the patient to the
doctor. Unfortunately documentation on this point was so incomplete that we
could not draw up a frequency table covering individual items.

We therefore recorded only the straightforward alternatives:
whether out-patient psychiatric treatment had been received in the six months
before the crime - irrespective of how often - or not.

Since the non-violent patients had been treated in specialised
hospitals more frequently than the violent offenders, it was to be expected
that this would be true also of the last six months before the crime and also
of out-patient forms of care. It turned out, however, that there was no
significant difference between the two groups in respect of out-patient or
in-patient psychiatric treatment in the period in question (Table 43). About
68% of the violent offenders had received no form of psychiatric treatment
during the six months preceding the crime. The corresponding figure for patients
in the control group was a little higher, though not much (about 72%). The
difference can be explained by the fact that in-patient treatment during this

period was slightly more frequent in the violent group, i.e. it does not mean
that they had been receiving specialist care outside the clinic.

It is worth remembering (cf. Table 40) that 90% of all the 533
offenders had been ill for more than six months before the crime. Nevertheless
out-patient treatment was rare for both groups (about 10%), even though we
counted as 'treatment' not only continuous therapy but also even one single
visit within the six months to a psychiatrist or neurologist.

There is one more finding to report, although, as has been said,
we could not quantify it: it was our impression that in about 40% of the violent
cases mention was made of some kind of general medical and/or social care
during the six months in question. About one-third of these patients had sought
help from general practitioners and social workers purely on account of
difficulties or disturbances which were not considered to be an expression of
psychological symptoms. This confirms the finding of Gurin, Veroff & Feld (1960)
in the USA that mentally ill patients attend a general physician more often

Table 43. *Out-patient and in-patient psychiatric treatment in violent and
non-violent patients in the six months preceding the crime or admission
to hospital*

	Violent patients		Non-violent patients		Difference
	n	%	n	%	%
No psychiatric treatment	361	67.9	378	72.3	+ 4.4
Out-patient psychiatric treatment only	56	10.5	48	9.2	- 1.3
In-patient psychiatric treatment[a]	115	21.6	97	18.5	- 3.1
Total	532	100.0	523	100.0	

Significance test:

Whole group χ^2 = 2.4603   df = 2   Null hypothesis not refutable

[a] For the violent offenders this included those patients who had been treated
in hospital during the six months preceding the crime, irrespective of whether
they had been discharged before the crime or were still in hospital at the
time it was committed.

than a specialist, although by training and experience the former is often
not able to do much for them.

Nature of discharge after the last stay in hospital before the crime or admission

It might be assumed that patients who later become violent would
have already caused difficulties through their significantly greater tendency to aggressive and antisocial forms of behaviour (especially the schizophrenics and the mentally defective: see section 7.2, p.113) and that this
would have been apparent to some extent also during their hospital stay.
Since such difficulties might be interpreted as indicators of impending
violence, we looked for any information concerned with premature interruption of hospital stay (discharge under pressure from the patient or his
relatives, absconding). This would also provide an indication of symptoms
or persisting anomalies of behaviour that had received inadequate treatment.
Although this covered intricate forms of behaviour which were subject to the
influence of other persons, e.g. relatives, the items in question were of a
kind that might be expected to provide information that could be used to
detect imminent risk.

It will be seen from Table 44 that 219, or 88.3%, of those
violent offenders who had already been treated in hospital were discharged
in the ordinary way; in 17 cases, approximately 7%, there had clearly been
doubts about their fitness for discharge. This proportion, like that of the
absconding patients (12, or about 5%), is significantly higher than that
found in the control group of non-violent patients (7 cases, or 2.4%). Taken
together, this means that about 12% of the future violent offenders had left
hospital without the consent of the medical staff.

Once more the finding applies with particular force to the
schizophrenics: 23 offenders (14.5%) as compared with 4 non-violent patients
(2%) had broken off in-patient treatment in this way. About 15% of the
offenders who had been in-patients are thus seen to be at risk. The difference,
in comparison with the non-violent group, may be connected with the higher
number of delusional patients in the violent group and with the paranoid
patient's well-known lack of insight into his illness. Possibly also the
tendency to break off treatment by absconding is less easy to detect in time
because of the capacity of these patients for dissimulation.

The problem of allowing patients out on leave, which is particularly difficult where paranoid patients are concerned, is also relevant here.
In some cases we formed the impression that this measure, which is of great

Table 44. *Nature of discharge for violent and non-violent patients after the last stay in hospital before the crime or before re-admission to hospital*

	Whole group		Schizo- phrenia		Affective psychoses		Mental deficiency	
	n	%	n	%	n	%	n	%
Violent patients								
Regular discharge	219	88.3	135	85.5	16	88	20	91
Discharged against advice [a]	17	6.9	14	8.8	1	6	0	–
Absconded	12	4.8	9	5.7	1	6	2	9
Subtotal	248	100.0	158	100.0	18	100	22	100
In hospital at the time of the crime	16		8		0		5	
No previous hospital admissions	264		116		19		40	
Not known	5		2		0		1	
Total	533		284		37		68	
Non-violent patients								
Regular discharge	287	97.6	187	98.0	20	100	32	94
Discharged against advice [a]	1	0.4	1	0.5	0	–	0	–
Absconded	6	2.0	3	1.5	0	–	2	6
Subtotal	294	100.0	191	100.0	20	100	34	100
Transferred from another hospital	31		22		0		4	
No previous hospital admissions	208		80		29		31	
Not known	1		0		0		1	
Total	533		293		49		70	

[a] Discharge against the express advice of the doctors treating the patient, the relatives usually having to sign a statement to this effect.

importance if the patient is to be gradually restored to his previous milieu,
was not always preceded by adequate co-ordination of all concerned and was not
always carried out and monitored with sufficient care. In such circumstances
some violent crimes were committed during periods of leave, as the following
case illustrates:

Case no. 423: Schizophrenia

A mechanic, born 1929; a shy, gentle child whose upbringing
presented no difficulties; of below average intelligence, unmarried,
lived a solitary life with his parents, became ill in 1952 with an acute
schizophrenic psychosis with paranoid hallucinatory symptoms. In an
excited state he threatened his mother with a knife. After in-patient
treatment with psychotropic drugs and insulin he was discharged home
well and until 1956 worked regularly and without incident. After changing
his place of work in 1957 he suffered a catatonic relapse: he wandered
away from home in a state of great unrest, waded across a river and finally
broke into a strange house in order to get dry clothes. He got into a
quarrel with the people who lived in the house, threatened them with
various objects, threw a stone at them and was then himself knocked down
and taken to a surgical clinic with severe concussion and an injury where
he had been struck. As he was very disturbed, he was admitted after two
weeks to a clinic for nervous disorders, where he remained inaccessible
and seemed to be under the influence of anxious ideas of persecution.
He would clench his fists, complain about disturbances of thought, wander
up and down in restless anxiety. It was not possible to discover the
precise content of his delusion. After a series of electroconvulsive
treatments the catatonic state of excitement subsided and the patient was
again discharged to live with his parents, under instructions to take
two mg Serpasil daily.

Fourteen days later he made a direct assault on his father,
seriously maltreating him. The father had forced him to come to eat, and
the son answered with fisticuffs. A few days previously he had seemed to
become restless and tense. On 25 April 1957 he was admitted to a regional
mental hospital, where a further catatonic episode was diagnosed. Tearful
and bewildered, he said he would never again be properly well: he had
attacked his father 'because the wind drove him to it'.

He was treated with chlorpromazine and soon appeared to be
calm and orderly again, though his affective level was low. Three weeks
after admission his parents and sister, as well as the patient himself,
began to press for his discharge.

The hospital doctors wrote in his notes as follows: '...
the patient was then put to work in the colony and worked here for
the next two weeks regularly and without incident. Towards his
relatives, who visited him regularly, he behaved in a friendly and
sympathetic way. He constantly denied psychotic experiences, both to
the ward doctor and to another psychiatrist who had assessed him from
the point of view of responsibility at the time of the housebreaking
episode and who again examined him two days before the trial discharge,
which took place at the repeated insistence of his relatives.'

After this examination on 25 May 1957, at which the patient
said he felt 'considerably better', he was allowed home on trial discharge for an indefinite period. He took up no work, lived an isolated
life and only very occasionally helped in the garden.

In spite of the previous history of violence and the repeated
attacks of illness, there was no specialist or social care during this
period.

On the night of 6 June 1957 the patient, who could not sleep,
went into the kitchen, laid out three knives, and stabbed his sleeping
mother in the throat with one of them. He did not say a word and was
trembling all over. The injury was so severe that the victim bled to
death. In the ensuing tumult he assaulted his father, who broke a
leg in the struggle. When his sister and neighbours rushed to help, he
defended himself with the knife until finally he was overpowered.

Interval between last discharge and the crime or readmission

Breaking off in-patient treatment or committal procedures against
medical advice is thus presumably a risk factor. A further question then arises,
namely, whether in-patient psychiatric treatment that is regularly carried
out and continued till completion has a favourable influence on this risk.
This could be evidenced in a comparatively longer violence-free interval after
discharge. In other words, it might be expected that if the patient is discharged with medical approval after a period of intensive therapy carried out
in a specialist hospital, there will be a longer period of remission with a
lower risk of violence.

We therefore asked how many patients committed violent crimes - or
were readmitted to hospital - at various intervals after their last discharge
from hospital. The comparison (Table 45) did not confirm the hypothesis that the
rate of violence would be less in the first six months following discharge, as
an expression of successful treatment. Violent crimes reached about 39% in the

Table 45. *Interval between last discharge from hospital and crime or readmission, for violent and non-violent patients respectively*

	Whole group		Schizo-phrenia		Affective psychoses		Mental deficiency	
	n	%	n	%	n	%	n	%
Violent patients								
Up to 6 months	99	39.3	59	36.9	11	61	7	30
6 months to 1 year	36	14.3	24	15.0	2	11	5	22
1-5 years	76	30.2	49	30.6	3	17	8	35
5 years and over	41	16.2	28	17.5	2	11	3	13
Subtotal	252	100.0	160	100.0	18	100	23	100
Not discharged[a]	280		124		19		45	
Not known	1		0		0		0	
Total	533		284		37		68	
Non-violent patients								
Up to 6 months	66	22.7	49	26.1	4	20	6	18
6 months to 1 year	43	14.8	26	13.8	3	15	5	15
1-5 years	128	44.0	83	44.2	8	40	15	44
5 years and over	54	18.5	30	15.9	5	25	8	23
Subtotal	291	100.0	188	100.0	20	100	34	100
Not discharged[a]	238		102		29		35	
Not known	4		3		0		1	
Total	533		293		49		70	

Significance test:	$\chi^2 =$	df =	$\alpha =$
Whole group	19.55	3	0.001
Schizophrenia	6.88	3	0.05
Affective psychoses	5.091	1	Null hypothesis
Mental deficiency	0.0343	1	not refutable

(In the case of affective psychoses and mental deficiency only two classes were tested: 'up to 6 months' and 'more than 6 months'.)

[a] For the violent patients the class of 'not discharged' covered 264 patients who had never been in a psychiatric hospital and 16 patients who were violent while in a psychiatric hospital (Total 280). And for the non-violent patients it covered 207 patients who had had no previous admission to a psychiatric hospital and 31 patients who had been transferred direct from other psychiatric hospitals and institutions (Total 238).

first six months after discharge, while readmissions in the control group
amounted to about 23% of all relevant patients who had been treated in hospital.

Table 46 shows the diagnostic distribution of the violent offenders
(n = 99) and control readmissions (n = 66) who had been discharged in the six
months preceding the crime or readmission. It can be seen that there is an
increased proportion of depressives and 'unclassifiable endogenous psychoses'
(which include many depressive syndromes as well as mixed psychoses with
depressive traits) among those who committed a crime within six months of being
discharged: this is true also when comparison is made with the readmissions of
non-violent patients with the same diagnosis. The differences, which could only
be of limited predictive value because risk of readmission and risk of violence
are scarcely comparable, are all in all not significant.

The period after discharge from a psychiatric hospital is one in
which the risk of violence is high: this represented one of the most important
findings in our study. How is it to be explained? Even the non-violent patients
show a slightly increased readmission rate in the first six months after discharge as compared with the ensuing period (23% as against 15% in the second
six months). Genuine relapses account for only part of this rate. A further
proportion is associated with social difficulties not accompanied by any fresh
outbreak of illness, or may be due to the fact that the discharging doctor has

Table 46. *Diagnoses of violent and non-violent patients whose crime or readmission took place within six months from discharge from in-patient treatment*

	Violent patients		Non-violent patients	
Diagnoses	n	%	n	%
Unclassifiable endogenous psychoses	8	8	2	3
Schizophrenias	59	60	49	74
Affective psychoses	11	11	4	6
Mental deficiency	7	7	6	9
Cerebral organic deterioration	2	2	0	–
Late-acquired cerebral damage	4	4	3	5
Epilepsy	7	7	2	3
Other disorders	1	1	0	–
Total	99	100	66	100

Significance test: χ^2 = 2.2076   df = 2   Null hypothesis not refutable underestimated the disturbances that arise when remission is not complete. The high rate of violent crimes which we found in the first six months after discharge from hospital can hardly be explained by a high rate of relapse into illness.

If we also take into account that mentally disturbed violent offenders – the mentally defective are not comparable in this respect – show more chronic and persistent forms of illness and fewer exacerbations of symptoms before the index event (crime or admission to hospital) than the non-violent patients in our control group, then the part played by genuine relapse into illness in this period becomes still less important. We must also bear in mind that only a small proportion of the violent crimes committed in the first six months after discharge from hospital coincided with a relapse or a genuine recurrence of the illness.

This raises a further question of practical importance, namely whether the doctors responsible were able in any way to recognise the risk of violence in the patients whom they discharged; an answer to this question will still not explain, however, the difference found in our study. We could in any case not obtain a precise answer from our material, though one of our findings permits us to draw a limited conclusion: out of 17 patients discharged against medical advice, eight committed a violent crime within the first six months, while out of 12 patients who absconded a further eight committed a violent crime within the same period (four of them on the very day they absconded); six of these eight offenders were diagnosed as schizophrenic.

We may conclude from this that there is a limited group of mentally disturbed patients whom the hospital psychiatrist does not wish to be discharged, probably because he recognises an increased risk of violence towards others. We still know little about the grounds or criteria which cause him to hold this opinion: according to our findings, most of the patients to whom it applied had already shown serious aggressive forms of behaviour and this was often mentioned in the medical objection to discharge. From the point of view of diagnosis, paranoid schizophrenics seemed to head the list. The numbers are too small, however, to permit any reliable conclusion.[9]

For most of the patients who committed their crime within six months of discharge, it must be assumed that their doctors were not in a position to assess the increased risk. It can hardly be expected that these ·patients (83 out of 99 offenders) would have been discharged with medical approval if the danger had been recognised. There is therefore an urgent need for more knowledge about indicators of increased risk.

In considering our interpretation of this risk period we have tacitly assumed that the reasons for it are the same for all diagnostic groups. This assumption, however, applies reliably only to the prediction that relapse into illness is not of decisive importance.

If we look first at the mentally defective group only, we see that they contribute little to the rise in violent crime after discharge. With about 30% committing violent crimes in the first six months as against 22% in the second six months, the figure is, however, considerably above the average of 4% for the next eight six-monthly periods (i.e. the first five years after discharge). Compared with the affective psychoses, with 61% of violent crimes in the first and 11% in the second six months, and schizophrenia with 37% in the first and 15% in the second six months, there is, however, a perceptible difference. From the outset the diagnosis of mental deficiency differs from the others because of the association found here between the crime and the 'fact of illness': in mental deficiency there are no exacerbations or relapses.

Since in this group the risk of violence is closely linked to factors of personality and behaviour, we may provisionally assume that the influences which produce high-risk periods here probably lie in the same area as those which produce similar risks in schizophrenic offenders. At the same time we must assume that their effect is not so serious, and that this may be explained, for example, by a higher susceptibility on the part of schizophrenics to these influences, or a lower susceptibility on the part of mental defectives.

Passing now to the schizophrenics who, with their 59 offenders in the first six months out of a total of 160 who committed their crime at any time after being discharged from a mental hospital, must be considered the most important group, we may advance three possible areas of explanation. Factors which increase the risk of violence may lie (1) in the area of the patient's personal, family, professional or social situation after discharge (problems of reintegration); (2) in the area of the effects of hospital admission and stay; (3) in the possibly false assumption that the timing of an admission to hospital is independent of the timing of a later violent crime; or (4) in a combination of two or three of the above grounds.

Let us begin by discussing the third possibility. If it alone were true, then this would mean that the risk period has nothing to do with the effects of hospital stay or the period after discharge. It is conceivable that the chances of being admitted to hospital in the period before a violent crime are high. One could explain this hypothesis by saying that a violent crime is usually preceded by a period of increasing anomalies of behaviour,

particularly aggressive acts or crimes. These could cause an increase in the
frequency of admission to hospital. At the same time one would have to assume
that this mounting risk, or whatever forms the basis of it, would not be
arrested by the hospital treatment of subsequent offenders, and would possibly
even be accelerated. The timing of a crime would thus be only superficially
determined by the timing of admission to hospital. In fact the timing of the
hospital admission would be influenced by the timing of the crime, or, to
put it more precisely, by the anomalies preceding it, which would have to be
regarded as symptoms of the same process which finally culminates in the crime.

It is not possible to confirm or reject this explanation on the
basis of our data; we must state, however, that some of our findings indirectly
argue against rather than in favour of this hypothesis. For one thing, the
general assumption of a process in which a progressive increase in anomalies
culminates in an act of violence becomes dubious if it is supposed to apply to
very different diagnoses, for example to mental deficiency as well. Anomalies,
in particular aggressive forms of behaviour or previous crimes, are moreover
already much in evidence in abnormal offenders a long time before the crime.
We were admittedly not able to study the lifelong distribution of such symptoms -
this could hardly be reliably achieved in a retrospective enquiry - but behaviour
in the six months before the crime, which we did cover in our survey, showed
relatively high quotas in this respect both for discharged offenders and for
those who had never been in hospital. In the control group of non-violent
patients anomalies classified as 'abnormalities' were by far the most frequent,
while in the violent group there was a slight predominance of threats outside
the circle of family and intimate associates (19% of the offenders) and violence
(15%). In the affective psychoses the rate of threatened suicide (39%) and
attempted suicide (25%) was high among the offenders, but a little above
average also among the non-offenders (12% threatened, 27% attempted).

It is thus probable that in the affective psychoses a proportion
of the 61% discharged offenders who committed their crime within six months
of discharge had been admitted to hospital on account of the very illness
which finally led to the crime: this is less likely to be the case in the
other diagnostic groups. Suicidal behaviour, which presumably played a certain
part in bringing about admission, is also likely to be in some cases a symptom
of the depressive phase which gave rise to an extended suicide after discharge.

In the group of offenders as a whole and in the schizophrenic
group, however, it was the less acute anomalies which predominated in the six
months before the crime and which, as mentioned, had also been much in evidence
before this period. In mental deficiency aggressive forms of behaviour were

the most common. If we consider, finally, how seldom there was an exacerbation
of the illness before the crime, then the assumption that the admission to
hospital was often the result of warning signs of violence is of only very
limited validity.

The last argument is in keeping with the fact that the great
majority of the offenders in question were discharged from hospital in the
ordinary way. If we accept a connection between reason for admission and crime,
then we have to assume that the risk of violence, or at least the need for
treatment, was on the earlier occasion judged by non-specialist physicians or
even by laymen to be more serious than the discharging psychiatrist considered
it to be closer to the crime. This possibility cannot necessarily be excluded,
even when the risk of violence and the severity of the symptoms of illness do
not run parallel as we must assume they do in depressed offenders. But as an
assumption that has to apply to all diagnostic groups, even to the high-risk
chronic paraphrenics and to the mentally defective in whom the fact of illness
in the narrower sense has little or no chance of changing with clinical treatment, it is still very improbable.

It therefore follows that only in the affective psychoses can the
same distinct phase of illness frequently trigger both the crime and the
hospital admission which precedes it. For the other diagnostic groups we
believe that only a modest proportion of the increased risk in the post-
discharge period can be attributed to the fact that the timing of admission
is affected by a progressive morbid process which in the long run helps to
determine also the timing of the crime.

The next question - and here we exclude the affective psychoses -
concerns the significance of the other factors which operate in the post-
discharge period. In fact the period following discharge, which so far has
been studied mainly in schizophrenics, is for the mentally ill one of
increased risk of relapse and readmission (Wing *et al.*, 1964; Häfner, 1968).
This was borne out by the high readmission rate of 23% in the non-violent
patients of our control group. As already mentioned, it also seemed that in
this group there were significantly more 'acute exacerbations of symptoms'
than in the groups of offenders, in whom clear changes in morbid state played
a far less important part.

The general explanation for this risk period lies, if we judge
by the schizophrenics, in difficulties in occupational, social and family
reintegration: because of his stay in a mental hospital the patient has been
labelled mentally ill, with the negative prejudices that this implies on the
part of those around him. However, this played only a limited part. As will

be shown later, we examined the frequency of possible causes of violence in
the form of external stresses and clearly found that, even if the results are
of only limited reliability, crude occupational or social difficulties, or
severe personal losses caused perhaps by death or separation, did occur but
had limited significance. We assumed, therefore, and our case analyses also
bore this out, that in schizophrenic offenders in particular the interaction
between social and especially family and intimate relationships on the one
hand and modes of reaction that are specific to the patient's personality and
illness on the other, form the most important combination of factors that
increase the risk of violence.

Brown *et al.* (1962) showed that family relationships are of paramount importance in the rehabilitation of schizophrenics. Discharged schizophrenics who live in families in which emotional relationships are intense,
particularly if the patients themselves have a tense relationship with one
other family member, show higher rates of relapse and readmission.

The schizophrenic offenders suffered to a large extent from
chronic systematic delusions which were usually centred on one or more people.
They felt their lives were endangered by these people, with whom they frequently
had a family or other intimate relationship. Such relationships are often not
only emotionally fervid and tense, but are also affected on one side by
delusionally augmented anxiety and hostility. The danger inherent in them -
and this seems clear enough - thus progresses in a dimension which in its
dynamics and motivation is governed by aggressiveness, rather than in a dimension of the illness in the narrower sense.

The delusional situation of feeling threatened, in danger of one's
life, always 'from behind one's back' and without open hostility, combined
with the characteristic suspiciousness observed in this group of offenders,
naturally makes them particularly vulnerable to any form of discrimination
and especially to any concealed or veiled rejection or hostility. It is thus
understandable, for example, that a patient with delusional jealousy can have
his jealousy and delusional fears increased even by the separation caused by
his absence in hospital. The morbidly jealous patient, as well as other
paraphrenics, looks on his 'normal' partner, who collaborates or even just
tolerates his admission to hospital, as acting 'to get rid of him' or to
deceive him. Discrimination experienced in this way is often taken as confirmation of paranoid fears. It can increase the social isolation of the future
offender and thus lessen the effect of what is really an attempt to counter
his growing paranoid hostility.

Finally, many discharged paranoid patients find that their

partners really have altered: the long separation from a delusional partner sometimes strengthens the 'normal' partner's orientation to reality. If, however, the pathological association continues, at a distance so to speak, then this can cause a further rise in the patient's delusional anxiety and hostility. All this indicates that the period after discharge does entail stresses that increase the risk of violence in patients who are so inclined.

The above considerations contain a good many conclusions based on analogies, as well as generalisations based on clinical experience but not empirically tested. They should therefore be treated with particular critical care.

The last possibility which we have to discuss is: Can in-patient psychiatric care increase the risk of violence in certain patients? In the light of what has been said, this would mean only a contribution to the increased risk, not its exclusive cause.

Most of the violent patients in question had been treated in mental hospitals. We have no adequate information about the relationship between voluntary admission as opposed to compulsory committal. It can only be said that most of them, and particularly most of the schizophrenics, had been committed to a closed ward as a result of a judicial decision or a special order: the law concerning this was not the same in all federal regions.

An increase in aggressive behaviour in such a situation has been to a varying degree assumed and sometimes also empirically confirmed. Folkard (1956, 1960) showed, for example, that withdrawal of freedom and extreme restriction of personal territory cause an increase in aggressive behaviour in some patients newly admitted to a psychiatric hospital. Many other authors have demonstrated that in long-stay patients there is an association between aggressive patterns of behaviour and the extreme lack of scope found in mental hospitals described as custodial or, by Goffman (1961), as 'total institutions' (Belknap, 1956; Caudill, 1958; and others). This finding, however, again applied to only a small number of the inmates. The syndrome of institutionalism is in most patients characterised by unproductive, passive forms of behaviour (Wing & Brown, 1961; Rosenberg, 1970).

Stierlin formed the impression that violence committed within the walls of psychiatric hospitals was less frequently reported in well-run institutions with psychologically trained staff and more frequently in hospitals with staff who were poorly trained and too authoritarian.

It is therefore worth considering whether compulsory admission to a hospital which has the hallmarks of a total institution helps to increase the risk of violence in a small, circumscribed proportion of patients. The

small number of offenders (16 out of 533) who committed their crime while they
were in-patients in a psychiatric hospital tells us little, for various
reasons.

     If we consider that a substantial proportion of our offenders
belonged to this risk group, and for the above reasons might have experienced
an increase in their aggressiveness while in hospital, then in order to
explain the subsequent risk period we must further assume that this increase
in aggressiveness has at times persisted long after the patient has been discharged. This is possible, but not very plausible.[10]

     We would therefore in conclusion suggest that in schizophrenic
offenders in particular, the increased risk in the post-discharge period is
connected chiefly with such family and social stresses as are reinforced after
discharge from a psychiatric hospital. We further assume that these patients
are in their personality as well as in their illness specifically vulnerable
to tensions which are centred particularly on the area of close and often
delusionally altered emotional relationships. The vulnerability and the
paranoid aggressive mode of reaction that goes with it seem not only to
contribute to an increase in tension but also to be responsible for channelling
this tension into suspicion, anxiety and hostility, and for its substantiation
in feelings of being menaced and violent acts.

     In some respects, i.e. in so far as delusion is involved, these
assumptions do not apply to the mentally defective; in other respects they
apply only in a diminished form. In mental deficiency it would seem that
material and occupational difficulties are more significant, as well as
difficulties in secondary social relationships: but the small number of cases
does not permit us to generalise. For the same reason we cannot make any
definite statement about the other diagnostic groups, apart from the affective psychoses.

     We have already referred to the special position occupied by the
last-named group. The offenders with this diagnosis who committed crimes
within six months of discharge were all depressives. The same was broadly
true of those, mainly suffering from depressive psychoses, who came from
the group of 'unclassifiable endogenous psychoses': the crime was almost
exclusively extended suicide or an attempt at this violent act. The close
association between the crime and the illness is also shown by the fact that
threatened suicide was the most common cause of admission for this category
of offender. Any attempt at explaining the risk period must therefore examine
also the risk of suicide in depressed patients.

     Stengel & Cook (1958) showed that the suicide rate for depressed

patients reaches its maximum after the most serious clinical phenomena have
subsided, namely the state of inhibition and the depressive delusions. This
is explained by regarding the delusion and the inhibition as a form of
pathological defence or self-protection, the removal of which liberates the
patient's self-destructive activity, particularly when he is faced once more
with the stress of personal problems and of the daily environment. Stengel &
Cook found that suicides were indeed more frequent in depressive psychoses in
the post-discharge period. The same explanation can almost certainly be applied
to this risk period in depressed offenders who commit extended suicide.
Compared with schizophrenic and mentally defective offenders, moreover,
depressed patients commit their crime more frequently in the first three months
after discharge. The hypothesis formulated above, namely that in depressive
offenders the same phase of illness affects both the timing of admission to
hospital and the period of heightened risk after the peak of the illness has
passed, is hardly open to doubt.

Whatever factors may be responsible for the increased risk of
violence after discharge from hospital, the lack of specialist and general
medical or social care in this risk period remains a serious problem. If
preventive measures are to be effective, and if a period of increased risk is
to be regarded as a special point at which these should be applied, then the
first requirement is contact with persons who are in a position to carry out
or arrange for such measures.

Summary

The important fact which emerges was that in spite of the long
duration of their illnesses half of all the abnormal offenders - in contrast
to only 39% of all the non-violent control group - had up to the time of the
crime never received in-patient psychiatric treatment.

If we concentrate our attention on the six months before the crime
and include also out-patient forms of care, then we find that 68% of all the
violent offenders and about 72% of the non-offenders did not receive any
psychiatric help. Our impression was that general medical and social care
during this period could also be regarded as inadequate. (Exact figures cannot be given because of incomplete documentation.)

The great majority (88%) of the 248 offenders who had been in
hospital at any time before the crime had been discharged in the ordinary way,
that is to say with medical consent. Of the 17 (about 7%) who were discharged
against advice, i.e. about whom the doctors had doubts, eight committed serious
crimes of violence within six months of breaking off their in-patient treatment, as did eight of the 12 patients (about 5%) who absconded from hospital.

This first period of six months after the end of in-patient treatment is one of increased risk: 23% of the non-violent patients had to be readmitted, and almost twice as many violent offenders (about 39%) committed
their crime during this time.

It is only in the case of the depressive psychoses that the
increased risk of violence in the post-discharge period seems to be an
immediate consequence of one continuous morbid process governed by its own
laws. In most of the schizophrenic offenders, and to some extent also in the
mentally defective group, there seems to be a complex interaction between the
discharged patient and his environment, often associated with tensions in his
personal or social relationships. It seems probable that paranoid schizophrenics in particular show a specific vulnerability to such stresses and
that this is connected with their personality or illness: the same may be
true, though to a much lesser extent, of those mentally defective patients
who are of a violent disposition.

In this period of increased risk a relatively high proportion of
our patients were given no appropriate medical or social support. In only
41 cases or 18.7% of the 219 violent offenders who had been discharged from
hospital in the ordinary way, did the record contain any mention of specialist
contact in the six months before the crime.

7.5 Social situation and behaviour during the six months preceding the crime

Since the aim of our study is prevention, this section is
particularly relevant. In it we look for factors which we hope may provide
indicators of a high risk of violence, and which may also contribute to our
understanding of the genesis of violent crime. Some of the findings have
already been included in our discussion of the risk period that follows
discharge.

We were interested in items concerned with relationships with the
environment (secondary social relationships) within the last six months
before the crime and also in items concerned with contacts with the family
and other intimate associates (primary social relationships). We looked in
particular for anomalies, especially modes of behaviour which might point
to an aggressive attitude towards other people that was in existence before
the crime. A high proportion of the offenders were married and we wished
above all to see whether there was an association between conflict with, or
aggressive behaviour towards, partners and other members of the family and
subsequent violent crime. We also wished to test the correctness of the

widespread and disquieting stereotype of the violent offender as one who in a
blind rage runs amok and attacks random victims 'out of the blue'. The specific
problem was to determine how many violent crimes were preceded by no anomalies
of behaviour.

We enquired whether the patient lived alone or with his family,
whether he shared a dwelling with friends or whether he had been admitted to
a residential home or hospital. In order to determine also the influence of
life events which might be possible causes of the crime, we included in our
study such stressful events as loss of a partner, material or occupational
misfortunes, etc.

By comparing our two groups in respect of these items we hoped to
obtain pointers of varying significance which might throw light on the
motivation and immediate cause of the crime and which could later be tested
or amplified by analysis of the offender-victim relationship (see p.232) and
by examination of the subjective reasons put forward by the offenders for their
crimes (see p.253).

The completeness and reliability of the data we collected on family
and social behaviour and on external stress factors was limited and at times
inadequate. Apart from a few hard items of information such as living arrangements, all the factors examined in this section depend to a moderate or marked
degree on value judgements. Thus the responses given by a patient's relatives
to questions about his disturbing or socially isolating behaviour cannot be
compared directly in different cases, since the threshold of tolerance for
socially deviant and aggressive conduct varies in different social classes,
different areas (e.g. town and country) and at different educational levels
(Sellin, 1938; Christiansen, 1968).

Descriptions of social behaviour before the crime were provided
in the main by witnesses of the crime, colleagues at work, employers, neighbours and others. The data recorded also included the equally subjective
opinions of different medical examiners and assessors. Even if we ourselves
had interviewed relatives and colleagues of the offenders this would have
been on an average six to seven years after the crime, and we would not have
obtained more reliable data. Gross anomalies were no doubt more or less
reliably recorded and we therefore based our study mainly on these.

Living arrangements

Our original assumption that the mentally abnormal violent
offenders would include a high proportion of solitary individuals with few
or no attachments, had already been proved wrong, since so many of the

Table 47. *Living arrangements of violent and non-violent patients in the six months preceding the crime or admission to hospital*

	Whole group		Schizo-phrenia		Affective psychoses		Mental deficiency	
	n	%	n	%	n	%	n	%
Violent patients								
In the family	369	69.2	193	68.0	37	100	31	46
Alone	85	15.9	51	18.0	0	–	17	25
With friends, relations	27	5.1	14	4.9	0	–	5	7
In homes, camps	32	6.0	17	6.0	0	–	6	9
In mental hospitals[a]	20	3.8	9	3.1	0	–	9	13
Subtotal	533	100.0	284	100.0	37	100	68	100
Not known	0		0		0		0	
Total	533		284		37		68	
Non-violent patients								
In the family	350	66.3	190	65.0	41	86	39	57
Alone	102	19.3	56	19.2	4	8	13	19
With friends, relations	25	4.7	14	4.8	3	6	3	4
In homes, camps	32	6.1	20	6.9	0	–	5	7
In mental hospitals[a]	19	3.6	12	4.1	0	–	9	13
Subtotal	528	100.0	292	100.0	48	100	69	100
Not known	5		1		1		1	
Total	533		293		49		70	

Significance test:

	χ^2 =	df =	α =
Whole group	2.1272	4	Null hypothesis not refutable
Schizophrenia	0.8151	4	Null hypothesis not refutable

[a]The figures for this item ('living in mental hospitals') do not tally exactly with those for 'Crime committed while in hospital' and 'transfers'. This is because on the one hand patients were counted as 'transfers' when they came from residential homes, such patients being counted as coming from 'homes' so far as the above table was concerned. On the other hand, the table records the living arrangements which applied for the longest period of time during the six months covered, and these were not necessarily the same as those which were recorded at the time of the crime.

offenders were married (about 45% of the offender group against about 36% of
the control group: see p.122). In order to obtain basic information about the
social milieu in which the patients lived before the crime, we now determined
whether the patients had during the last six months lived within the family
(parental or conjugal), with friends or relations, in homes, camps or hospitals,
or whether they had lived alone.

Table 47 shows that more than two-thirds (about 70%) of all the
violent offenders were living within the conjugal or parental family, that is
to say under the eyes of close relatives. Only about 16% were living alone
without a partner. The depressed patients, who were mostly married women,
were all living with their families, while the same was true of less than half
of the mentally defective offenders, who were mainly unmarried.

As the proportions found in the control group were not significantly
different, the item covering living arrangements does not provide any indication of the risks of violence. This finding recalls the results of our test
of parental family intactness: there, too, there was no difference between
the two groups in regard to 'broken homes', and no risk factor could be
inferred.

Social circumstances, as measured by the crude but fundamental
index of 'living arrangements', were thus much the same for the violent
offenders as for the non-violent patients. This does not tell us, of course,
whether from a psychological point of view the milieu was predominantly
favourable or unfavourable. In order to obtain some orientation on this
question, we next tried to build up a qualitative picture of the contacts
made by our patients with their fellow men.

Contacts

Personal relationships can, of course, be of many different kinds.
In studying them we drew a broad distinction between contacts with the
parental (primary) family, with marriage partners and children - what might
be called the intimate circle - on the one hand, and contacts with colleagues
at work, superiors, neighbours, etc. - what might be called secondary
relationships - on the other. The concept of contacts covered not only
personal relationships in everyday life but also visits or lasting contact
through letters, etc.

With the intimate circle

Where the many patients who lived with their parents or with their
spouse and perhaps children were concerned, it seemed to us that the quality

of their relationship with members of the family was vital to any consideration of the dynamics of the crime. We limited ourselves to enquiring whether
there was much or little tension and conflict in the conduct of family life,
although we realised, of course, that the reliability of the answers recorded
might be very small. As mentioned at the outset, information on such matters
could only be incomplete and affected by the subjective judgement of those
who originally examined the patients.

We therefore formulated only a very general rating of the quality
of relationships, distinguishing between 'good relationships', i.e. experienced by the relatives and patients as essentially good (this being understood as regularly maintained contact without persistent conflict or tension)
and 'bad relationships', under which we included contacts associated with
much conflict and persistent tension.

With the primary family

The primary family was defined as the family of natural or foster
parents from which the patient originally came. Our findings are shown in
Table 48.

With spouse or other intimate partner

Under this heading we included contacts with those partners with
whom the patients had cohabited. Widowed and divorced patients were counted
as 'not married'. Our findings are shown in Table 49.

With own children

By 'own children' we understood all legitimate and illegitimate
issue. If the patient's children were no longer living, this was counted as
'no children'. Our findings are shown in Table 50.

When we look at the figures given in Tables 48 to 50, the first
feature which strikes us is the *quantitative* difference between the two cohorts in regard to the frequency of their contact with parents, intimate
partners and children. Understandably, not all patients did have contact with
persons in these three categories.

So far as contact with the primary family is concerned, the violent
offenders as a whole lived with their parents less often (n = 153) than the
patients in the control group (n = 182). This presumably stems from the fact
that the offenders were more often married. No such difference is found in the
schizophrenic and depressed groups, but it is again prominent in the mental
defectives.

Table 48. *Existence and quality of contacts with the primary family for violent and non-violent patients in the six months preceding the crime or admission to hospital*

	Whole group		Schizo- phrenia		Affective psychoses		Mental deficiency	
	n	%	*n*	%	*n*	%	*n*	%
Violent patients								
Living with the family:								
relationship good	94	61.4	63	65.6	4	67	11	55
relationship bad	59	38.6	33	34.4	2	33	9	45
Subtotal	153	100.0	96	100.0	6	100	20	100
No primary family or not living with them	370		185		27		48	
Not known	10		3		4		0	
Total	533		284		37		68	
Non-violent patients								
Living with the family:								
relationship good	123	67.6	72	63.2	8	100	25	69
relationship bad	59	32.4	42	36.8	0	–	11	31
Subtotal	182	100.0	114	100.0	8	100	36	100
No primary family or not living with them	312		161		35		29	
Not known	39		18		6		5	
Total	533		293		49		70	

Significance test:

1. Existence of relationships: 'living with family' v. 'not living with family or no primary family':

	χ^2 =	df =	α =
Whole group	6.6240	1	0.01
Schizophrenia	3.1412	1	Null hypothesis not refutable
Affective psychoses	0.0023	1	Null hypothesis not refutable
Mental deficiency	9.1934	1	0.01

2. Quality of relationships: 'good' or 'bad':

	χ^2 =	df =	α =
Whole group	1.3768	1	Null hypothesis not refutable
Schizophrenia	0.1391	1	Null hypothesis not refutable
Affective psychoses	Could not be tested because the values anticipated were too small		
Mental deficiency	1.1720	1	Null hypothesis not refutable

Table 49. *Existence and quality of contacts with spouse or other intimate partner for violent and non-violent patients within the six months preceding the crime or admission to hospital*

	Whole group		Schizo-phrenia		Affective psychoses		Mental deficiency	
	n	%	n	%	n	%	n	%
Violent patients								
Living apart [(a)]	20	8.4	13	11.6	0	0	0	–
Living together: [(a)]								
relationship good	107	45.2	44	39.3	25	74	2	22
relationship bad	110	46.4	55	49.1	9	26	7	78
Subtotal	237	100	112	100	34	100	9	100
No marital/intimate relationships	295		172		3		59	
Not known	1		0		0		0	
Total	533		284		37		68	
Non-violent patients								
Living apart [(a)]	10	5.3	5	6	0	–	0	–
Living together: [(a)]								
relationship good	137	73.3	60	72	28	80	4	100
relationship bad	40	21.4	18	22	7	20	0	–
Subtotal	187	100.0	83	100.0	35	100	4	100
No marital/intimate relationships	342		210		12		66	
Not known	4		0		2		0	
Total	533		293		49		70	

Significance test:

1. Existence of relationships: 'marital or other intimate relationship present' v. 'no marital or other intimate relationship':

	$\chi^2 =$	df =	$\alpha =$
Whole group	9.3553	1	0.01
Schizophrenia	7.9537	1	0.01
Affective psychoses	4.2912	1	0.05
Mental deficiency	2.2791	1	Null hypothesis not refutable

2. Quality of relationships: 'living apart', 'good' or 'bad':

	$\chi^2 =$	df =	$\alpha =$
Whole group	34.2770	2	0.001
Schizophrenia	20.9118	2	0.001
Affective psychoses	0.4084	1	Null hypothesis not refutable
Mental deficiency	Could not be tested because the values anticipated were too small		

[(a)] In our questionnaire we also asked whether the separation occurred at the initiative of the patient or of the partner, and whether, if the relationship were bad, the external form of the marriage was maintained or had already been abandoned. Because the numbers were so small, we have not detailed the answers here.

Table 50. *Contacts with own children for violent and non-violent patients during the six months preceding the crime or admission to hospital*

	Whole group		Schizo-phrenia		Affective psychoses		Mental deficiency	
	n	%	n	%	n	%	n	%
Violent patients								
Living together:								
relationships good	166	86.5	82	92	30	94	5	83
relationships bad[a]	26	13.5	7	8	2	6	1	17
Subtotal	192	100.0	89	100	32	100	6	100
No children or not living with them	334		193		4		62	
Not known	7		2		1		0	
Total	533		284		37		68	
Non-violent patients								
Living together:								
relationships good	120	87.0	57	86	30	97	3	100
relationships bad	18	13.0	9	14	1	3	0	-
Subtotal	138	100.0	66	100	31	100	3	100
No children or not living with them	364		218		14		66	
Not known	31		9		4		1	
Total	533		293		49		70	

Significance test:

1. Existence of relationships: 'living with children' v. 'no children or not living with them':

	$\chi^2 =$	df =	$\alpha =$
Whole group	9.5725	1	0.01
Schizophrenia	4.9233	1	0.05
Affective psychoses	4.6285	1	0.05
Mental deficiency	Anticipated values too small		

2. Quality of relationships: 'good' or 'bad':

	$\chi^2 =$	df =	
Whole group	0.0173	1	Null hypothesis not refutable
Schizophrenia	1.3673	1	Null hypothesis not refutable
Affective psychoses	Anticipated values too small		
Mental deficiency	Anticipated values too small		

[a] Under bad relationships our questionnaire included also bad relationships combined with maltreatment (refusal of care, hard blows, cruel upbringing). Here again, because of small numbers and inadequate documentation, we could make no comparisons between the groups. (Maltreatment of children occurred in nine cases in the violent offender group.)

Marital and other intimate relationships (even when there was no cohabitation) were significantly more frequent among the violent offenders (n = 237) than in the control group (n = 187), which bears out what we have already postulated, namely that the violent offenders are clearly much more capable than the non-violent patients of pursuing active social contacts and intimate relationships. Such contacts were mentioned more frequently even in the records of the mentally defective offenders (n = 9) than in those of their non-violent controls (n = 4).

The possibility of associating with one's own children is determined to a large extent by marriage rates and more such contacts were therefore made by the violent offenders (n = 192) than by the control group (n = 138): this applied to all the main diagnostic groups, though the difference was most marked in the patients with affective psychoses.

Turning now to the quality of existing contacts, we found that contrary to expectation - the offenders who lived with their primary family did not have 'bad' relationships with their parents or foster-parents much more often than the relevant group of controls (about 40% as against about 32%). This result surprised us because when we coded the offender-victim relationships (see Chapter 8) we found that the victims included a relatively high proportion of parents and siblings (about 18%), so that we expected to find more clear-cut differences in the inter-group comparisons of violent and non-violent patients.

Since the violent schizophrenics, who constitute the largest proportion of all abnormal offenders, hardly differed from the non-violent patients with the same diagnosis, we would suggest that they must in fact more frequently live in a state of family tension which is concealed or denied. A family atmosphere described by those involved as low in tension cannot, at least in the families of schizophrenics, be counted as 'proof' of well-balanced relationships. It may equally well amount to denial, or reflect a 'pseudo-mutuality' (Wynne, 1958) which conceals serious latent tensions. It is possible that a proportion of the schizophrenics who later became violent grew up in families where tensions were rife but concealed or denied, so that this would not be recorded in our questionnaire.

Depressed and mentally defective offenders showed, surprisingly, more bad relationships than their control groups, so that one might suppose that the tendency to conceal them was less. The small numbers, however, preclude any statistical predictions. The frequency of bad relationships between the violent offenders and their marital or other intimate partners was striking: conflict between partners was more than twice as frequent for the

whole group of offenders of all diagnoses (about 46%) than for the control
group (about 21%). The ratios for the schizophrenics were similar, but the
proportion of those living apart was somewhat higher. Only about a quarter
to a fifth of both the violent and non-violent depressed patients had a bad
relationship with their marital partner, contacts in most cases being fairly
free from conflict. The mentally defective violent offenders were, like their
controls, mostly unmarried, but where there was a record of an intimate
relationship, it was almost always (seven cases out of nine) full of tension.

When we came to interpret this finding, our first thought was
that there might be a systematic error: data on 'bad relationships' had
usually been obtained from the marital partner (if alive) and other informers
immediately after the crime, while they were still influenced by what had
happened, and might therefore reflect an assessment of the relationship that
was distorted in reaction to the crime. This psychological fact would, however, also apply to the positive assessments of the offender's relationship
with his primary family, in other words to the majority of the assessments;
moreover it clearly did not produce the same proportion of negative assessments in the relatives of the depressed patients.

A more likely explanation is that the proportion of open tension
and conflict in the conjugal family was in fact higher. This does not
necessarily mean that, counting concealed conflict, tense relationships must
be less common in the primary family. The denial or concealment of tension
must be more difficult to achieve when equal and adult partners are living
together in intimate relationship and with shared responsibility for contacts
with the outside world as well as for home and children than, for example,
in relationships between adult offspring and parents, which are governed more
clearly by unilateral possibilities of dependence, of passivity and of avoidance of close emotional ties and open conflict.

It is also possible that dependence on parents - which is seen
often in young adult schizophrenics - tends to increase marital conflict, if
the partner wishes to break away from primary relationships or the patient
himself tries to break away and founders. The example of jealousy (see case
no. 329, p.139) and the comments made in the following section on 'threatened
loss of the intimate partner' illustrate the tensions which can arise when
separation anxiety or a strong ambivalent emotional tie dominates the marital
relationship. Rivalry over the children's love or arguments about their upbringing, or conflicts in marital roles, etc. (Lidz *et al.*, Richter) may in
actively belligerent personalities with fears of passivity and severe often
paranoid disturbances, lead more often to open altercation than to denial.

The high percentage of marital and other intimate partners among
the victims (about a quarter of all the offenders attacked persons who stood
in this relationship to them) confirms the risk of their being endangered and
lends probability to the thesis that this danger is associated both with the
tensions that often persist and with the delusional component which, as already
mentioned, is often present in these relationships, especially among schizophrenic offenders.

In so far as contacts with their children existed, these were
generally (about 87%) described in both groups as good; there were no
significant differences between groups. One cannot therefore talk of open
tension or disturbances in the relationships between most of the violent
offenders and their children. (Nevertheless children were victims in a fifth
of all cases.) The finding is, however, subject to the same reservations as
applied to contacts with the primary family; there is possibly an even stronger
tendency to deny bad relationships with (and maltreatment of) one's children,
since such behaviour encounters considerable social disapproval. Where depressed
female offenders committed acts of extended suicide, their relationship towards
their children calls for special assessment. This relationship was described
overwhelmingly (94% as against 97% in the control group) as good. Our case
studies showed clearly that these female offenders had mostly had a very close
relationship - not entirely free of contradictory and sometimes hostile feelings - with their children. Not uncommonly one had the impression that this
relationship could truly be described as 'symbiotic'. The motivation of the
extended suicide, which was mostly governed by the delusion that the children
were under the same threat of illness, poverty and destruction as the abnormal
offender herself, was in most cases a delusional deliverance by means of a
shared death. Such a motive of delusional identification or incorporation is
associated more with particularly close, symbiotic relationships than with
those that are full of conflict and disunity. Here again the motivation and
the crime of depressed offenders seem to be governed by a characteristic
depressive psychopathology.

Secondary relationships

In addition to contacts with close relatives, which we have
described above, we were also interested in the quality of contacts with other
people outside the intimate family group. We had supposed, for example, that
the mentally defective group would find themselves more frequently in conflict
outside the family, i.e. in dealings with friends, neighbours, colleagues,
superiors, fellow inmates of homes, etc., all of which were grouped together

as 'secondary relationships'. This assumption was in line with statements in the literature (e.g. Werner *et al.*) as well as with our own preliminary clinical studies.

For the reasons already mentioned, we again gave up the idea of using a rating scale for difficulties in making contacts or for degree of conflict, using only the alternatives 'little conflict' and 'much conflict'.

Table 51. *Secondary relationships for violent and non-violent patients during the six months preceding the crime or admission to hospital*

	Whole group		Schizo- phrenia		Affective psychoses		Mental deficiency	
	n	%	*n*	%	*n*	%	*n*	%
Violent patients								
Relationships showing:								
little conflict	318	61.3	180	64.6	33	89	25	37
much conflict	201	38.6	99	35.4	4	11	42	63
Subtotal	519	100.0	279	100.0	37	100	67	100
Not known	14		5		0		1	
Total	533		284		37		68	
Non-violent patients								
Relationships showing:								
little conflict	363	74.4	204	73.9	38	97	37	54
much conflict	125	25.6	72	26.1	1	3	31	46
Subtotal	488	100.0	276	100.0	39	100	68	100
Not known	45		17		10		2	
Total	533		293		49		70	

Significance test:

	$\chi^2 =$	df = 1	$\alpha =$
Whole group	19.161		0.001
Schizophrenia	5.315		0.025
Mental deficiency	3.314		Null hypothesis not refutable

(No test could be carried out for the affective psychoses because the anticipated values were too low.)

It can be seen from Table 51 that secondary relationships in which conflicts were rife were recorded significantly more often for the violent than for the non-violent patients. The numerical differences in frequency were, however, not so great here as in the area of intimate partner relationships.

For the schizophrenic offenders the difference between the two groups was smaller, which can again be taken as an indication that in this diagnostic group relationships within the close family circle are much more important.

In the group of depressed offenders there is a small disparity in favour of relationships with much conflict (four out of 37 as against only one case out of 49 in the non-violent depressed group); but the low numbers involved make it impossible to carry out any test of significance. The relatively small proportion of secondary relationships in which there was much conflict, as compared with the other diagnoses as a whole, can be interpreted as reflecting the characteristic conformity of depressed patients to social rules and their tendency to internalise external conflicts.

As we had expected, the contacts of the mentally subnormal offenders showed a high proportion of conflict. There was, however, no significant statistical difference between them and their non-violent control group. This finding reflects the selection problem presented by this group, which has already been discussed: bad relationships with the environment and social difficulties are among the few real grounds for admitting mental defectives to a regional mental hospital. The negative statistical finding has thus little meaning and the high proportion of bad relationships, which is far above the average for the group of abnormal offenders taken as a whole, must be taken seriously. This is borne out by the fact that exactly half of all the persons assaulted by mentally defective offenders came from outside the circle of family members or intimate partners.

The following case history exemplifies a social situation of conflict which formed the background of a mental defective's violent crime:

Case no. 492: Low-grade mental defect

Abnormal reaction, with delusions developing as a reaction to sexual humiliation and social conflicts. According to his mother, this building worker (M.), born in 1931, had a forceps delivery, after which he suffered from infantile convulsions and was late in learning to walk and speak.

In his primary school he twice had to repeat classes; he left without any certificate of education and because of his low intelligence proved incapable of learning a trade. He worked first on his parents' farm and after the age of 21 as a builder's mate.

Although according to the local police he was considered to be a 'feeble-minded but decent lad', who attended work regularly and gave an impression of tidiness, he had from his schooldays been teased by his village companions and was known as the 'village idiot'. He frequently suffered because of his awkward approach to girls.

While at home he was regarded as willing and obedient, he reacted with growing irritability and distrust to the humiliations inflicted upon him in the village. At times he could be quick with his fists. In 1958 his unstable mixture of anxiety and anger developed into delusional fears that the village youths wanted to force him to be castrated, otherwise he would be chased out of the village. He believed he heard these threats uttered behind his back, on the street and in the church. At this period he bought himself an air-rifle with his savings and set up a practice target in the garden. In August of that year he violently broke through the barriers of fears and inhibitions which isolated him from the opposite sex and one night in a very drunken state he attacked from behind a woman he did not know, tearing off her clothes in order to assault her breasts and genitals. The woman was able to escape. As he was not recognised in the darkness, nothing further happened.

At the end of October he made a second serious assault, upon a butcher's boy who had, he believed, been jeering at him for a long time because of his inability to get himself a girl.

For a long time M. had been planning a surprise attack on this opponent, who was more than a match for him in strength. To this end he lay in wait for him, armed with a cudgel, and on the day of the crime injured him seriously with a blow on the head from behind.

Because of his low intelligence he was referred by the court for a psychiatric assessment. While under observation he several times got into a threatening and excited state and was afraid he was going to be caught in a net and burned. He thought the attendants were teasing him and threatening him with injections. He gradually grew calmer and after being in hospital for several years he was discharged home to his mother in 1963.

The example speaks for itself. It makes clear how understandable motives can induce someone with a substantial degree of defect to commit a violent crime, which he hopes will compensate for wrongs he has suffered in the social field. The psychodynamics of the crime may well be similar in the case of many other mental defectives.

Life events as stress factors which increase the risk of
violence

In formulating our hypotheses we were guided by the idea that
violent crimes may also be caused by stressful events which have occurred in
the lives of the offenders during the six months before the crime and which
have been largely independent of their personality and illness.

We had in mind relatively gross stresses such as are generally
held to be momentous, which might cause an individual to lapse into aggression
or at least to lose a precarious mental balance. In order to define such
stress factors globally and according to their quality we divided them into:
'occupational/material stresses', defined as loss of job, demotion, shortage
of money, housing worries, receiving notice, etc; and 'loss or threatened
loss of intimate partners', which we defined as including death of or divorce,
separation or threatened separation from partners with whom the patients lived
or had lived in close association. Stress in other areas of life was not
included, because the difficulties of identifying and classifying such stresses
increase considerably if the definition is broadened.

In almost 11% of the violent offenders and about 6% of the control
group, that is to say in only a small proportion of all categories of patient,
were there external stresses, in the terms of our definition, that could be
associated with the crime or the readmission.

'Occupational/material' stresses were only slightly more frequent
among the violent offenders than among their controls. One might have expected
occupational problems to be a more frequent source of stress, considering, for
example, the difficulties in readaptation that follow discharge from a psychiatric hospital. We had, however, recorded stress events in two important areas
only; and they were mentioned in the files only if they had made a marked
impression on those who originally examined the patients.

'Loss or threatened loss of an intimate partner' was on the whole
infrequent, though it happened more often (5.4%) in the violent offenders than
in the control group (2%). The importance of stress in the area of marital
and other intimate partnerships in the previous history of homicidal offenders
is thus underlined. The noteworthy finding that this kind of stress is highest
for mentally defective offenders (at 7%, as against the expected 3% for non-
violent offenders), followed by 4.6% for schizophrenic offenders, is not
capable of one single interpretation. Presumably one group, whose victims are
mostly persons from outside the offender's intimate circle, reacts to loss or
threatened loss of a partner in a different manner from those offenders whose
victims come mainly from that intimate circle. One may postulate that in the

case of the mentally defective offenders loss of close associates leads more to
lack of restraint and weakening of control over instinctive aggressive impulses,
such control being often linked to external influential figures.

In the case of the schizophrenics it is very difficult to make a
differentiated interpretation. Presumably there is a great difference between
threatened losses which involve absence of the partner - for example imminent
divorce - and losses such as illness or death which are not in any way connected
with the often very tense relationships between the partners. We did not
distinguish between the two kinds of loss, so that some of these stresses are

Table 52. *Fortuitous life events in the six months preceding the crime or
admission to hospital, in violent and non-violent patients*

	Whole group		Schizo-phrenia		Affective psychoses		Mental deficiency	
	n	%	n	%	n	%	n	%
Violent patients								
Occupational/ material stresses	28	5.3	10	3.5	1	3	5	7
Loss of intimate partner	29	5.4	13	4.6	1	3	5	7
No such influence	476	89.3	261	91.9	35	94	58	86
Total	533	100.0	284	100.0	37	100	68	100
Non-violent patients								
Occupational/ material stresses	20	3.8	6	2.0	2	4	6	9
Loss of intimate partner	11	2.0	3	1.0	2	4	2	3
No such influence	502	94.2	284	97.0	45	92	62	88
Total	533	100.0	293	100.0	49	100	70	100

Significance test:

	$\chi^2 =$	df =	$\alpha =$
Whole group	10.12	2	0.01
Schizophrenia	8.08	2	0.025
Mental deficiency	0.126	1	Null hypothesis not refutable

(Because of the small values anticipated, we again did not carry out a test
for the affective psychoses. In the case of mental deficiency we tested only
two classes: life events present or not.)

governed by the same factors as affect the future offender's behaviour or his
illness. They are therefore not 'fortuitous life events' as defined by us at
the outset.

From study of the cases we formed the impression that threatened
separation or temporary or partial absence of the partner might at times be a
contributory cause of the crime. It seemed that the crime was liable to occur
both in the separation period and in the phase of resumption of relations,
both of which stages are usually fairly conducive to conflict, ambivalence and
tension. An extended or partner-suicide seems sometimes to be the pathological
reaction of a schizophrenic to such a conflict, governed by fear of the
separation or desire for union, as well as by an inability to achieve a genuine
restitution of the relationship. One must, however, remember that the proportion
of schizophrenic offenders who underwent such stresses before their crime was
only about 3% higher than the control rate (loss or threatened loss of partner
in non-violent patients), which is a minimal figure. Quantitatively, therefore,
loss or threatened loss of a partner is hardly significant as a cause of
violence in schizophrenics.

In depressed offenders the figures are too small for generalised
conclusions to be drawn. The fact that such events were recorded less frequently
among the offenders than among the non-violent depressed patients argues
against rather than for the hypothesis that loss or threatened loss of a
partner plays a part in causing violence in the group of depressed offenders.
This view gains in probability if we anticipate a finding which will be
reported later: the typical crime committed by these mainly female offenders
was extended suicide in which they included their own children and to a lesser
extent their marital partners. The possibility that loss of a partner might
provide the impetus to this action cannot be ruled out - it might be a
contributory cause of the depression itself - but this is not very likely.

Case no. 417: Schizophrenia

A 23-year-old artisan who in puberty had for several months
suffered from a state of nervous exhaustion and had therefore left school
early, later developed into a very shy young man who was inhibited
particularly in his dealings with girls but who nevertheless earned a
decent living as a lithographic printer. Four years before the crime he
became acquainted with a girl on the firm's outing, after which he met
her from time to time and eventually, two years later (1955), had intimate
relations with her when she stayed in his room over the Easter holidays.
In his inexperience he felt uncertain about maintaining regular sexual
relations with her, although he had long wanted to do so. In the autumn

of the same year he succeeded in having sexual relations twice with
another girl whom he gave up in the following year because she was
'too sensuous'.

Shortly afterwards he took up with his first girlfriend
again and spent Christmas with her parents. The girl's mother thought
he was 'modest and polite' and he became a welcome visitor.

About the time he resumed this friendship he began to feel
not so well again: his concentration deteriorated, his work was less
satisfactory and his employer reprimanded him. In contrast to his
previous behaviour, he became liable to react angrily. The girl also
reproached him for not earning enough money. In the end he said he
wanted to give notice, but he withdrew this and remained undecided.
His firm then suggested that, from the New Year of 1957, he should
look for another job, but he did not do this. Instead he asked,
inexplicably, for a rise in wages.

In February 1957 his colleagues at work noticed his nervous
state, his brooding, and his strange wish to have the printing machine
taken to pieces and repaired, though he could give no reason for this
demand. At the end of February his friends urgently advised him to
see a doctor, because he was clearly under 'a nervous strain'. His
mother, who visited him in his room on 3 March, found him 'confused'
and talking incoherently. She was worried, told the patient's father
about it, and asked him to take his son to a specialist.

On the following day the father fetched him from his place
of work. The patient complained of his depressed mood and of general
exhaustion which was caused by self-indulgence. He reproached himself
on this account. In tears he said he had become a Nazi, because he had
read Hitler's book *Mein Kampf*. He was not taken to see a specialist.

On 8 March he went again to his general practitioner who
found him 'calm, coherent and sensible'. On the same day the patient
asked his girlfriend's mother on the telephone to send her to him the
following evening; he had to speak with her as he was 'completely
confused'.

On 9 March, the day of the crime, his father called on him
at midday, but came home with his mind at rest, as his son seemed to be
all right and had conversed calmly with him. Towards evening the patient
wandered restlessly through the city, and ate a good meal in a restaurant
before meeting his friend at the bus stop. He then went with her to his
room.

His attempts to make sexual contact with her were neither rejected offhand nor accepted readily; the girl, as he later stated, had been in turn tender and reluctant, letting him, for example, unbutton her blouse but then pushing his hand away, and finally saying she was bored, there was no point in it all, he had no money, he only got into difficulties at work and could offer her nothing. She wanted to have no more to do with him. The patient was above all conscious of his lack of sexual success with her and got into a state of increased inner tension.

Finally the idea came to him that he should kill the girl and himself die with her. After trying for several minutes to reject this thought, he strangled the girl who was lying beside him on the bed and in a state of violent excitement bit her several times in the face and breast. Then he pulled her shoes off, straightened her legs on the bed, covered the body and left the room.

In his landlady's kitchen (she was not in at the time) he turned on the gas taps and was later found unconscious on the landlady's return.

On psychiatric examination he was diagnosed as schizophrenic, on the grounds of hypochondriacal delusions and unfounded ideas of reference as well as on grounds of a considerable disturbance of association, the first attack of the disorder having occurred in 1949.

This short case history illustrates the connection discussed above between schizophrenic disturbances of personality, inability to form a satisfactory love relationship, threatened loss of a partner and tense, unsuccessful attempts to resume the relationship. The crime seems to have its cause and at least part of its motivation in this background of strong, complex and clearly ambivalent tensions and fears of loss and defeat. The conversion of disappointed erotic aggressiveness into violence, and of thwarted desire for union into a wish to share a common death, might be a plausible interpretation of this pathological reaction to a conflict determined partly by personal pathology.

Such motivation recalls the examples described by Rasch of 'killing the intimate partner'. In his interpretation, homicide is the last intimate and most intense form of communication offered as the partnership founders. The act is understood here, even when committed by sane individuals, as the despairing outcome of an unsuccessful conflict-laden 'intimate relationship'.

In conclusion it may be said that our findings suggest that

external stress is of little quantitative significance in causing violent
crime. So far as such stress does play a part it consists, in schizophrenics,
rather of tensions within close human relationships, especially where these
are characterised by conflict-laden, ambivalent attempts at separation or
reunion. In depressed offenders stress of this kind seems to have no significance whatsoever as a causal factor. In mentally defective offenders such
stress is likewise rare, though it is encountered more frequently in this
than in any other diagnostic category. So far as external stress has a
causal effect it may be postulated that analogous motivational connections
operate only in a proportion of the schizophrenic offenders. Our study of
cases suggests that in these patients loss of a partner may increase the risk
of violence partly because of the resultant rootlessness or loss of ties and
the effect this has on behaviour.

Behaviour anomalies during the six months preceding the crime
As already discussed above (p.152), mentally abnormal patients
have the reputation of being liable to switch suddenly from seemingly normal
behaviour to violent acts, without arousing any suspicion at all in the minds
of those around them that their mental state has deteriorated to the point of
making them dangerous.

We encountered this stereotype in a surprisingly large number of
reports by assessors, judges and relatives, and made it the basis of a hypothesis which we wished to test. At the same time we looked for warning signs
of impending violence, which might provide a foundation on which to build
possible preventive measures. Accordingly we enquired how often during the six
months preceding their crime the offenders had seemed to those around them to
show 'no anomalies of behaviour'. We coded the complex category of 'anomalies'
under the following headings.

1. Decrease in social contacts, especially isolation,
   autism, falling into a state of neglect.
2. Change in relationships, especially abnormal, and
   particularly aggressive, behaviour towards others.
3. Expressions of auto-aggression (suicidal threats).

Signs of social isolation
Withdrawal from contact with one's fellow men is an important
indicator of various mental disorders, not least of mounting intrapsychic
tension and fears in psychoses of a depressive or schizophrenic nature.
In our questionnaire we tried to formulate a four-point scale

ranging from social contacts that were undisturbed or little affected to complete isolation. The demarcation is naturally imprecise. In Table 53 and in the statistical test the first two points in the scale have been amalgamated.

Table 53. *Ratings of social withdrawal for violent and non-violent patients during the six months preceding the crime or admission to hospital*

	Whole group		Schizo-phrenia		Affective psychoses		Mental deficiency	
	n	%	n	%	n	%	n	%
Violent patients								
Little or no social isolation	347	66.5	150	53.4	30	88	57	86
Considerable social isolation	92	17.6	55	19.6	4	12	8	12
Autism (complete isolation)	83	15.9	76	27.0	0	–	1	2
Subtotal	522	100.0	281	100.0	34	100	66	100
Not known	11		3		3		2	
Total	533		284		37		68	
Non-violent patients								
Little or no social isolation	309	59.0	128	44.3	41	89	53	76
Considerable social isolation	71	13.5	42	14.5	3	7	9	13
Autism (complete isolation)	144	27.5	119	41.2	2	4	8	11
Subtotal	524	100.0	289	100.0	46	100	70	100
Not known	9		4		3		0	
Total	533		293		49		70	

Significance test:	$\chi^2 =$	df =	$\alpha =$
Whole group	21.2948	2	0.001
Schizophrenia	12.8536	2	0.001
Mental deficiency	0.1331	1	Null hypothesis not refutable

(It was not possible to carry out a test on the affective psychoses, since the numbers anticipated were too small. For the mentally deficient we tested only the class 'no isolation' against 'considerable isolation present'.)

Examination of the findings shows that in 33.5% of the offender
group as a whole there had been during the six months preceding the crime a
moderate to complete withdrawal from human contact. The proportion of patients
showing more severe signs of social isolation was slightly higher in the control
group (at 41%), considerably more patients in this group showing autism, that
is to say a complete withdrawal from the surrounding world (27.5% as against 16%).
This difference is significant.

Autism was particularly common among the non-violent schizophrenics.
One reason for this is presumably that the patients in this group generally have
fewer symptoms, which tends to make them more remote and withdrawn than those
with productive paranoid-hallucinatory forms of the illness. On the other hand
one must seriously consider whether autistic withdrawal from contact with
others may not be a form of defensive behaviour, which protects the patient
from open altercations. One might interpret it as a defence against anxiety,
vulnerability and external aggression directed at the patient. In schizophrenic
offenders, whose intimate relationships are often fraught with tension, this
autistic remoteness might contribute to a blunting of tension and might thus
decrease rather than increase the risk of conflict resulting in violence.
Viewed in this way, the violent schizophrenic's less marked tendency to isolation might be interpreted as an expression of his stronger inclination to
altercation which, as we have already seen, was reflected in the personality of
schizophrenic (and mentally defective) offenders by a history of previous violent
crime and antisocial forms of behaviour (cf. sections on personality factors,
social behaviour, etc.).

Even if there is some tendency for the violent group as a whole
to be socially isolated, this social encapsulation is clearly not a symptom
which correlates positively with violence. Nevertheless such a withdrawal from
social contacts was found in about a third of the cases in both groups and can
be seen as an indicator of a high degree of social disturbance. It was noticed
not only by those who knew the non-violent patients but also by those who knew
the offenders during the six months preceding the crime.

Abnormal behaviour, particularly aggressiveness
This must be of particular interest to the investigator, since it
is the focal point for any study of clear or specific signs of aggressiveness before the crime.

Since we had already found that a history of previous delinquency,
particularly if associated with aggressiveness, was significantly more common
in the violent group (see pp. 125-9), it was to be expected that the two

groups would also show clear differences in respect of antisocial and aggressive behaviour during the six months preceding the crime or the admission to
hospital. We tried, therefore, to draw up a scale of abnormal behaviour, that
is to say behaviour which struck those around the patient as morbid or
inexplicable, which would range from slight anomalies to open violence. The
first point on this scale was defined as 'abnormal'. We included here modes of
behaviour which made other people suspect mental illness or struck them as
conspicuous and aroused their attention: for example bizarre motor behaviour
(grimacing), peculiar new habits, strange claims and utterances on the part
of the patient.

Aggressive threats and similar changes in behaviour were not
included here but in the next category of 'threatening behaviour' which stopped
short of actual violence. (Phenomena related to social isolation, however
conspicuous, were excluded since they came under their own special heading:
they have already been discussed above.)

In order to determine where and how clearly abnormal/aggressive
behaviour was noticed in the environment, we made a distinction between such
behaviour directed towards intimate partners and signs of aggressiveness that
were observed also in a wider social circle.

The following significant differences were found between the two
groups (Table 54). Threats and violence towards other persons (from any area
of the patient's life) were found in about 48% of the violent offenders, but
only in about 28% of the non-offenders: violence as such occurred only in
2.3% of the control group but had been documented in rather more than 15% of
the violent group.

At the same time conspicuous aggressive behaviour extending beyond
the intimate circle had been observed significantly more often in the violent
group than in the control patients (threats and violence 'outside the intimate
circle' were recorded for about 25% of the violent offenders and about 10% of
the non-violent patients). This difference is a certainty for the group as a
whole: in the case of the schizophrenics and the mentally defective it shows as
a tendency and could not be statistically confirmed.

This finding may be affected by the more precise history obtained
in the case of the offenders. If, however, we bear in mind that during the six
months preceding the crime only 8.5% of all the offenders and only 5.7% of the
violent schizophrenics were reported as showing no abnormalities of behaviour,
then the result of this test deserves attention. It serves to weaken the
hypothesis that mentally abnormal violent offenders are 'unpredictable' and are
inconspicuous until they commit their crime. The finding also provides an

Table 54. *Frequency of abnormal and aggressive forms of behaviour in violent and non-violent patients during the six months preceding the crime or admission to hospital*

	Whole group		Schizo-phrenia		Affective psychoses		Mental deficiency	
	n	%	n	%	n	%	n	%
Violent patients								
Nothing conspicuous	45	8.5	16	5.7	3	8	15	22
Abnormal only towards intimate partner	75	14.2	40	14.2	12	33	1	1
Abnormal also outside the intimate circle [a]	156	29.4	92	32.6	18	50	16	24
Threatening only towards intimate partner	74	13.9	44	15.6	1	3	7	10
Threatening also outside the intimate circle [a]	100	18.9	50	17.7	0	−	16	24
Violent only towards intimate partner	46	8.7	22	7.8	1	3	5	7
Violent also outside the intimate circle [a]	34	6.4	18	6.4	1	3	8	12
Subtotal	530	100.0	282	100.0	36	100	68	100
Not known	3		2		1		0	
Total	533		284		37		68	
Non-violent patients								
Nothing conspicuous	58	11.1	15	5.2	8	17	8	12
Abnormal only towards intimate partner	160	30.5	87	30.1	35	73	6	9
Abnormal also outside the intimate circle [a]	163	31.0	102	35.3	3	6	31	44
Threatening only towards intimate partner	86	16.5	50	17.3	2	4	14	20
Threatening also outside the intimate circle [a]	45	8.6	29	10.1	0	−	8	12
Violent only towards intimate partner	5	1.0	3	1.0	0	−	1	1
Violent also outside the intimate circle [a]	7	1.3	3	1.0	0	−	2	3
Subtotal	524	100.0	289	100.0	48	100	70	100
Not known	9		4		1		0	
Total	533		293		49		70	

impressive indication of the need for and reasonableness of providing preventive or therapeutic measures for those mentally abnormal individuals who make
themselves conspicuous by aggressive behaviour or just by aggressive tensions.

Suicidal behaviour

Another form of anomalous behaviour which may be an indicator of
violence is aggressiveness directed against the self: suicide threats and
overt suicide attempts. Since several authors have described a fluctuation
between aggressiveness against the self and against others (von Hentig, East,
West, Wolfgang), and other writers have regarded failed suicide attempts as
indicating a special risk of later homicide (Macdonald), this point called
for special attention.

Table 54 *(contd.)*

Significance test:

As the numbers in these seven classes were too small (the affective psychoses
could not be tested at all), we tested only three classes of behaviour
disturbance:

1. No aggressive behaviour (inconspicuous and abnormal behaviour)
2. Threatening behaviour
3. Violent behaviour

	$\chi^2 =$	df =	$\alpha =$
Whole group	67.054	2	0.001
Schizophrenia	35.260	2	0.001
Mental deficiency	8.440	2	0.025

In a second series of tests we studied those patients whose behaviour was
marked by threats or violence, to determine whether:

1. This was only in family or partner relationships (intimate circle)
2. Aggressive behaviour was observed also outside the intimate circle (at
    work, towards neighbours, etc.)

	$\chi^2 =$	df =	$\alpha =$
Whole group	9.226	1	0.01
Schizophrenia	3.088	1	Null hypothesis not refutable
Mental deficiency	3.421	1	Null hypothesis not refutable

Note:

[a] These categories include all cases in which the conspicuous behaviour was
noticed outside family and partnership relationships, irrespective of
whether it was observed at the same time within the family and partner
relationships - which was usually the case.

We recorded under the heading of suicidal behaviour only threats
and actions which were considered by other people to be suicidal: suicidal
thoughts were thus covered only if they were somehow expressed as suicide threats
and accepted as such by those who heard them.

Table 55. *Suicidal behaviour observed in violent and non-violent patients
during the six months preceding the crime or admission to hospital*

	Whole group		Schizo- phrenia		Affective psychoses		Mental deficiency	
	n	%	*n*	%	*n*	%	*n*	%
Violent patients								
None	402	76.6	230	82.7	13	36	61	90
Suicide threats	72	13.7	33	11.9	14	39	1	1
Suicide attempts	51	9.7	15	5.4	9	25	6	9
Subtotal	525	100.0	278	100.0	36	100	68	100
Not known	8		6		1		0	
Total	533		284		37		68	
Non-violent patients								
None	453	85.0	262	89.4	30	61	63	90
Suicide threats	26	4.9	10	3.4	6	12	0	-
Suicide attempts	54	10.1	21	7.2	13	27	7	10
Subtotal	533	100.0	293	100.0	49	100	70	100
Not known	0		0		0		0	
Total	533		293		49		70	

Significance test:

The test was limited to only the presence or absence of suicide attempts, since
the recognition and documentation of such attempts was presumed to be more
reliable and complete than would be the case in respect of suicide threats or
indications of suicidal thoughts.

	$\chi^2 =$	df =	
Whole group	0.015	1	Null hypothesis not refutable
Schizophrenia	0.488	1	Null hypothesis not refutable
Affective psychoses	0.008	1	Null hypothesis not refutable
Mental deficiency	0.003	1	Null hypothesis not refutable

As Table 55 shows, suicide attempts were made by about 10% of both groups during the six months preceding the crime. They were a little more frequent among the non-violent patients than among the offenders, but the difference was not significant.

There were, however, clear differences in the frequency of suicide threats: they occurred only in 26, or about 5%, of the non-violent patients, as against 72, or 13.7%, of the patients in the violent group. Whether this is a real difference, or an artefact due to differences in documentation of the previous history, is difficult to determine. Since it is easier to regard threatened suicide as a form of openly aggressive behaviour towards others than it is to apply the same interpretation to the predominantly auto-aggressive suicide attempt, this finding is basically in line with the high proportion of directly aggressive forms of behaviour found in the violent offenders.

Summary

Our study of living arrangements, social contacts with various groups of associates, life events that caused stress or otherwise contributed to the crime, and anomalies of behaviour occurring during the six months preceding the crime, yielded some findings which are suggestive but which are not, however, all equally capable of generalisation.

The social adaptation of the violent offenders was found to be relatively favourable, or at least not less favourable than that of the control group: about 70% of the offenders lived in a family setting, either with their parents or with their spouses.

The family contacts of the offenders with their parents and with their children was depicted as being relatively harmonious and free from conflict, but relationships with the marital partners were mostly described as bad. This was particularly the case with the schizophrenic offenders. To what extent the 'good' relationships with the primary family actually existed, or were only an expression of mutual denial or transference, could not be reliably determined. The latter possibility was to some extent supported by a series of case studies of schizophrenic offenders.

The depressed offenders described their contacts with all members of the immediate family and with intimate partners as good. This result can be interpreted in terms of the tendency of depressed patients to intensify social norms. It remains an open question whether the absence of overt conflict in family and partner relationships reflects an unusually low degree of aggressiveness and a high capacity to adapt to partnership, or whether it is the effect on the one hand of a denial, or on the other of an exceptionally strong self-control developed as a reaction to the patient's own aggressiveness.

So far as relationships outside the family were concerned, for example with colleagues, superiors or neighbours, those of the violent offenders as a group were somewhat more often disturbed than those of the controls. This was particularly marked in the case of the mentally defective offenders, in whose secondary relationships conflict was often very rife.

The hypothesis that violent crimes are to a considerable extent triggered by events that are 'extraneous to personality and to illness, such as crises at work or death of a close associate, was not confirmed. External stresses occurring independently of the behaviour of the patient seemed to play a subordinate role: only about 10% of the violent offenders, as against 6% of the control group, had been affected by such experiences during the six months preceding the crime. This small difference may, moreover, be partly or wholly due to the more detailed case histories and documentation that were available for the violent offenders. In the psychosocial process which in certain personalities can culminate in a violent crime, personal entanglements in close human relationships clearly play a more important part, particularly in schizophrenics. Here a particularly high risk seems to be attached to associations which are continued in spite of ambivalence, feelings of hatred and delusional change. From several particularly well documented cases of schizophrenic offenders we formed the impression that the stimulation of strong and especially erotic emotions can be a causal factor. One young paranoid-hallucinatory schizophrenic, for example, who was being analysed by a woman lay psychotherapist, killed her by stabbing her several times with a knife, the cause of the crime being an extremely intense and partly delusional transference situation. Such an assumption could not, however, be confirmed or rejected by our findings. It is nevertheless of importance, as it would agree with the findings of other writers who suggest that schizophrenic relapses are often caused by strong emotional stresses (Brown *et al.*, 1962; Brown & Birley, 1970; Stevens, 1973). The finding does not apply to depressed patients: here the illness itself and its dependent course seem to be more significant. Nor does the finding apply to mentally defective offenders, where serious difficulties of social adaptation appear to be more in the forefront. In the area of family relationships, lack of ties and lack of balance are more important in this group than conflicting relationships.

The results with regard to warning signs during the six months preceding the crime are of particular significance. The main findings were as follows. Only 9% of the offenders were retrospectively described as showing no conspicuous anomalies of behaviour during this period (for schizophrenic offenders the figure was as low as about 6%). Almost half of the offenders - as against only 28% of the non-offenders - were described as behaving in a threatening or openly aggressive manner, such behaviour being observed to a considerable extent not only within the family and by intimate partners but also by other people (colleagues at work, acquaintances, friends, neighbours, etc.). At the same time the offenders were less frequently described as aut- istic and withdrawn than the control group of non-violent patients: this fits in with their tendency, which we have already mentioned, to show partial social adaptation and to be active, aggressive and quarrelsome.

A final point of difference was that the offenders contained more individuals who had made suicide threats, though they did not differ from the control group in regard to the number who had actually attempted suicide.

An increase in aggressive behaviour during the six months pre- ceding the crime (such as threatening other people and particularly violence on the part of a mentally abnormal person towards those around him) provided serious warning signs. The assumption that the mentally abnormal are basically 'unpredictable' and that their outbursts of violence cannot be foreseen, proved to be a prejudice, at least in this generalised form. There is much to be said in favour of the view that it is more often possible to make a fairly reliable estimate of the risk of violence in the mentally abnormal - by looking at the particular nature of the illness, the personality and the previous history, as well as at any accumulation of conspicuous anomalies of behaviour - than it is to assess the analogous risk of violence in the mentally normal.

Subgroup comparisons of violent patients

So far we have analysed differences between violent and non- violent patients in regard to heredity, personality, illness, previous treat- ment and the background of the crime. In what follows we shall investigate differences within the violent group itself. Inter-group comparisons have already shown that patients in the three diagnostic categories studied, namely schizophrenia, manic-depressive psychoses and mental deficiency, differ in regard to personality traits, social contacts, family relationships, and previous crimes. We shall now test and interpret such diagnosis-linked differ- ences, again in respect of the main factors in the five areas mentioned. Each section will show the test results in tabular form. We carried out three chi-square tests for each item, each test comparing two diagnoses.

7.6 Heredity

As we have already seen in section 4.3, many criminologists
(Brückner, Duncan & Frazier, S. & E. Glueck) and psychiatrists (Macdonald,
Guze *et al.*) have regarded severe impairment of the completeness or cohesiveness of the primary family as an important predictor of later antisocial
behaviour. Our results so far have shown that the parental family of the
violent patients was not significantly more often affected by mental illness
or by loss of one or both parents (broken home) than that of the non-
violent controls. On the other hand the parental families of the abnormal
offenders were very often burdened by the behavioural problems of suicide,
criminality and alcoholism, while inter-group comparison of offenders and
non-offenders showed a similar diagnosis-linked pattern of behaviour. This
pattern was now tested for significant differences within the group of
violent offenders, as shown in Table 56.

There were no significant differences between the diagnostic groups
with regard to mental disorders occurring in Grade 1 relatives. When we turn
to anomalies of behaviour and loss of parents (broken home) in the primary
family, however, a different picture emerges. The mentally defective offenders
came more often (almost half the cases) than the other abnormal offenders
from primary families who had histories of suicide, criminality and alcoholism.
The greatest difference in this respect was between them and the schizophrenic
offenders. The primary families of the mental defectives also showed a higher
percentage of broken homes, again amounting to more than half the cases,
whereas four-fifths of the offenders suffering from schizophrenia or depression
came from primary families that were at least superficially intact. Here
again it is significant that the mental defectives form a special group,
differing in both these dimensions from the offenders with functional psychoses.

7.7 Previous history

We hoped that the many personal items recorded would contain some
indices which might help to show whether the tendency to commit violent crimes
depends more on modes of behaviour that are linked to the personality or on
factors that are related to the illness. We had already found that the
depressed offenders were almost indistinguishable in these respects from their
non-violent controls, but that the schizophrenic and mentally defective offenders
differed clearly from their matched counterparts. We now wished to test whether
there were any diagnosis-linked differences between the three groups of
offenders (Table 57).

Antisocial behaviour appeared by far the most frequently in the

209

Table 56. *Genetic and social heredity of violent patients in three diagnostic groups*

Item	Schizophrenia		Sig. test v.		Affective psychoses		Sig. test v. mental deficiency	Mental deficiency	
	n	%	Affective psychoses	Mental deficiency	n	%		n	%
Severe mental disturbance in primary family	82	30.6	-	-	14	40	-	25	42
Aggressive/auto-aggressive behaviour (incl. alcoholism) in primary family	46	17.6	-	**	9	26	(+)	28	51
Broken home in primary family	55	20.7	-	**	6	19	*	35	54

Table 57. *Personality traits of violent patients in three diagnostic groups*

Item	Schizophrenia		Sig. test v.		Affective psychoses		Sig. test v. mental deficiency	Mental deficiency	
	n	%	Affective psychoses	Mental deficiency	n	%		n	%
Antisocial/psychopathic traits	23	8.2	(/)	**	1	3	(/)	48	74
Alcoholism	22	7.8	-	*	3	8	-	14	21
Did not complete normal education	60	21.5	(/)	**	0	0	(/)	61	90
Marital status single at time of crime	144	50.7	(/)	**	1	3	(/)	57	84
Not employed	76	27.0	(/)	-	1	3	(/)	17	25
Previous history of serious violent crime	95	33.6	**	**	3	8	**	40	59
Previous history of other crimes:									
with threats	119	41.9	(/)	**	4	11	(/)	28	41
without threats	21	7.4	(/)	**	0	0	(/)	24	35

Key:

- = not significant
(+) = slightly significant (α = 0.05)
* = significant (α = 0.01)
** = highly significant (α = 0.001)
(/) = not tested because of small number of cases

previous histories of the mentally defective offenders. Alcoholism was also
more frequent in this group (a fifth of the cases) than in offenders with
endogenous psychoses (3, or 8%). The difference *vis-à-vis* the schizophrenic
offenders was significant.

The fact that most of the mentally defective offenders (61 out of
68) failed to complete their normal schooling is self-explanatory. As we have
already mentioned (section 3.2, p.58), patients with *Propfschizophrenien*
(concurrence of mental defect and a schizophrenic psychosis) were included in
the group of schizophrenic offenders, which is one reason why about 20% of the
schizophrenic group had failed to complete their schooling. (It cannot, of
course, be ruled out that some of the schizophrenic illnesses that began in
adolescence may have caused a falling-off in performance or a deterioration
in intelligence during school years.)

Four-fifths of the mental defectives were unmarried, as were half
of the schizophrenics, but only one of the 37 depressed offenders was not
married. This item, of course, is very closely linked to the patient's sex:
the violent women of all diagnoses were much more often married than the men
($\alpha = 0.001$). This in turn is associated with the fact that women in the GFR
marry at an earlier age than men.

When it came to occupation, we investigated the male patients
only. Those with affective psychoses, who were predominantly female, were for
this reason excluded.[11] The male schizophrenic and mentally defective offenders were out of work or incapable of work to an almost equal extent - about
a quarter of the cases. Three-quarters of the mentally defective were unskilled
workers, only one out of the 57 having learned a skilled trade. Only about a
third of the male schizophrenics, on the other hand, were unskilled workers,
a further third being skilled workers or salaried employees.

Previous offences against life and limb (bodily harm, attempted
homicide, sexual assaults) had been recorded in almost two-thirds of the
mentally defective offenders, in one-third of the schizophrenics but only in
3 out of the 37 depressed offenders. This item, too, is linked to sex: a
previous history of violent crime was much more common in the men than in the
women ($\alpha = 0.001$).

All but a quarter of the mental defectives had a previous history
of 'other crimes' (indecent offences without violence, abuse, defamation,
threatening behaviour). But half of the schizophrenics and all but 4 of the
37 depressed patients had no such previous history. It is of interest to note
that 'crimes accompanied by threats' were almost as common among the schizophrenics as among the mentally defective offenders (about 42% of the schizophrenics, as against 28 of the 68 mental defectives).

7.8   The illness

There was no point in comparing the distribution of individual symptoms in the different diagnostic groups. We therefore looked only for differences between the two main groups of psychoses in regard to the duration of the illness up to the time of the crime.

Table 58 shows that there was a slightly significant difference between the two groups. In about a third of the depressed cases the crime had taken place within the first six months after onset of the illness, i.e. probably in the first phase of the illness. Only 8.7% of the schizophrenics had committed their crimes within the same interval from onset of illness. Most of the schizophrenics had been ill for a long time (about half of them for five or more years before the crime). If we consider the prevalence of delusional subgroups among the schizophrenic offenders, and take account also of the fact that it often requires several years for systematic delusions, e.g. delusional jealousy, to develop (Mowat), this might provide a possible explanation of the difference. At the same time 64% of the offenders with affective psychoses had been ill for at least a year before the crime, and 31% for at least 5 years.

Table 58. *Duration of illness in schizophrenic offenders as compared with those suffering from affective psychoses*

Duration of illness	Schizophrenia		Affective psychoses	
	n	%	n	%
Up to 1 month	8	2.9	4	11
1-6 months	16	5.8	8	22
Up to 1 year	21	7.6	1	3
1-5 years	96	34.7	12	33
5-10 years	68	24.5	4	11
10 years and over	68	24.5	7	20
Subtotal	277	100.0	36	100
Not known	7		1	
Total	284		37	

Significance test:

(For purposes of the calculation the first three classes were taken together.)

$$\chi^2 = 9.6517 \qquad df = 3 \qquad \alpha = 0.05$$

7.9   Previous treatment

We next wished to determine whether the diagnostic groups differed
in regard to the surprising fact that in spite of often year-long illnesses,
and in spite of the high proportion of offenders in whom abnormal aggressive
behaviour was observed during the six months preceding the crime, only a few
received specialist treatment (68% of the abnormal offenders had received
neither in-patient nor out-patient psychiatric treatment in the last six months).
For example it was conceivable that the schizophrenic offenders, with their
tendency to more productive symptoms such as delusions, hallucinations and
thought disorders, would differ from the depressed and mentally defective
offenders because of more frequent and more lengthy therapeutic contacts.

In fact significant differences did emerge (Table 59): the
mentally defective offenders had naturally received the least treatment: 40
of the 68 had never been in a psychiatric hospital before the crime. About
half of those with affective psychoses (19 out of 37) had never been in
hospital, while this was true of only about 40% of the schizophrenic offenders.
(Nevertheless even this percentage is surprisingly high.)

If we consider only those patients who had received psychiatric
treatment before the crime, and take only those of them whose in-patient treatment had been of longest duration, then we find a significant preponderance
of mentally defective offenders: a fifth of them had been in hospital for five
years or more before their crime, as against only about 3% of the schizophrenics.
None of the manic-depressive offenders had been in hospital for so long a
period.

Turning to the interval that elapsed between discharge from
hospital and committal of the crime, depressed patients seem more liable (11
out of 18) to commit a violent crime within six months of discharge than
schizophrenics (about 37%) or mental defectives (7 out of 23).

In regard to the frequency of specialist psychiatric treatment
during the six months preceding the crime, irrespective of whether this was
in-patient or out-patient, there was no significant difference between the
two groups of psychoses. The mentally defective offenders made somewhat fewer
contacts with the psychiatric services than the patients with affective
psychoses, but the difference was only slightly significant.

7.10   Social situation and behaviour during the six months
preceding the crime

Our inter-group analysis of living arrangements, contacts with
parents, marriage partners and children, as well as with persons outside

Table 59. *Previous treatment of violent patients in three diagnostic categories*

Item	Schizophrenia		Sig. test v.		Affective psychoses		Sig. test v. mental deficiency	Mental deficiency	
	n	%	Affective psychoses	Mental deficiency	n	%		n	%
No previous treatment in mental hospital	116	41.1	-	*	19	51	-	40	59
Hospital treatment 5 years and over	8	2.8	(/)	**	0	0	(/)	13	19
Committed crime within 6 months of discharge from hospital	59	36.9	(+)	-	11	61	(+)	7	30

Table 60. *Social situation and behaviour of violent patients in three diagnostic groups during the six months preceding the crime*

Item	Schizophrenia		Sig. test v.		Affective psychoses		Sig. test v. mental deficiency	Mental deficiency	
	n	%	Affective psychoses	Mental deficiency	n	%		n	%
Living with family	193	68.0	(/)	**	37	100	(/)	31	46
Conflicts with marriage/intimate partner	68	60.7	**	-	9	27	**	7	78
Conflicts in secondary relationships	99	35.4	**	**	4	11	**	42	63
Considerable or total social isolation	131	46.6	**	**	4	12	-	9	14
Threats and violence towards others	134	47.5	**	-	3	8	**	36	53
Suicide threats and attempt(s)	48	17.3	**	-	23	65	**	7	10

Key:

- = not significant

(+) = slightly significant (α = 0.05)

* = significant (α = 0.01)

** = highly significant (α = 0.001)

(/) = not tested because of small number of cases

the family, and of abnormal, particularly aggressive and suicidal forms of
behaviour, had already revealed diagnosis-specific differences, which we now
wished to test further by comparing the diagnostic groups in these respects.
It was not possible, however, to carry out tests on all the items in question
for all diagnostic pairs (for example to compare manic-depressive with
schizophrenic and mentally defective offenders in regard to living arrangements or contacts with their children), because the numbers were often too
small.

Our tests showed (Table 60) that all the depressed patients and
68% of the schizophrenics, but not even half of the mentally defective offenders, lived with their families. In the case of the mentally defective patients,
this mostly meant living with their parents. Their relationships with their
relatives were not described as worse than those of schizophrenics living with
their parents.

Relationships with the marital or other intimate partner were
described as full of conflict in about 60% of the married schizophrenics, but
in only about a quarter of the depressed offenders. Bad secondary relationships were very rarely recorded among the depressed offenders (only 4 out of
37 cases). For the schizophrenics the proportion rose to a third, and for the
mentally defective it was as high as two-thirds.

In assessing these records of good or bad relationships, with much
or little conflict or tension, we must repeat, however, the critical comment
already discussed (p.187), namely that relationships described as good are not
always the same as relationships in which there is little conflict. Apart from
keeping quiet about family tensions, denial of such a situation may be part
of the family pathology of schizophrenics, and perhaps also of depressives.

It is rare to find a severe degree of social isolation or autistic
withdrawal from society in the background of depressed patients who have
committed homicidal crimes, and the same is true of the mentally defective
offenders, in spite of their outwardly unfavourable social situation. Schizophrenics scored highly in this respect, with nearly 50%, and in this they
differ very significantly from the two other diagnostic categories. Even
although marked social isolation is a typical symptom in schizophrenia, this
does not detract from the value of this finding as a pointer to the risk of
violence: we have already discussed this in section 7.5.

Aggressive behaviour towards others (use of threats and violence)
occurred very rarely in the depressed offenders in the six months preceding
the crime (3 out of 37 cases), so that such behaviour cannot count as a
prognostic criterion. But it carries much more weight and is undoubtedly

of prognostic value in schizophrenic (47.5% of the cases) and in mentally
defective offenders (36 out of 68 cases).[12]

      As was to be expected, suicide threats and suicide attempts were
most common in the manic-depressives, occurring in 65% of the cases. There
was a highly significant difference between this group and the schizophrenic
(about 17%) and mentally defective offenders (about one-tenth of the cases).

8.   RESULTS V : THE CRIME AND THE VICTIM

So far we have tried to shed light on the effects of age, sex, family, personality and illness on the risk of violence by mentally abnormal offenders. By studying the symptoms of the illness, the behaviour of the offenders and the circumstances and stresses surrounding them before the crime, we have obtained our first pointers towards the motivation for the crime.

In the present section we shall concentrate on the nature of the crime, on its motivation, and on the characteristics of the victim. It remains to be seen how far this will provide further insight into the complex processes which give rise to such crimes. It should be mentioned again that our data are based on an evaluation of the records available on the crimes and the victims. Analysis of the genesis of the crime, and in particular of its motivation, therefore depends on the documentation available and on its degree of reliability. Some indications, which are based on indirect inferences drawn from hard data, will have a higher validity than others which are based on direct analysis of motives. We have assembled all this information in the hope that it may provide some clues as to which victims are particularly at risk at the hands of the offenders.

Von Hentig (1948) has already pointed out in regard to the crime of murder that in many cases the offender-victim relationships are more informative than the offenders alone, and in a later review of the same theme (1956) he recommended that one should speak not of motives for murder but of murder situations in which such offender-victim relations could be more concretely understood. We shall accordingly concern ourselves in the first instance with objective relationships, such as kinship and partnership, using these as a basis of interpretation (von Hentig, 1948).

A further question investigated was the contributory effect of other factors on the mental state of the offender: for example the effect of alcohol, of previous quarrelling, of sexual acts such as rape on the part of mental defectives, and other similar circumstances directly associated with the criminal act itself.

Another associated and very difficult problem was that of determining whether the mentally abnormal offenders were reacting to an unfore-
seeable 'short-circuit' or brain-storm arising explosively without any
recognisable warning from an undefined pressure (for example from an epileptic
disorder) or whether they were deliberately carrying out their attacks,
perhaps after lengthy preparation. Some of our patients - like Gaupp's paranoid murderer Wagner (see p. 7) - had worked for years on their homicidal
plans, motivated by fears of persecution or desire for revenge. They had a
precise concept of the purpose of their crime and its successful accomplishment
filled them with satisfaction. Others had committed the crime because they
were carried away in the heat of a belligerent quarrel with the victim or
because in a state of morbid despair they sought to kill themselves and their
families in a planned extended suicide.

In so far as the records contained details about motives for the
crimes, we were interested to see whether forms of motivation directly
associated with the illness, for example delusional jealousy or morbid
suspicion, suicidal thoughts in depressives, or delusional self-defence, were
more frequently advanced than motives which feature prominently in homicide
by the mentally normal, such as money (murder in the course of robbery),
concealment of punishable offences, removal of persons who are a burden, or
revenge for real wrongs. More or less reliable explanations could be found
in only a few cases, for example when the motive was part of the act itself,
as in the extended suicide of depressed patients.

In the sections which follow we report the frequency with which
certain characteristics were found in the crimes of the cohort of mentally
abnormal offenders as a whole, after which we give the results of tests
carried out to determine whether there is a correlation between these features
and (1) the sex of the offender and (2) the diagnostic group to which the
offender belongs (schizophrenia, affective psychoses or mental deficiency).
Where it seems feasible and useful, we shall also make a comparison between
convicted violent offenders who are considered to be normal and mentally
abnormal violent offenders, in respect of characteristics both of the crime
and of the victim.

8.1 The crime: manner of committal and accompanying circumstances

Violent crimes ending in death: influence of sex and diagnosis
of the offender

In the review of general data given in Chapter 4 we included a

preliminary analysis of the sex of the offenders who had committed homicide
and other violent offences ending, or not ending, in death: 279 (52.3%) of the
533 abnormal offenders had killed at least one victim, while in 254 cases
(47.7%) the crime had not resulted in death.

Among those whose crimes had not resulted in death, there were in
all 19 patients whose assault had not caused permanent injury to the victim.
Analysis of these 19 offenders according to their illness and sex gives the
results shown in Table 61. While the sex distribution of these 19 cases
corresponds roughly to that of the 533 abnormal offenders as a whole, the
diagnoses which are associated with intellectual defect (mental deficiency and
dementia) are found in more than half the cases (10 out of 19) and are thus
over-represented. Presumably failure to accomplish the crime is more likely
in this group than among mentally abnormal persons with no intellectual defect.

Turning again to the analysis of violent crimes according to fatal
or non-fatal outcome, we find a significant difference in sex distribution
for those crimes which resulted in death: men were much more frequently found
to be dangerously aggressive than women (the ratio was 410 to 123 for the
total group of violent patients) but in women the crime resulted significantly
more often in the death of the victim (about 63.4% as against about 43%).
This result is at first sight surprising, since it runs counter to expectation. But the analysis of the three main diagnostic groups in Table 62 throws
light on the question.

A glance at these diagnostic differences suggests the special
position of the affective psychoses, where there is a preponderance of the
female sex and of crimes resulting in death. Most of the crimes involved acts

Table 61. *Diagnosis and sex of 19 violent patients who neither killed nor
seriously injured their chosen victim*

| | Sex | | |
Diagnosis	Male	Female	Total
Unclassifiable endogenous psychoses	1	0	1
Schizophrenias	5	3	8
Mental deficiency	4	1	5
Cerebral atrophy, dementia	3	0	3
Late-acquired cerebral damage	1	1	2
Total	14	5	19

Table 62. *Violent crimes resulting in death or not resulting in death, in three diagnostic groups of violent patients*

	Schizophrenia		Affective psychoses		Mental deficiency	
Crime	n	%	n	%	n	%
Not resulting in death	142	50	9	24	45	66
Resulting in death	142	50	28	76	23	34
Total	284	100	37	100	68	100

Significance test:	$\chi^2 =$	df = 1	$\alpha =$
Schizophrenia v. affective psychoses	7.663		0.01
Schizophrenia v. mental deficiency	5.134		0.025
Affective psychoses v. mental deficiency	15.169		0.001

of extended suicide and most of the victims were children. It does not, however, seem to us justifiable to conclude from this that the outcome of the crime is most likely to be fatal in depressed patients, since as we explained in Chapter 3 we have to take into account a possible error in our data: namely, the possibility that a considerable proportion of attempts by depressed mothers to kill their children are not reported or punished, even though they may well lead to psychiatric treatment.

At the same time the suicide rate for depressives, which is clearly higher than in other psychiatric diagnoses (Pokorny, 1964; Pöldinger, 1968; Ringel, 1969), indicates a greater potential for self-destruction in these patients, and where mothers have a very close symbiotic relationship with their children this can escalate into extended suicide.

In schizophrenics, who according to the psychiatric and forensic literature are supposed to be particularly dangerous (see Chapter 2), half of the violent crimes resulted in death of the victim, the corresponding figure for the mentally defective being only a third.

Methods employed

Just as the means used to commit suicide are limited (see review by Ringel, 1969), so there is only a certain number of ways of committing aggression against other persons, and the choice of method is, again as in suicide, governed by availability (e.g. of fire-arms), by sex-linked inclinations to certain methods, and also by the intelligence of the aggressor.

Table 63 shows that the great majority of offenders of both sexes use blunt and sharp instruments (mostly axes and knives); next comes strangulation or choking of the victim. In male offenders the third most common method is to apply brachial pressure, without the use of a weapon, and in female offenders it is the use of poison or gas. The clearest difference between the sexes lies in the use of poison or gas and in drowning of the victim, both being used much more often by women.

Since the schizophrenic offenders include a higher proportion of men than the group of abnormal offenders as a whole, the distribution of methods used by this diagnostic group is fairly much in line with that for all male offenders: blunt and sharp instruments head the list, along with strangulation and choking. The use of fire-arms by schizophrenics comes just ahead of their use of brachial pressure. Poisoning or gas was recorded in only five cases.

The methods most commonly used by offenders with affective psychoses, who were mostly women, were poisoning and drowning, which were used in the typical crime for this group, namely extended suicide.

So far as the mentally defective offenders are concerned, most assaults were made with blunt and sharp instruments, only one mental defective using a fire-arm. (This diagnostic group included the only case of neglect, or denial of care: an imbecile took a 3-year-old child, who had been playing

Table 63. *Methods of aggression used by 533 mentally abnormal offenders, related to the sex of the offender*

Method of aggression	Male		Female		Whole group	
	n	%	n	%	n	%
Brachial pressure	30	7.3	8	6.5	38	7.1
Strangulation, choking	60	14.6	24	19.5	84	15.8
Blunt and sharp instruments	265	64.6	42	34.2	307	57.5
Fire-arms	26	6.4	3	2.4	29	5.4
Poison, gas	8	2.0	21	17.1	29	5.4
Drowning	1	0.2	17	13.8	18	3.5
Starvation, denial of care	1	0.2	0	−	1	0.2
Combination of two or more of the above	15	3.7	2	1.6	17	3.2
Other	4	1.0	6	4.9	10	1.9
Total	410	100.0	123	100.0	533	100.0

with his portable radio, for a walk. After a few hours he came back but had left the child behind, alone, although it was completely exhausted and crying. The child died during the night from cold.)

From time to time one still finds reports in the press which fit in with the earlier prejudices we have mentioned about the unpredictable aggressiveness of the mentally ill and which suggest that violent crimes by the mentally abnormal are marked by particular brutality and ferocity: some previous investigators have, however, been unable to confirm this (e.g. East, Gibbens & West, who compared the methods used by sane and insane murderers). We had included in our data sheet a question about 'particular savageness' in carrying out the crime (e.g. sadistic torturing or gruesome mutilation of the victim, skulls brutally smashed in), but we found that an answer could be given for only 65 of our 533 offenders, that is to say in 12.2% of the cases; and even so the answers admittedly depended very much on the attitude of the two investigators.

Suicide and attempted suicide by the offender in association with the crime

From the outset it was to be expected that we would find an association between violence against others and violence against the self, especially in the form of extended suicide by depressed patients. In addition to such behaviour, we also recorded suicidal acts which in intent and execution arose from the crime, no matter what the motivation was (remorse, fear of punishment, 'short-circuit' reaction, etc.).

In the light of what was said in section 5.4, it could be assumed that there would be marked differences between the sexes in regard to this item. As Table 64 shows, suicidal behaviour associated with the crime occurred in almost a quarter (23.5%) of the cases. Suicidal impulses arising at the time of or after the crime were recorded with almost the same frequency in both sexes, while the planned aggression of extended suicide was found significantly more often in women than in men (38.1 as against 6.2%). The diagnostic differences confirm the association discussed above between extended suicide and depressive symptomatology.

An analysis by diagnostic group (Table 65) confirms extended suicide as the typical violent crime of the affective psychoses or, to put it more precisely, of the depressions. Suicidal thoughts accompany also other aggressive acts against third parties in a large number of cases: only in

Table 64. *Suicide and extended suicide (including attempts) by 533 abnormal offenders as an adjunct to the crime*

	Male		Female		Whole group	
	n	%	*n*	%	*n*	%
No suicidal behaviour	337	83.2	63	53.4	400	76.5
Suicide after the crime (incl. attempts)	43	10.6	10	8.5	53	10.1
Extended suicide (incl. attempts)	25	6.2	45	38.1	70	13.4
Subtotal	405	100.0	118	100.0	523	100.0
Not known	5		5		10	
Total	410		123		533	

Significance test: $\chi^2 = 80.785$ df = 2 $\alpha = 0.001$

Table 65. *Suicide and extended suicide (including attempts) as an adjunct of the crime in three diagnostic groups of violent patients*

	Schizophrenia		Affective psychoses		Mental deficiency	
	n	%	*n*	%	*n*	%
No suicidal behaviour	232	82.6	9	26	61	91
Suicide after the crime (incl. attempts)	27	9.6	5	14	4	6
Extended suicide (incl. attempts)	22	7.8	21	60	2	3
Subtotal	281	100.0	35	100	67	100
Not known	3		2		1	
Total	284		37		68	

Significance test: $\chi^2 =$ df = 1 $\alpha =$

	χ^2	α
Schizophrenia v. affective psychoses	52.470	0.001
Schizophrenia v. mental deficiency	2.323	Null hypothesis not refutable
Affective psychoses v. mental deficiency	42.591	0.001

9 out of 35 cases in this diagnostic group was there no mention of suicidal impulses.

Conversely, all forms of serious violence, irrespective of whether this was directed against the self or against others, seem often to be followed by or associated with depression: West (1965), in a retrospective study of the incidence of murder followed by suicide carried out in Great Britain, compared two groups each comprising 148 murderers from London and its outskirts (from the years 1946 to 1962). One group (the 'murder-suicide sample') had committed suicide shortly after the crime and before being brought to trial, while the other (the 'murder sample') had been convicted of murder and had not committed suicide. In both samples the proportion of insane offenders (in the sense that they could be said to be not responsible or to have only diminished responsibility) was about 50%, but the illnesses from which they suffered were clearly different in the two groups, especially so far as the men were concerned. For the murder sample West does not give diagnostic tables; but in a carefully investigated subgroup of 78 offenders from the murder-suicide sample, 33 were found to be 'relatively normal', 28 depressed, 4 schizophrenic, 2 morbidly jealous, 4 psychopathic and 7 neurotic. After discussing forensic and psychiatric findings from the Institution for the Criminally Insane at Broadmoor, West concludes that the diagnosis of 'psychotic depression' applies to the majority of the mentally abnormal murder-suicide group, but is also found 'very frequently' in the murder group.

In our study violent crimes by schizophrenics were much less often accompanied by suicide (17.4% of cases), while homicidal acts which were planned to include the killer's own death were a more prominent feature (about 8%) in the schizophrenics than in the group as a whole.

At the bottom of the diagnostic list come the mentally defective offenders, with mention of suicidal behaviour in only 6 out of 68 cases; extended or attempted suicide played a very subordinate role, featuring in only 2 cases.

Sexual activity associated with the crime

In section 7.5 (p.195) we discussed the significance of threatened separation from the intimate partner and presented a case history (case no. 417) in which fear of separation and rage at being slighted changed a tender sexual approach to violent aggressiveness that ended in the girl's death. The association of sexuality and violence is, however, also found in psychological situations of a different complexion: some of our more severely handicapped mental defectives combined sexual interference with children with sadistic acts, injuring or killing them in sexual lust or 'in order to see how the blood flows', or also perhaps to satisfy a perverse curiosity which was not held in check by any capacity for sympathetic understanding of the victim or by any ethically motivated self-control.

There is a widespread and uneasy notion that the mentally abnormal may be driven to homicidal acts by uncontrolled sexual desires and perversions. The figure of the 'sex murderer' and 'instinct-driven killer' is frequently combined with the concept of the mentally ill and the 'abnormal' individual in one and the same'stereotype. For this reason it seemed useful to determine how often the violent crimes of our patients were accompanied

Table 66. *Crime and accompanying sexual activity in 533 abnormal offenders*

Crime	Men		Women		Whole group	
	n	%	*n*	%	*n*	%
No accompanying sexual activity	375	91.5	123	100.0	498	93.4
With accompanying sexual activity	35	8.5	0	–	35	6.6
Total	410	100.0	123	100.0	533	100.0

Significance test: $\chi^2 = 331.88$ df = 1 $\alpha = 0.001$

Table 67. *Crime and accompanying sexual activity in three diagnostic groups of violent patients*

Crime	Schizophrenia		Affective psychoses		Mental deficiency	
	n	%	*n*	%	*n*	%
No accompanying sexual activity	269	94.7	37	100	52	77
With accompanying sexual activity	15	5.3	0	–	16	23
Total	284	100.0	37	100	68	100

Significance test:

Schizophrenia v. mental deficiency $\chi^2 = 20.531$ df = 1 $\alpha = 0.001$

(No test could be carried out for the manic-depressive group because the values expected were too small.)

by sexual activity and which patients were most often involved.

Tables 66 and 67 show that accompanying sexual acts were found only in male offenders, and only in 35 cases (8.5%) of all diagnoses. They occurred most frequently in the mentally defective offenders (in a quarter of the cases). In those instances in which children were sexually assaulted it was our impression that it was not the sadistic element which played the chief part in triggering the crime but often the primitive idea of 'undoing' the sexual assault or concealing it by removing the most important witness.

The following case illustrates both motivational aspects: fear of punishment after rape and the association since puberty of sexual and aggressive drives and tensions in a middle-grade mental defective.

Case no. 415

S., a casual worker, born in 1938, grew up in a disturbed home. His father, who ran a small carrier's business, drank a lot and the marital relationship was bad. Because of considerable learning difficulties, S. left school after the third year; his work capacity was below average but he earned some money as a casual worker. His personality soon made him conspicuous and he got into trouble with the law because of his unbridled behaviour. Although he was normally good-natured and quiet, he could not stand any kind of contradiction. He would flare up in rage and occasionally grabbed hold of a knife. By the age of 13 he was already assaulting little girls violently. At 15 he attacked a 12-year-old girl with a pocket knife, 'in order to frighten her'. At 19 he tied a girl of the same age to a tree in the wood and cut her with a knife, for which he received a sentence of 1 year's juvenile detention.

In the summer of 1960, three weeks before the crime, he married a woman 15 years older than himself, with six illegitimate children, and moved in with his parents-in-law. His wife reported that she found him extraordinary because during the first few nights after the wedding he had seized her 'playfully' by the throat. She had also noticed his love of gruesome fantasies: before going to sleep he often told her primitive horror stories about women being raped and slashed with knives. The couple had daily sexual intercourse.

On 16 August 1960 S., under the pretext that he was an underground worker and had to take measurements, occupied himself down a manhole in the street. He got to know a 9-year-old girl who was watching him at work. Looking up from the shaft he became sexually excited by the sight of the girl's underwear and decided to take her

somewhere on his moped and assault her. By offering to take her to a
milk bar he persuaded the girl to get up behind him. He took her to
a lonely bit of woodland, tied her hands and tried to pull off her
clothes and get hold of her genitals. When she cried, he choked her
and finally attacked her throat with his pocket knife - he wanted to
kill her because she would later betray what he had done. Believing
that he had killed her, he left her lying and went away. The girl was
later able to drag herself on to the road and was saved.

Influence of alcohol

At the beginning of section 7.2 we examined the previous history
of the offenders, discussed in a preliminary way the relationship between
alcoholism[1] and violence, and tried to show, using case no. 480 as an
example, how alcohol may possibly induce an epileptic twilight state which
in turn discharges itself in violent crime. From many other case histories,
particularly among the men, we gained the impression that alcohol might by
virtue of its stimulating and disinhibiting effect cause aggressive tensions
to be discharged in an act of violence, in a way that is known to happen
also in the mentally normal. We turn now to the question of possible differences
between the diagnostic groups in this respect.

(We had originally included general items about 'clouding of
consciousness' at the time of the crime and about confusion or disorientation
induced by drugs or by organic cerebral disorders. A total of 421 offenders
were reported as showing no signs of toxic or organic disturbances of
consciousness, as against 111 in whom such impairment was present and 90 of
whose records contained mention of alcohol. Our present test is therefore
limited to the effect of alcohol only, other drugs such as hallucinogens or
opiates being of no significance during the decade in question so far as the
mentally ill were concerned.)

Table 68 shows that alcohol plays virtually no part in female
violence; in the male group, however, it was mentioned in 21.5% of the cases.
Only 2 of the 37 depressed offenders were under the influence of alcohol at
the time of their crime (Table 69). For schizophrenics the proportion is of
much the same order (10.4%). But the mentally defective offenders were much
more frequently drunk at the time of their crime (19 out of 68 cases). This is
above the average for all diagnoses (17.4% for both sexes).

8.2 The victim

The sections which follow are concerned with the circle from which,
and the reasons for which, mentally abnormal violent offenders select their

victims. Are there demonstrable relationships between offenders and victims
which might throw light on certain causes of violence, or is it more often a
question of a psychosis or some otherwise disintegrated or defective mode of
experience which leads to a blind 'release of latent readiness to commit
murder' (Schipkowensky), i.e. to a senseless and irrelevant discharge of

Table 68. *Influence of alcohol on the crimes of 533 violent offenders*

	Men		Women		Whole group	
	n	%	n	%	n	%
No alcohol	318	78.5	117	97.5	435	82.9
Alcohol associated with the crime	87	21.5	3	2.5	90	17.1
Subtotal	405	100.0	120	100.0	525	100.0
Not known	5		3		8	
Total	410		123		533	

Significance test: $\chi^2 = 22.164$ df $= 1$ $\alpha = 0.001$

Table 69. *Influence of alcohol on the crimes of violent patients in three diagnostic groups*

	Schizophrenia		Affective psychoses		Mental deficiency	
	n	%	n	%	n	%
No alcohol	251	89.6	35	95	49	72
Alcohol associated with the crime	29	10.4	2	5	19	28
Subtotal	280	100.0	37	100	68	100
Not known	4		0		0	
Total	284		37		68	

Significance test: $\chi^2 =$ df $= 1$ $\alpha =$

		Null hypothesis
Schizophrenia v. affective psychoses	0.434	not refutable
Schizophrenia v. mental deficiency	12.787	0.001
Affective psychoses v. mental deficiency	6.263	0.025

pathological tensions? Sensational cases, such as the Volkhoven flamethrowing
in 1964, in which eight schoolchildren and two women teachers were killed,
may well foster the belief that aggressive mentally ill patients chiefly
commit blind attacks on those who happen to cross their path or, like the
Volkhoven attacker, discharge their morbid hate on randomly selected victims.

As the data given in Chapter 4 showed, 293 people in all were
killed by the 533 violent abnormal offenders in our study and 362 injured.
Only 19 (3.6% of all the offenders) attacked three or more victims, while
only 9 offenders (1.7%) killed three or more people. A crime such as that
which took place in Volkhoven is an extreme rarity. It was committed by a
mentally disturbed patient, and in ten years in a population of about 42.5
million people over the age of 14, happened only once in the GFR with this
degree of seriousness. Multiple murders by the mentally ill are thus
extremely rare.

Children or adults as victims

As a first step we determined whether our offenders differed in
sex or in diagnostic category in regard to their tendency to select adult or
child victims (children were defined as persons up to the age of 14).

In about 75% of all the crimes investigated by us, the victims
were adults; about 25% of the violent crimes were directed against children
(Table 70). As might be expected in view of the correlation between diagnosis
and sex (e.g. in the group of the affective psychoses), the choice of an
adult or child victim is influenced both by the sex of the offender and by
the form of his or her illness. About 64% of the women chose child victims
(usually their own children, as will be demonstrated below). Most of the men,
on the other hand (86%), attacked only adults, though in 14% of the cases

Table 70. *Children or adults as the victims of 533 mentally
abnormal offenders*

	Men		Women		Whole group	
Victims	*n*	%	*n*	%	*n*	%
Only adults	353	86.1	44	35.8	397	74.5
Children as well	57	13.9	79	64.2	136	25.5
Total	410	100.0	123	100.0	533	100.0

Significance test: $\chi^2 = 125.449$ df = 1 $\alpha = 0.001$

the victims were children.

The sex difference is seen also in the diagnoses (Table 71). In schizophrenia and mental deficiency, where most of the offenders were male, the victims were mainly adult, while in the affective psychoses, where the offenders were mostly female, the victims were mainly children.

Table 71. *Diagnostic differences in the choice of adult or child victims by mentally abnormal offenders*

	Schizophrenia		Affective psychoses		Mental deficiency	
Victims	n	%	n	%	n	%
Only adults	232	81.7	8	22	51	75
Children as well	53	18.3	29	78	17	25
Total	284	100.0	37	100	68	100

Significance test:	χ^2	df = 1	α =
Schizophrenia v. affective psychoses	59.464		0.001
Schizophrenia v. mental deficiency	1.163		Null hypothesis not refutable
Affective psychoses v. mental deficiency	25.609		0.001

Table 72. *Sex of adult victims of 533 mentally abnormal offenders*

	Men		Women		Whole group	
Victims	n	%	n	%	n	%
Male adult	139	42.9	23	52	162	44
Female adult	185	57.1	21	48	206	56
Subtotal	324	100.0	44	100	368	100
Multiple adult victims of both sexes	44		4		48	
Only children	42		75		117	
Total	410		123		533	

Significance test: χ^2 = 1.027   df = 1   Null hypothesis not refutable

Sex of adult victims

The next question of interest was whether the sex of the offender
was in any way related to the sex of the victim. As a sex-specific choice of
victim is most likely to be found when an adult person, e.g. the marital
partner, is attacked, we limited our test to adult victims only.

Where the attack was on adults, more than half of the victims,
both of the male and the female offenders, were of the opposite sex (Table 72).
The difference was not, however, significant.

In order to exclude the effect of diagnostic differences we carried
out on the schizophrenics only a further test of the relationship between sex
of the victim and sex of the offender. Without reproducing the figures we can
say that the results were the same as for the group as a whole: there was a
slight preference for victims of the opposite sex, and this was the same for
the male and for the female offenders. There was no point in carrying out a
similar comparison for the other diagnostic groups because of the different
sex distribution in the groups in question and also because in the case of
the affective psychoses the number of adult victims was so small.

The findings as regards victims given above may be summarised as
follows. Taking the 533 abnormal offenders as a whole, most of the men had
attacked adult victims, most of the women had attacked children. So far as

Table 73. *Victims (by age and sex) of 178 sane (convicted) murderers
(incl. attempted murder) by sex of the offender*

Victims (age and sex)	Men		Women		Whole group	
	n	%	n	%	n	%
Only adults	152	95.6	15	79	167	93.8
Only children	7	4.4	4	21	11	6.2
Adults and children	0	−	0	−	0	−
Total	159	100.0	19	100	178	100.0
Male victims	85	53.5	8	42	93	52.3
Female victims	66	41.5	9	47	75	42.1
Both sexes	8	5.0	2	11	10	5.6
Total	159	100.0	19	100	178	100.0

diagnosis was concerned, the depressed offenders chose mostly child victims,
a quarter of the mentally defective offenders also chose child victims, while
the schizophrenics were to a large extent representative of the group as a
whole in choosing mostly adult victims. In regard to the sex distribution of
the (adult) victims, both the male and the female offenders showed a slight
but not a significant preference for victims of the opposite sex, the ratio
being approximately the same in both cases. (No diagnostic differences could
be confirmed.)

It is naturally of great interest to compare these findings with
analogous data on the victims of mentally normal violent offenders. There are,
however, no statistics available for the decade in question which would make
an exact comparison possible. Fortunately a study does exist of a two-year
sample of convicted murderers which contains some analogous findings. Even
although this sample was not selected according to strictly comparable criteria
and is not representative of the group of offenders defined by our study, it
still provides a useful orientation so far as comparison with the mentally
abnormal offenders is concerned. The data in Table 73 are taken from the
Murder Statistics of 1959 and 1963 published by the Federal Statistical
Bureau, Wiesbaden;[2] they cover 178 offenders held to be fully responsible
for their actions who were convicted of murder and attempted murder, and
include also details about their victims.

No tests of significance could be carried out, because of the
unequal numbers involved, but comparison shows the following differences.
Unlike the abnormal offenders, the 'sane' offenders mainly attacked adults –
the men almost exclusively, the women in more than three-quarters of the cases.
The mentally abnormal male offenders tended more to choose children, while
the victims of the abnormal female offenders were predominantly children. This
finding can be explained to a certain extent by a difference in marital status:
the sane offenders were for the most part young single men, while a higher
percentage of the abnormal offenders were middle-aged and married. Moreover
factors associated with the illness and with the personality of the offenders
had an important influence upon the choice of victim, particularly in the
depressive psychoses where the commonest crime was extended suicide, which of
course did not feature much among sane offenders.

Turning to the sex distribution of the victims of the sane
offenders, we see that the slight preference for the opposite sex which we
found in the abnormal offenders is not here confirmed: the male murderers

more frequently attacked men, the women more frequently women. Here again the
difference in marital status may be responsible: a high percentage of the
abnormal offenders chose marital partners as victims, morbidly distorted
emotions, such as delusional jealousy, often playing a part, within the setting of family relationships, in motivating the crime. So far as the dynamics
of the crime are concerned, the sane offenders are, on the other hand, clearly
influenced more by relationships and motives that lie outside the family (see
also in section 8.3).

The section which follows deals with the relationships recorded
as existing between offenders and victims at the time of the crime, study of
which may throw light on the choice of victim and the genesis of the crime.

Relationship between offenders and victims

In section 7.5 we tried to determine the social situation of the
offenders during the six months preceding the crime and to establish the
circles from which their personal contacts came. We hoped thereby to assemble
preliminary clues which might help to explain the motivation of the crime in
terms of the external circumstances and social relationships of the offender.
For example, the offenders had more frequently lived in conflict with their
marital partners and their relationships with colleagues, superiors and
neighbours had likewise shown more conflict than those of the non-violent
patients in the control group.

It was clear to us from the outset that one methodologically
acceptable way of studying motivation was to enquire further into the choice
of victim and the relationship between victim and offender: the first stages
of this enquiry have already been reported in the sections on the age and sex
of the victims. In the light of these findings it was to be expected that the
victims would have been selected from within a certain circle, perhaps from
intimate partnerships. In order to classify more precisely this circle or
these individuals, we divided them according to the kind of tie which linked
them to the offenders at the time of the crime:

1. *Strangers,* by which term we understood such victims as
   were personally unknown to the offender before the crime
   and represented for him anonymous strangers.
2. *Persons in authority.* Starting with the observation that
   conflicts with authority often played a part, particularly
   in the case of schizophrenic violent offenders, we included
   here those victims who because of their professional role
   were seen by the offenders as persons in authority. They

included employers or overseers, policemen, judges, lawyers,
doctors, directors of institutions, etc., irrespective of
whether they were known personally to the offender or not.

3. *Friends and acquaintances,* that is to say persons with whom
the offender had a more or less casual relationship: e.g.
neighbours, fellow inmates of a home or institution,
colleagues at work and so on.

4. *Parents and siblings* (including adoptive and foster parents).

5. *Marital and other intimate partners,* 'intimate partners'
being taken to mean persons with whom the offender had a
sexual relationship.

6. *Own children.*

7. *Own children and marital partner.* We introduced this class
in order to find out how often 'family tragedies' (so-called
family murders in the sense of Muralt, Näcke and Jacobi)
were recorded in our sample of offenders.

Our first task was to look again at sex differences between the
offenders in regard to choice of victim (Table 74). Most of the victims of
the abnormal violent offenders were chosen from the intimate circle, that is
to say from those with whom the offender had close family ties or intimate
partner relationships; only about 30% of the group as a whole attacked persons
who were not so close to them, and only in 9% of the cases was the victim
unknown to the violent offender (for example a passer-by).

Other authors have also found that relatives and intimate
partners are particularly at risk: Lanzkron (1963) reported that out of 157
victims of his 150 mentally abnormal murderers 73, or 47%, were members of
their families: 27% of all the victims were wives, 19% husbands. The Indian
investigators Varma & Iha (1966) reported figures for victims as high as 75%
marital partners and members of family (27.8% wives, 0.58% husbands), which
presumably is partly governed by the cultural factor of a society oriented
towards large families. Mowat (1966) quotes the comparison shown in Table 75
of the victims of 200 sane and 300 insane murderers, collected by East &
Fullerton from Broadmoor. In this cohort the insane murderers attacked their
wives much more frequently than did the sane, but attacked strangers much more
rarely. The study mentioned earlier of German murders in the years 1959 and
1963 (Federal Statistical Bureau, Wiesbaden) also gives some analogous figures
covering the relationship between 178 sane murderers and their victims (Table 76).
These percentages, like the data quoted from Broadmoor for the sane offenders,
show a preference for victims from the area of secondary relationships. A murderous

assault on relatives, marriage partners or children occurred in only a fifth
of all cases in the group as a whole: only the female offenders attacked
nearly as many persons from the immediate family as from the area of secondary
relationships, though of course the numbers here are very small. When we
compare the figures with those for abnormal offenders, we find that a strikingly
higher percentage of sane male offenders attacked persons in authority,

Table 74. *Relationship between 533 mentally abnormal violent offenders
and their victims, by sex of the offender*

Classification of victim	Men		Women		Whole group	
	n	%	n	%	n	%
1. Strangers	47	11.5	1	0.8	48	9.0
2. Persons in authority	34	8.5	5	4.1	39	7.3
3. Friends and acquaintances	115	28.0	10	8.1	125	23.4
4. Parents, siblings	80	19.3	14	11.4	94	17.6
5. Marital and other intimate partners	103	25.1	15	12.2	118	22.3
6. Own children	20	4.9	76	61.8	96	18.0
7. Children and marriage partner	11	2.7	2	1.6	13	2.4
Total	410	100.0	123	100.0	533	100.0

Significance test: $\chi^2 = 211.586$ df = 6 $\alpha = 0.001$

Table 75. *Relationship between victims and offenders
in 200 sane and 300 insane murders, in relative
percentages*

Classification of victim	Sane (%)	Insane (%)
Stranger	17.0	7.3
Acquaintance or friend	21.0	32.3
Lover	16.5	3.6
Wife	17.0	29.3
Girlfriend	15.5	5.3
Other relationship	16.0	32.6

particularly policemen (about 17% as against 8.5% for the mentally abnormal
male offenders).

Turning again to our cohort of mentally abnormal offenders, we
see that the female offenders in this group also chose their victims much
more often from the intimate circle (87%) than did the sane female offenders,
the victims in the most cases (62%) being their own children. Only one woman
attacked a complete stranger. Diagnostically, too, she was exceptional, being
a patient suffering from acute mania who at a beer festival hit the person
sitting next to her on the head with a beer measure.

The abnormal male offenders, on the other hand, directed their
violent attacks almost as frequently outside the intimate circle, and in 11%
of cases their victims were total strangers. In so far as they did attack
members of their families (52% of all male offenders), the victims were in
about half of the cases marital partners.

The circle composed of friends, acquaintances and colleagues
claimed a high proportion of victims, particularly where the male offenders
were concerned (28% in our study), while for the sane offenders this group of
victims reached a much higher percentage, coming in fact at the top of the
list; in female offenders the ratio was much less, at 8%.

Table 76. *Class of victim and sex of offender for 178 sane (convicted)*
murderers (incl. attempted murder)

Classification of victim	Men		Women		Whole group	
	n	%	n	%	n	%
Stranger	30	20.0	3	16	33	19.5
Person in authority [a]	26	17.3	0	–	26	15.4
Acquaintance	69	46.0	8	42	77	45.6
Acquaintance and relation	1	0.7	0	–	1	0.6
Relation, marital partner, children	24	16.0	8	42	32	18.9
Subtotal	150	100.0	19	100	169	100.0
Not known	9		0		9	
Total	159		19		178	

[a] These were exclusively policemen or penal officers.

Contrary to expectation, the percentage of persons in authority
who were attacked was very small, about 7% in the group as a whole, which was
lower than the figure for the sane offenders: there was also less sex differentiation here than we had first supposed.

Table 77, with its statistical test results, shows that the choice
of victim is also clearly influenced by the form of illness. This is particularly
marked in the case of patients with affective psychoses, who chose their victims
almost exclusively from within the intimate circle (35 out of 37 cases). The
result is influenced by the fact that 29 of the 37 offenders were women (they
are of course not identical with the 29 depressed patients who attacked their
children).

Table 77. *Diagnostic differences in the choice of victim by 533
mentally abnormal offenders, by relationship to victim*

Classification of victim	Schizo-phrenia		Affective psychoses		Mental deficiency	
	n	%	*n*	%	*n*	%
1. Stranger	24	8.5	1	3	17	25
2. Person in authority	31	10.9	-	-	3	4
3. Acquaintance or friend	64	22.5	1	3	27	40
4. Parents, siblings	63	22.2	1	3	6	9
5. Marital and other intimate partners	64	22.5	4	10	12	18
6. Own children	35	12.3	29	78	3	4
7. Children and marital partners	3	1.1	1	3	-	-
Total	284	100.0	37	100	68	100
Victim from outside the intimate circle	119	41.9	2	5	47	69
Victim from within the intimate circle	165	58.1	35	95	21	31
Total	284	100.0	37	100	68	100

Significance test:	$\chi^2 =$	df =	$\alpha =$
Schizophrenia v. affective psychoses	17.044	1	0.001
Schizophrenia v. mental deficiency	15.234	1	0.001
Affective psychoses v. mental deficiency	36.563	1	0.001

As already mentioned, extended suicide emerges as the typical crime
in our group of depressed offenders. This is in line with the findings of
other authors. Hopwood (1927), studying a large sample of offenders from
Broadmoor, found that depressive syndromes were particularly common among
166 women who had killed their babies (defined as murder before the end of
the lactation period), while in 60% of the cases suicidal thoughts were at
the root of the decision to commit the crime.

West (1965) carried out a careful study of 78 murderers who
committed suicide before final judgement was passed on them and who included
39 cases of serious mental illness, among them 21 depressed women. His
statistical analysis of this murder-suicide sample included 60 women of whom
55 had killed their children or their husband and children, and he emphasised
the great frequency of depressive conditions.

A symbiotic tie between parent and child is experienced in
particular by the mother and is strongest in the period immediately following
the birth: it is probably less marked in the father and it is therefore
understandable that depressed fathers - when they do commit extended suicide -
more commonly not only involve their children but include the whole family
in their own death (Zumpe, Langelüddeke, Popella, Resnick). But it seems to
us that an equally important aspect of motivation for extended suicide lies
in the fact that in our culture the mother feels responsible first and foremost for her children, while the father feels responsible for both wife and
children. If a depressed patient feels unable to discharge his responsibility,
and if his delusional fears of destruction are extended to include everyone
who should be in his care, then the danger of extended suicide applies also
to all those whom he sees as directly dependent on him and directly threatened by the same disaster. In the case of a woman this tends to mean her
children, and in the case of a man his wife and then the children. In fact
about two-thirds of the female patients, but only 7.8% of the male patients,
had directed their violent attacks against their children. The men had more
frequently included their wives in their extended suicide. The percentage of
men who had attacked the whole family (children and partner) was only minimal
(2.7%) and not significantly higher than the corresponding figure of 1.0% for
the women.

The victims chosen by our schizophrenic offenders came in 58% of
the cases from their intimate circle, parents and siblings being somewhat
more frequently represented here than in the group as a whole (22.2% as
against 17.6%). This is not surprising, since according to the findings of
family psychiatric research (see in section 7.5), bad relationships within

the family (for example strong emotional tension) are frequently encountered in the primary family, that is to say in the patient's dealings with his parents and siblings, and may often even contribute to the outbreak of the psychosis.

Schipkowensky (1938) found that 10 of the 15 offenders who were clinically rated as schizophrenic and whom he described in detail in his book *Schizophrenie und Mord (Schizophrenia and Murder)* had attacked members of their intimate circle. The same applied to 6 of the 11 delusional murderers whose case histories were presented by Brandt in 1948 and who suffered mainly from schizophrenic psychoses.

Nevertheless the proportion of victims from outside the intimate circle who were attacked by our schizophrenic offenders stood at almost 42%, which was considerably above the corresponding figure for depressives. They showed a slightly greater tendency than the group as a whole to attack persons in authority (10.9% as against 7.3% for the whole group): this may be connected with the tendency already mentioned for relationships with parents to be full of tension, since it might be the expression of a transference to other 'father figures' of feelings originally experienced towards the father. The somewhat higher percentage of similar victims chosen by the sane offenders, however, which is presumably associated with motives such as ensuring one's escape by killing a policeman, is a warning that this interpretation should be viewed with critical scepticism. In Wilmanns' case studies (1940) of 26 murderers and other violent offenders who were schizophrenic or at least were considered by the author to be schizophrenic, the victims in 11 instances were strangers of whom 8 were persons in authority (almost all political crimes); in another 11 instances the victims came from the intimate circle. We cannot, however, use this material as a basis of comparison: there was much bias in its collection and in some cases there are doubts about the diagnosis, at least at the time of the crime.

We must, however, give serious consideration to the possibility that delusional schizophrenics, who tend to project their own feelings, may have a warped view even of complete strangers, because of the distortion of their own experiences or because of their morbid fancies, seeing them, for example, as objects of their projected hatred. The following case may serve to illustrate what we have in mind:

Case no. 337

A 26-year-old student, born into a family of teachers with a marked history of schizophrenia and other mental illnesses, interrupted his course in electrical technology, entered a Jesuit

college and then developed acute schizophrenia with anxiety and
delusions of reference. In later psychotic attacks his delusional
ideas centred round his father whom in his hallucinations he saw
as God the Father. He believed that the direction his further
studies should take depended on an audience with the Pope, whose
gestures (he had been able to see him from a distance when he visited
Rome) he had interpreted as a command to return to the Technical
High School.

Shortly after resuming his studies he had another
delusional episode in which he took a train south from the place
at which he was studying, with the vague intention of travelling
again to Rome. On the way there he left the train, hired a taxi and
asked to be taken to the Black Forest, where his parents lived. Half-
way there he became very restless and asked the driver to increase
his speed because he felt he was being followed by the car behind.
In a sudden state of panic he fell upon the taxi driver, beside whom
he was sitting, and tried to strangle him. The driver was able to
stop the car and fetch help.

When asked in the clinic about his motive for attacking
the driver he described his anxious and delusional certainty that
the Devil himself was sitting at the wheel of the car and that it
was a matter of life and death. At the same time he had experienced
a conviction that his father, whom he was on the way to visit, was
dead.

There were no details in the records that might shed further light
on the motivation of this patient, who committed suicide a short time
afterwards in the psychiatric hospital, but his case suggests that the
attack on the completely unknown taxi driver was closely connected with
the patient's delusions about his father.

The most marked tendency to attack persons outside the family
and the intimate circle is found in the mentally defective offenders, of
whom more than a third (27 out of 68) attacked acquaintances, fellow-
inmates or neighbours, while a quarter (17 out of 68) made violent assaults
on complete strangers. In spite of (or perhaps because of?) their subordinate social situation, they were less liable than the schizophrenics to
attack persons in authority (only 3 out of 68 cases), although one might
have expected them to have many opportunities for conflict in their dealings
with such persons as their superiors at work, the directors of institutions,
or the police.

Their inability to come to terms with society outside the family is correlated with their origins - the mentally defective offenders frequently came from very seriously disturbed primary families (almost half of them were from broken homes) - and with their antisocial personality traits, which were significantly more prominent in this than in the other diagnostic groups (48 out of 65 cases).

8.3 The offender's view: subjective antecedents of the crime

So far we have tried to analyse and interpret the crime-victim relationship according to more or less objective features such as the place, the method, the number of victims, and obvious ties between the offender and his victim. In what follows now we shall concern ourselves exclusively with the offender and the subjective forms of experience associated with the crime.

We were interested in the entire complex of motivation and inner genesis of the crime. Was it planned in advance or did it occur on impulse after a quarrel or even with no obvious cause? Had the victim played a special, perhaps delusionally governed role in the offender's inner experience? Which motives were advanced by the offender himself when he was first questioned?

It is important to remember that every interpretation of these 'soft' data, which had already been subjected to the distorting judgements of the original assessors and affected by the methods of enquiry used, must be more problematic than analogous interpretations of the 'hard' items which we have so far discussed.

Impulsive or planned violence

Dramatic case studies in the literature suggested that it would be worth finding out how often mentally abnormal offenders make long-term plans for carrying out their violent crimes. One has only to recall the delusional mass-murderer Wagner (Gaupp) or Volkhoven flamethrower who attacked the schoolhouse (Kiehne) and who is included in our sample: both had spent months or years developing plans for their attack. It is also of interest to determine whether this kind of planning and preparation is more common in certain illnesses, say in delusional schizophrenia.

Our first task was to examine differences between the sexes (Table 78). The most striking finding here is that the proportion of female offenders who planned their crime is considerably higher (about 64.5%) than

the corresponding proportion of male offenders (43.5%): planning with intent
to kill predominated in the female group. Looking at the cohort as a whole,
about half the crimes were recorded as being planned in advance, while in
more than a quarter of the cases the act seemed to be committed impulsively,
without any recognisable cause.

One must, however, ask whether a certain amount of bias may have
operated in these 'crimes without cause'. It is conceivable that where
overtly psychotic offenders are concerned, who are certain to be dealt with
under Section 51, para. 1, and who may not come to trial or whose prosecution does not call for serious effort, questions of motive and intent may
not be precisely elucidated, especially if the patient does not reveal his
thoughts. Many judges, examining authorities, and even psychiatrists, assume
that the behaviour of psychotic and particularly of schizophrenic patients is
not open to elucidation, since all understandable motivational aspects of the
crime will have been shattered by the 'senseless eruption' of the psychosis.
This may well account for the relatively high percentage of crimes regarded
as 'impulsive, with no apparent cause'.

Quarrels featured more frequently in male than in female offenders
as the immediate cause of violence. Even when the crime was planned, the men
did not 'mean it as seriously' as the women. Attacks which aimed at the death
of the victim (and did not fit into the category of 'teaching him a lesson' -

Table 78. *Sex distribution of impulsive and planned crimes of violence
in 533 mentally abnormal offenders*

Crime	Men		Women		Whole group	
	n	%	n	%	n	%
Impulsive, with no apparent cause	112	27.6	26	22.0	138	26.4
After a quarrel	117	28.9	16	13.6	133	25.4
Planned, but without intent to kill	44	10.9	5	4.2	49	9.4
Planned with intent to kill	132	32.6	71	60.2	203	38.8
Subtotal	405	100.0	118	100.0	523	100.0
Not known	5		5		10	
Total	410		123		533	

Significance test: $\chi^2 = 31.724$ df = 3 $\alpha = 0.001$

a concept which cropped up in many of the male offenders' own accounts of the
crime) occurred in 60% of the women but only in 32% of the men.

Looking back to the section at the beginning of this chapter, on
violence resulting in death, we find that from the statistical point of view
the number of fatal results in women corresponds roughly to their intentions,
while assaults committed by men often have a worse outcome than they allegedly
intended.

It can be seen from Table 79 that the violent crimes of depressed
patients are predominantly planned and prepared in advance and are intended
to end in death. Only in 9 out of 35 cases were the crimes of depressed
offenders recorded as unplanned. About 47% of the violent crimes of schizophrenics were reported as having been planned, and most of these (38% of all
the schizophrenic crimes) were intended to end in death. About 53% of the
attacks were unplanned, and of these half arose from a quarrel; in the remaining cases no cause could be ascertained from the patient's records.

Of the three diagnostic groups studied, the mental defectives had
the smallest proportion of crimes planned to end in death (17 out of 67 cases).

Table 79. *Diagnostic differences in impulsive and planned crimes of
violence by the mentally abnormal*

Crime	Schizo-phrenia		Affective psychoses		Mental deficiency	
	n	%	*n*	%	*n*	%
Impulsive, with no apparent cause	73	26.2	7	20	22	33
After a quarrel	74	26.5	2	6	20	30
Planned, but without intent to kill	26	9.3	0	–	8	12
Planned with intent to kill	106	38.0	26	74	17	25
Subtotal	279	100.0	35	100	67	100
Not known	5		2		1	
Total	284		37		68	

Significance test:	χ^2 =	df =	α =
Schizophrenia v. affective psychoses	10.524	2	0.01
Schizophrenia v. mental deficiency	3.894	3	Null hypothesis not refutable
Affective psychoses v. mental deficiency	13.827	2	0.001

Two-thirds of the violent crimes were unplanned; this is a somewhat higher rate than that of the schizophrenics, though the difference is not significant. In interpreting this finding we must bear in mind that mental defectives are, because of their lack of intelligence, less often in a position to anticipate their actions than are those with normal intellectual endowments. They may also be subject to more frequent aggressive mood disorders and unrestrained sexual impulses that are more or less beyond their control and can often end in sudden bursts of violence.

Delusional relationships with the victim

Apart from objective relationships based on kinship or marriage or associated with home or work, many of our offenders also described strong emotional ties between themselves and their victims, which often arose without any real communication between the two and were built on a purely intrapsychic and delusional foundation. Since in severe psychoses one often finds forms of communication that have little or no basis in reality, it seemed probable that the relationships between our mentally abnormal offenders and their victims might, particularly in the case of the schizophrenics, often be similarly distorted by powerful emotions or transformed by delusions.

Analysis of the records showed that many offender-victim relationships which seemed to the outside observer to be ordinary and even free from tension, had in fact often been severely and pathologically 'loaded' before the crime by the patient's paranoid ideas. Gestures or remarks made by the

Table 80. *Frequency of delusional relationships between mentally abnormal offenders and their victims*

	Men		Women		Whole group	
	n	%	*n*	%	*n*	%
No delusional relationship	198	50.1	51	43.2	249	50.5
Delusional relationship with victim	197	49.9	67	56.8	264	49.5
Subtotal	395	100.0	118	100.0	513	100.0
Not known	15		5		20	
Total	410		123		533	

Significance test: $\chi^2 = 1.469$ df = 1   Null hypothesis not refutable

victim, which to a normal person would be of no consequence, had provided many delusional patients with 'proof' of dangerous enmity or threats, against which they believed they had to assert themselves, either in revenge or in self-defence. This delusional relationship could also make the patient his potential victim as someone who shared an imaginary danger (for example depressed mothers might believe a child was threatened by an incurable illness or inescapable misery and had to be 'released' in shared death).

As Table 80 shows, in half of the cases it was recorded that the offender's attitude to the victim was distorted by an inner experience that was not based or not fully based on reality, in other words by delusional misinterpretation of existing or imagined relationships. The distribution of delusional relationships with the victim was the same for both sexes.

Since the mixture of diagnoses in the group as a whole makes it an unsuitable sample on which to base predictions about delusional relationships, we carried out another test on sex differences in the schizophrenics alone (Table 81). As we had assumed, violent schizophrenics selected their victims predominantly under the influence of delusional relationships, which in turn were to a significant extent based on delusions of enmity.

While half of the entire group of mentally abnormal offenders were recorded as having delusional relationships with their victims, this proportion rose in the schizophrenic subgroup to 68%, while in the affective psychoses it amounted to two-fifths of the cases. In the mentally deficient offenders, however, delusional relationships played no part at all.

The frequency of delusional relationships to the victim was about the same for schizophrenic men and women. But the nature of the relationship was very different in the two sexes: around three-quarters of the schizophrenic men saw their victims as enemies (predominant motive: revenge and self-defence, see section 7.3, (pp. 133-41), while this applied to less than half of the delusional schizophrenic women. Most of the women had 'other delusional relationships' with their victim. The following is an example of the form these tended to take:

Case no.334

L.F., aged 40 at the time of her crime. She was born in 1916, the illegitimate daughter of a factory worker in Central Germany, and was brought up in institutions. There was nothing in her case notes to suggest psychiatric illness in her blood relations.

She finished school in the eighth grade and worked unobtrusively until the age of 19 in a children's home in her native town. In 1935 she had her first schizophrenic attack but after two

Table 81. *Diagnostic differences in data about delusional relationships between mentally abnormal violent offenders and their victims*

	Schizo- phrenia		Affective psychoses		Mental deficiency	
	n	%	n	%	n	%
No delusional relationship	82	31.7	21	60	68	100
Delusional relationship with victim	177	68.3	14	40	0	-
Subtotal	259	100.0	35	100	68	100
Not known	25		2		0	
Total	284		37		68	

Significance test:

Schizophrenia v. affective psychoses $\chi^2 = 9.671$ df = 1 $\alpha = 0.01$

(a) Sex differences in the delusional relationships of schizophrenic offenders with their victims

	Men		Women		Whole group	
	n	%	n	%	n	%
No delusional relationship	68	32.2	14	29	82	31.7
Delusional relationship with victim	143	67.8	34	71	177	68.3
Subtotal	211	100.0	48	100	259	100.0
Not known	21		4		25	
Total	232		52		284	

(b) Delusional threats experienced by schizophrenic offenders v. other delusional relationships to the victim (e.g. often 'a fellow-sufferer, also being persecuted')

	Men		Women		Whole group	
	n	%	n	%	n	%
Victim as delusional enemy	109	76.2	14	41	123	69.5
Other delusional relationships	34	23.8	20	59	54	30.5
Total	143	100.0	34	100	177	100.0

Significance tests on sex differences in schizophrenics:

	$\chi^2 =$	df = 1	$\alpha =$
Frequency of delusional relationships	0.057		. Null hypothesis not refutable
Delusional enemy	14.305		0.001

months' treatment in a university psychiatric clinic she was able to
resume work. The scanty information which was available from 1935 to
1942 provided no picture of her personality and behaviour.

In 1943 she married a gardener from the Sudetenland who
shortly afterwards was sent to the front. The first child of this
marriage, a daughter, was born in 1944.

While her husband was away, Frau F. began an extramarital
relationship which led to a breakdown in the marriage. For this reason
the husband did not return to his wife till 1953 - she had meantime
moved to south-west Germany and he, after being a prisoner of war,
had spent some years in the Foreign Legion. Finally, however, he
forgave her lapse and they lived together again as man and wife. A
second child, a son, was born in 1953. The husband worked as a porter,
and the wife earned extra money cleaning. In her absence her mother
looked after the children, to whom Frau F. was known to be very attached.

Her husband described her at that time as full of religious
ideas of purity and all kinds of reforms. He found the sexual relationship unsatisfactory because she was cold and frigid. Because of this,
she read a book shortly before the crime on 'Carezza' technique, but
she could not accept the suggestions made in it.

In November 1955 she again fell ill, experiencing feelings
of change and alienation and complaining about her fears of disaster
and about the 'dead, empty atmosphere' which surrounded her. Although
she belonged to the Evangelical Church she consulted the Catholic priest
and made her confession to him. In a distressing dream she saw her son
lying dead in the cellar and herself in prison. Finally she attempted
suicide by drinking benzene, but in spite of all this she was not given
psychiatric treatment. Her relationships with her family fluctuated
between lavish friendliness and withdrawal.

In February 1956 she thought she possessed 'God's holy
magnetism' and in the days preceding the crime she heard imperative
voices commanding her to kill her son. She felt that he was not blessed
by God because she had conceived him 'in horrible sin'; she had a
mission from God to sacrifice this child as atonement for her former
marital lapse.

On the day before the crime she dreamt of her grandmother
and saw her nodding her head. From this she understood that the grandmother approved of the proposed sacrifice. On the other hand, however,
she struggled inwardly against the final decision, but felt herself

more and more strongly under the pressure of menacing voices which
threatened her with physical tortures and all kinds of punishments
if she did not carry out their commands.

On Sunday morning, 26 February 1956, she carried her son,
under the pretext that she wanted to show him something nice, into the
coal cellar and strangled him there with a nylon stocking which she held
for several minutes bound tightly round his neck. The little boy smiled
before she did this, which made her certain that he too agreed he should
be sacrificed. She then carried the body to his cot and told her husband
his son was now dead and that she had done it in order to help the
husband. To the neighbours who were called in she said she should be
left in peace, she would appear before the Final Judgement. After the
crime she heard God's voice telling her 'You have done what was right'.

When detained for questioning she said that her 12-year-
old daughter Rosemary was also under an evil star and had 'pieces of
wood' in her spine. She was really her husband's mother, who had come
back to earth and always protected him in a mysterious way. She had to
remove her daughter's clitoris; she was driven by an inner threat to
new acts of violence.

In the psychiatric hospital she said that God had brought
the dead child to life again; he would return on a certain day, in
good health. She believed she could already feel the 'magnetic current'
which flowed through her and the body of the child.

Table 82. *Frequency of imperative voices ordering the offender to commit
the crime, in 284 violent schizophrenics*

	Men		Women		Whole group	
	n	%	n	%	n	%
No imperative voices	174	82.5	37	77	211	81.5
Imperative voices ordering the crime	37	17.5	11	23	48	18.5
Subtotal	211	100.0	48	100	259	100.0
Not known	21		4		25	
Total	232		52		284	

Significance test: $\chi^2 = 0.436$ df = 1   Null hypothesis not refutable

This example shows clearly the sacrificial motive which chiefly
drove her to kill her son. The crime also illustrates, however, the influence
of auditory hallucinations and commands (imperative voices) and we decided
to re-examine this statistically.

In section 7.3 (p.143), we stated that auditory hallucinations
had been part of the symptomatology of about 66% of all our violent schizophrenic offenders (172 out of 284 cases) and that in about 26% of these (45
out of the 172 cases) the hallucinations had taken the form of imperative
voices. Table 82 gives the result of our analysis of the frequency of imperative voices immediately associated with the crimes of all our schizophrenic
offenders. In both sexes, therefore, about a fifth of all the schizophrenic
offenders were under the influence of imperative voices at the time of the
crime. The difference is not significant.

Motives

In a retrospective enquiry the difficult question of motivation
can be answered only in very broad outline and even then not without some
falsification. The complicated motives which drove them are not always clear
even to the mentally ill offenders themselves and have moreover been influenced
and distorted by preliminary examiners, eye witnesses and by the patients' own
rationalisations of their acts.

Our first objective was to determine how often the files on our
mentally abnormal offenders contained any mention of a motive for the crime.
(By 'a motive' we meant the dominant reason for action, the *Leitmotiv*, in
conjunction with which there would doubtless also be other contributory
forces operating and helping to bring about the crime.)

According to Jaspers' concept of the 'lack of understandability'
(*Uneinfühlbarkeit*) in endogenous psychoses (see also Gruhle's *Ursache, Motiv,
Grund, Auslösung (Cause, Motive, Reason, Immediate Occasion)*, 1947), and also
in the opinion of many laymen and jurists, motiveless and therefore apparently
'senseless' crimes are more frequently encountered in mentally abnormal than
in mentally normal offenders (Rasch). The actions of the mentally ill are
sometimes contrasted with those of 'motivated' offenders, and are regarded as
forming an independent group and requiring no mention of motive at all. [3]

As has already been mentioned, many careful statistical analyses
and enquiries were influenced by this bias. As De Boor, however, showed by
the examples given in his detailed study *Über motivisch unklare Delikte
(Crimes of Unclear Motivation)* (1959), penetrating psychological and in
particular psychoanalytical examination can uncover the convincing, if masked

and largely unconscious, motives which lie behind many crimes that at first
sight seem to be motiveless. It is also more clearly recognised today that
many of the actions of normal individuals cannot be explained outright by
empathy, 'understanding', or 'putting oneself in the other man's position'
(Häfner).

The methodological approach which we selected for tackling the
problem of motivation in the mentally abnormal does not allow for any subtle
analysis. We shall limit ourselves in the first place to a tabular representation of cases according to whether a motive was recognised, or recorded as
absent, noting also those in which no mention of motive was made. As Table 83
shows, violent crimes for which no motive was registered are thus in the
minority, being recorded in only about a fifth of the cases in both sexes
(with no significant difference between sexes). When a test of diagnostic
differences was carried out (Table 84), there was likewise no undue proportion of crimes which seemed to be motiveless. About 80% of the crimes were
registered as motivated, and there was basically no significant difference
in this percentage in the three diagnostic groups.

Our next aim was to determine which were the main motives documented in our cohort as a whole. From the psychiatric literature one gains
the impression that strong emotions very often lie at the root of violence
on the part of the mentally abnormal: jealous, suspicious, angry, despairing
or fearful emotions with which the patients can no longer cope. Whether such
emotions are aroused by real, imagined, or delusionally misinterpreted
experiences, is of course of great interest, but cannot always be satisfactorily

Table 83. *Sex distribution of the motives of 533 mentally abnormal*
violent offenders

	Men		Women		Whole group	
	n	%	n	%	n	%
No recognisable motive	70	17.4	26	22.0	96	18.5
Motive recorded	331	82.6	92	78.0	423	81.5
Subtotal	401	100.0	118	100.0	519	100.0
Not known	9		5		14	
Total	410		123		533	

Significance test: $\chi^2 = 1.32$ df = 1   Null hypothesis not refutable

determined in the individual case (e.g. murder from motives of revenge and
jealousy). It was easier to distinguish between delusional and non-delusional
motivation when the motive of self-defence was given, particularly by a
schizophrenic (on the basis of the paranoid relationship to the victim).

Lanzkron (1963) estimated that of his 150 mentally ill murderers
32.6% were driven by such motives as rage, revenge and jealousy, 'which can
also influence the mentally normal', while 40% were assumed by him to have
'killed as a direct consequence of a delusion'.

Gibbens (1958) carried out a retrospective study in New Jersey,
USA, of 115 mentally abnormal homicidal delinquents who committed their crimes
before 1950 and were at some time treated in the New Jersey State Hospital.
He reported the main motive for the crime to be delusional phenomena in 29
cases, quarrels in 29 cases, and jealousy in 21 cases. Murder accompanying
robbery was found in only 7 cases.

If we turn, however, to the motivational spectrum reported in the
criminological literature in normal violent offenders, e.g. murderers,
'materialistic' motives, that is to say those concerned with gain, personal
advantage, avoidance of punishment (so-called crimes of concealment), and

Table 84. *Diagnostic differences in data on motivation for violent
crimes by the mentally abnormal*

	Schizo-phrenia		Affective psychoses		Mental deficiency	
	n	%	*n*	%	*n*	%
No recognisable motive	52	18.8	8	24	10	15
Motive recorded	225	81.2	25	76	58	85
Subtotal	277	100.0	33	100	68	100
Not known	7		4		0	
Total	284		37		68	

Significance test: $\chi^2 =$ df = 1 $\alpha =$

Schizophrenia v. affective psychoses   0.269   Null hypothesis
                                                                  not refutable

Schizophrenia v. mental deficiency   0.368   Null hypothesis
                                                                  not refutable

Affective psychoses v. mental deficiency   0.805   Null hypothesis
                                                                  not refutable

motives concerned with the satisfaction of sexual and other drives seem to play a more important part than they do in mentally abnormal offenders. German authors, in particular, stress the importance of this group of motives.

Roesner (1938) published a careful and mainly statistical analysis of the penal files of 169 individuals convicted of murder (Section 211 of the Penal Code) in the German courts, excluding Saarland, in the years 1931 to 1933. The motives most frequently advanced were:

1. 'Desire for financial or economic gain': in 61 cases (36.1%), of which 46 were cases of murder accompanying robbery.

2. Sexual murders: 29 cases (17.2%), of which 21 (12.4%) were 'lust murders' and 8 (4.7%) 'murders following sexual crimes'. Revenge, hate and quarrels were reported in only 22 cases (13.0%); jealousy, family dissension, despair in 10 (5.9%); and 'love for another' in 8 cases (4.7%). 'Fear of being reported for a punishable offence' was recorded in 13 cases (7.7%).

Brückner (1961) examined the crime of murder in the Oberland judicial regions of Stuttgart and Karlsruhe and published personal data on 80 convicted murderers who had mostly committed their crimes (74 cases) between 1945 and 1956. Of these 42 (52.5%) were described as 'murderers for gain', 13 (16.3%) as 'murderers for concealment', 5 (6.2%) as 'sexual murderers' and only 20 (25%) as 'conflict murderers', driven by a 'passionate upsurge of feelings'. The author quotes Bader (1949), according to whom murder accompanying robbery 'was clearly the murder of the post-war period'. Von Hentig too, who in 1931 published German data on murder victims, put robbery at the top of his list of motives. (A new, short review of the distribution of motives for murder was published by Göppinger in 1971.)

A classification of the motives of 178 convicted murderers and attempted murderers was examined in more detail by Rangol (Federal Statistical Bureau, Wiesbaden) on the basis of court verdicts in the two years 1959 and 1963 (see p.230): Table 85 shows the broad distribution he gave. Here again 'material motives', such as gain, or removal of burdensome persons or those who represented a risk of discovery or arrest, come easily at the top of the list.

Of course the sane convicted violent offenders, particularly those guilty of homicide, also included many who had acted under the influence of strong emotions (Lorentz, 1932). Various attempts have been made to arrive at a typology of such individuals, who have been described by Gast (1930) as 'passion murderers', by von Hentig (1956) and Brückner (1961) as 'conflict murderers' and by Steigleder (1968) as 'affect offenders'. It is interesting to note that Anglo-Saxon criminologists, reporting for example on American murderers, have found a much higher proportion of offenders in this category than has been reported in Germany.

Gibbens described 120 sane individuals convicted of murder or man-slaughter in New Jersey, USA, between 1947 and 1949. The records of a further 15 murderers who received the death sentence and who included some cases of murder accompanying robbery, were not, however, available to him. In the cases he examined he found that murders motivated by gain were rare, while those motivated by quarrels (often under the influence of alcohol), revenge and jealousy were in the majority. Wolfgang (1958) obtained a similar result from his thorough investigations of all criminal homicides confirmed by the police in Philadelphia, USA, between January 1948 and 31 December 1952 (588 cases in all), which he analysed by characteristics of the crime, the criminal and the victim. (Since he used police information and not court records of

Table 85. *Motives of 178 sane (convicted) murderers (including attempted murder) by sex of the offender*

Motive	Men		Women		Whole group	
	n	%	*n*	%	*n*	%
Robbery (gain); removal of burdensome persons; concealment of a punishable offence; defence against threatened arrest	124	78.5	15	79	139	78.5
Jealousy (incl. fear of or anger at threatened separation from partner)	12	7.6	1	5	13	7.4
Revenge	10	6.3	0	–	10	5.6
Sexual drive; lust	6	3.8	0	–	6	3.4
Other motives (e.g. sectarian, political)	6	3.8	3	16	9	5.1
Subtotal	158	100.0	19	100	177	100.0
Not known	1		0		1	
Total	159		19		178	

convicted individuals, his findings are broadly based.) In his statistics of
motivation, homicides arising from often trivial quarrels, insults, arguments,
etc., head the list with 35%, followed by domestic conflicts (14.1%),
jealousy (11.6%) and disputes about money (10.5%). Robbery as a motive was
found in only 6.8% of all cases. Wolfgang quotes von Hentig's study of murder
and homicide in New York City between 1936 and 1940, according to which
altercations were the most common motive, accounting for 34% of cases,
followed by family disputes which accounted for 26%. According to a report
on more than 500 homicides published by the Metropolitan Life Insurance
Company in 1939, 30% were caused by domestic quarrels and jealousy and
'practically all homicidal crimes were committed under the emotional pressure
of fear, hate, anger, jealousy or envy' (Wolfgang, 1958, p. 196).

The reasons for such variations in the distribution of motives
may well lie in different cultural and socio-economic factors (such as the
ease with which weapons may be acquired, the standard of living, or the
tolerance of aggression in different social groups) which cannot be fully
discussed here.

In our study we continued to receive the impression that motives
of gain, removal of burdensome persons and concealment of punishable offences
tended to be less frequent in mentally abnormal than in normal violent
offenders. We therefore collected such motives in one common category which
was kept separate from the other categories encountered. As a glance at
Table 86 shows, our expectation was confirmed. In our cohort of mentally
abnormal offenders emotional motives - of which the main one in the male
offenders was revenge and in the female offenders a desire to release the
victim from feared suffering or illness - far exceeded the materialistic
and egoistic aims which motivated so many of the convicted sane murderers.

Even if, as shown above, the proportion of motivated crimes was
about the same in both sexes (approximately four-fifths of the cases), the
individual categories of motive were distributed in a very different way.
The men were motivated mostly by revenge or self-defence, or their actions
were governed by disappointment in love or by jealousy. The frequency of the
'release' motive in the women is correlated with the fact that their victims
were mostly children; the motive itself bears the stamp of the nihilistic
fears of delusions of poverty that occur in psychotic depression. Delusional
self-defence played a very small part in motivating the female offenders.

Comparing the omnibus category of materialistic motives (the
first in Table 86) with all the other motives, in both sexes, we find that
the rate for the omnibus category is slightly higher for the male than for

the female abnormal offenders: χ^2 = 4.3777, df = 1, α = 0.05. When we test the distribution of the motives classes as 'revenge' as against those classes as 'release from feared suffering', we find a highly significant sex difference: χ^2 = 53.4564, df = 1, α = 0.001.

It will be seen from Table 87 that in the affective psychoses, with their predominance of female offenders and child victims, the desire for release was, as already mentioned, the decisive motive (19 out of the 25 patients in this group for whom a motive was recorded). In the schizophrenic offenders, on the other hand, feelings of revenge are well to the fore (39.1%); delusional self-defence and jealousy (together accounting for about 31%) form the largest group of motives. Reasons which aim at improvement of one's own situation (gain as in murder accompanying robbery; concealment of other crimes such as sexual assault; removal of burdensome persons) are found most frequently in the mentally defective group of offenders (38 out of the 58 in

Table 86. *Motives advanced by 533 mentally abnormal violent offenders by sex of the offender*

Motive	Men		Women		Whole group	
	n	%	*n*	%	*n*	%
Gain; removal of troublesome persons; concealment of punishable offence (incl. sexual assault), etc.	72	21.8	11	12	83	19.6
Jealousy (incl. delusional jealousy and disappointed love)	49	14.8	9	10	58	13.7
Revenge	126	38.1	24	26	150	35.5
Delusional self-defence	46	13.9	4	4	50	11.8
Release from feared suffering	19	5.7	40	44	59	14.0
Other motives (e.g. religious motives)	19	5.7	4	4	23	5.4
Subtotal	331	100.0	92	100	423	100.0
No ascertainable motive	70		26		96	
Not known	9		5		14	
Total	410		123		533	

this group whose motive was recorded). In this group, too, acts of vengeance
are fairly prominent; they may be explained partly by the numerous humiliating
experiences to which the mentally defective are often subjected (see Case no.
492, p.191).

To conclude this chapter, let us look once more at those crimes
which seem to be unmotivated. It is only in the schizophrenic group that it is
possible to pursue the investigation further, for example by studying the
pattern of distribution on the psychopathological subgroups. In the other
diagnostic categories the number of cases is too small to permit any
closer analysis of the so-called motiveless crime.

There were 52 schizophrenics who apparently had become violent for
no comprehensible reason. They included, as Table 88 shows, more patients with
simple forms of the illness, somewhat more catatonic patients, and

Table 87. *Motives advanced by 533 mentally abnormal violent offenders
in three diagnostic groups*

	Schizo-phrenia		Affective psychoses		Mental deficiency	
	n	%	n	%	n	%
Gain; removal of troublesome persons; concealment of punishable offence (incl. sexual assault), etc.	27	12.0	2	8	38	66
Jealousy (incl. delusional jealousy and disappointed love)	33	14.7	2	8	3	5
Revenge	88	39.1	1	4	15	26
Delusional self-defence	36	16.0	0	–	0	–
Release from feared suffering	21	9.3	19	76	0	–
Other motives (e.g. religious motives)	20	8.9	1	4	2	3
Subtotal	225	100.0	25	100	58	100
No ascertainable motive	52		8		10	
Not known	7		4		0	
Total	284		37		68	

distinctly fewer paraphrenics than the schizophrenic group for whom motives were recorded. If we compare this distribution with that of the non-violent schizophrenics (Table 88) we find a striking correspondence between the ostensibly unmotivated violent schizophrenics and the control group of non-violent schizophrenics admitted to the Regional Psychiatric Hospital of Wiesloch and matched for sex, age and diagnosis of schizophrenia.

We next compared the apparently unmotivated schizophrenics (*n* = 52; hereafter referred to as 'group B') with motivated violent schizo-phrenics (*n* = 225; 'group A') in respect of 18 items from their previous history and in respect of items connected with the crime. The results are presented here briefly, without the statistical analysis. It was found that the duration of illness was shorter for patients in group B (level of significance 0.05) and that patients in this group were also less often delusional than those in group A (significance level 0.001). Moreover the proportion of those with a previous record of violence was lower in group B

Table 88. *Distribution of psychopathological subgroups in violent schizophrenic offenders with and without ascertainable motives, and in their non-violent controls*

| | Schizophrenic offenders | | | | | | |
| | With motive | | Without motive | | Not known | Schizophrenic non-offenders | |
	n	%	*n*	%	*n*	*n*	%
Clinically quiet	31	13.8	16	31	3	85	29.0
Catatonia	21	9.3	6	11	0	33	11.3
Paranoid-hallucinatory schizophrenia	132	58.7	27	52	5	157	53.6
Paraphrenia	41	18.2	3	6	0	18	6.1
Total	225	100.0	52	100	8	293	100.0

A test of the distribution confirms the impression conveyed by the figures:

$$\chi^2 = \qquad df = 1 \qquad \alpha =$$

	$\chi^2 =$	$\alpha =$
Violent offenders with motive v. offenders without motive	11.856	0.01
Violent offenders without motive v. non-violent schizophrenics	1.57	Null hypothesis not refutable

than A (one-fifth as against one-third: significance level 0.05).

The following other tendencies were observed, although in no case was the significance level of 0.05 reached. The schizophrenics in group B were somewhat younger, and were more frequently unmarried; if married, they were less likely to allege bad relationships with their marriage partners. They tended either, on the one hand, never to have received in-patient psychiatric treatment, or on the other hand to have been in-patients in such hospitals for longer periods of time. In the six months preceding the crime they had seemed to those around them to be more autistic and less aggressive. This mosaic of data is also very reminiscent of that found in the non-violent control group.

So far as the crimes were concerned, those committed by group B tended to be impulsive acts with no apparent cause (significance level 0.001) and to a lesser extent this group tended to hear imperative voices telling them to commit the crime (significance level almost 0.05).

These findings seemed to justify an attempt to develop different typologies for the schizophrenic offenders in groups A and B. The smaller number of psychotic patients in group B, who apparently made violent attacks without any motive, clearly represent a selection of schizophrenics who, to outward appearance, can be described as 'harmless' (less aggressive before the crime, with fewer symptoms, less often delusional) and 'better adapted' (better relationships with their marital partners), though at the same time they are 'more withdrawn', and consist of younger individuals who have not been ill for so long. Their violence, which is impulsive, occurs without any understandable cause or ascertainable motivation and comes as a surprise to those around (and often also to the patients themselves): it may represent a discharge of mounting tension that had been concealed behind a facade of apparently ordinary behaviour.

The offenders in the much larger group A are in many respects just the opposite. They are often older, more often married, have been ill for a longer time and have made themselves more conspicuous before the crime by their symptoms and aggressive behaviour; in other words they are more 'disturbing' and expansive schizophrenics whose marked tendency to systematic delusions indicates a 'mad' but more active and more thoroughgoing discord with the world around them. Their violence, too, seems - more distinctly than that of patients in group B - to be part of this often ineffectual discord, and it is not surprising that reports of open marital conflict are more common in this group.

In fact all the motives so frequently encountered in the violent

crimes of schizophrenics (revenge, delusional self-defence, jealousy; as well
as the motive of release) presuppose the existence of a defined object to
which the patient must have some kind of a relationship, even if a delusional
one. The development of such motives clearly requires that this relationship
should have existed for a fairly long time and this in turn is correlated with
a fairly long duration of illness (Mowat confirmed this in his study of morbid
jealousy and murder). This interpretation has the therapeutic implication that
one can and should intervene and help in the relationships of these patients
with their 'defined objects' (which, as already stated, often means their
relationships with the members of their immediate families).

8.4 Committal after the crime

To conclude our enquiry we investigated the manner of committal,
that is to say we asked how many offenders had as a result of the crime been
committed to a psychiatric hospital for treatment or detained in a penal
institution. Many of our mentally abnormal offenders had been admitted to a
specialised hospital after a stay in prison, some because the severity of
their mental illness was not recognised immediately, others because of a
combination of measures (for example many mentally defective offenders were
sentenced to penal confinement under Section 51, para 2, of the Penal Code

Table 89. *Committal measures after the crime in 533 mentally abnormal
violent offenders*

	Whole group		Schizo-phrenia		Affective psychoses		Mental deficiency	
	n	%	n	%	n	%	n	%
No measures taken	17	3.6	5	2.0	2	8	5	7
Detention only (prison or long-term prison)	14	3.0	1	0.4	0	–	6	9
Detention and committal to mental hospital	101	21.2	41	16.0	2	8	27	42
Mental hospital only	343	72.2	209	81.6	22	84	27	42
Subtotal	475	100.0	256	100.0	26	100	65	100
Died at time of crime (suicide)	19		8		5		0	
Not known	39		20		6		3	
Total	533		284		37		68	

but because of considerations of public safety were finally committed to a
regional psychiatric hospital under Section 42b of the Penal Code).

It can be seen from Table 89 that about three-quarters of our
offenders were admitted to psychiatric hospitals immediately after the crime
(they were mostly patients who were dealt with under Section 51, para 1 of
the Penal Code which here usually also involved Section 42b). Fourteen
offenders were, however, sentenced to prison only and no treatment or
committal was found necessary, although they were in fact mentally abnormal
(in most cases mentally defective). In more than a fifth of all the cases
where details were recorded of the measures adopted, committal to a psychiatric
hospital was preceded by a period in prison.

It was a surprise to find the relatively high figure of 17
patients (3.6%) for whom no measures of any kind were documented. This is
partly connected with successful suicide after the crime. In our questionnaire
we enquired about the course of illness after the crime and found that 26
offenders had 'died uncured' in the period between the crime and the enquiry.
Nineteen patients (3.6% of all the mentally abnormal offenders) died at the
actual time of the crime.

Looking at the main diagnostic groups, certain differences emerge
in regard to the measures taken. Patients with psychoses were usually
committed to psychiatric hospitals, mostly without previous imprisonment.
Those suffering from depression tended to be discharged earlier (13 out of
22 had been discharged by the time of our enquiry), while the schizophrenics
nearly all stayed in hospital for a long time (only 20 out of 209 had been
discharged). This difference holds good, even although it had to a certain
extent affected the make-up of the cohort (significance level 0.001).

The mentally defective offenders were rarely sent for in-
patient psychiatric treatment directly after the crime: 41% of them were
committed to mental hospitals without sentence being carried out, as
against 81% of the schizophrenics (significance level 0.001). Perhaps this
is because mental deficiency, in contrast to mental illness, can more easily
be understood as a 'characteristic that can respond to punishment' and
because mentally defective offenders in many ways resemble the 'normal'
violent offenders.

9.   RESULTS VI : QUALITATIVE ANALYSIS OF SMALL
     DIAGNOSTIC GROUPS

9.1   Epileptic violent offenders

In this chapter we shall deal with the main characteristics of
those diagnostic groups whose small numbers or heterogeneous nature made
statistical analysis impossible. They comprise the violent offenders suffering from epilepsy, from late-acquired brain damage and from cerebral atrophy.

Taking first those offenders who were diagnosed as epileptic, and
considering again the findings quoted in our review of the literature (Section
2.2), we may expect to find in these patients not only the characteristics of
their convulsive illness but also certain other features such as mental
deficiency or decline in intelligence, alcoholism and similar personality
disorders (Alström; Hill & Pond), or psychiatric complications such as cerebral degeneration, personality changes (Alström) or psychotic episodes (Janz),
all of which serve to distinguish violent epileptics from non-aggressive
epileptic patients. Among the psychiatric complications it is the epileptic
twilight state which in the earlier psychiatric literature in particular
carried with it a reputation for dangerousness.

The violent acts in question are described in many textbooks and
earlier case studies as explosive and to a large extent unpredictable and
unaccountable emotional outbursts which are discharged against persons who
happen to cross the patient's path. With this assumption in mind, we carried
out a brief analysis of the crimes and the victims of violent epileptic
offenders.

We shall begin by describing some important demographic characteristics of the 29 violent epileptic offenders in our cohort.

Sex

The predominance of male offenders was even more marked than in
the group of mentally abnormal violent offenders as a whole: the violent epileptics consisted of 27 men and 2 women.

Table 90. *Age distribution*
of violent epileptic offenders

Years	No.
14-19	4
20-29	12
30-39	4
40-49	4
50-59	4
60 and over	1
Total	29

Age

Compared with the group as a whole, for which the peak age lay
between 30 and 40, the epileptic offenders were younger (peak between 20 and
30 years of age: Table 90). Only 5 patients were aged above 50.

Marital status

The high number of unmarried offenders corresponds to the predominance of lower age groups. More than half (*n* = 16) were unmarried, as
against 45% in the group as a whole. Seven of the remaining epileptic
offenders were married at the time of the crime, the remainder being divorced,
separated or widowed.

Occupation at the time of the crime

At the time of the crime none of the offenders held a position
higher than that of **skilled** worker, low-grade clerical worker or low-grade
civil servant. Twelve were out of work or incapable of work, 11 were
auxiliary workers, 1 was in training and 2 were housewives. The proportion of
those who were untrained or at best skilled workers (*n* = 12) was higher than
in the group as a whole, where the corresponding figure was only a third.
This is probably due to features of personality and illness which are
discussed below.

Personality traits

The first finding of note was that more than half of the epileptic
offenders (*n* = 16) were of below-average intelligence (ranging from the

slightly handicapped to the mentally defective). In the group of offenders as
a whole only 37% fell into this category. For the purposes of our enquiry the
level of intelligence was determined mainly by the test or other investigation that was carried out in closest temporal proximity to the crime, and it
must therefore be assumed that any lack of intelligence due to cerebral
degeneration, in other words the process of dementia, would be covered by such
procedures. The result in any case confirms the tendency found by Alström as
well as by Hill & Pond for mentally defective epileptics to be more prone to
aggressive behaviour than those with normal intellectual endowments.

Antisocial psychopathic traits were found in the basic personality
of only a seventh of the epileptic offenders (n = 4), all of whom were also
of low intelligence. The proportion of antisocial personality disorders is
here less than that found in the group as a whole, which was about 20%.

Alcoholism and other addictions were found in 8 cases, being
thus more common here than in the group as a whole (14.4%). In so far as the
small numbers permit comparison, this result is in line with the reports
cited in our review of the literature.

Heredity

Even for the group of mentally abnormal offenders as a whole and
for the main diagnoses of schizophrenia, affective psychoses and mental
deficiency, the information available in the files was too incomplete to
permit us to predict the effect of an adverse family history of mental illness and antisocial behaviour except in respect of very broad characteristics, and even then with reservations. Such predictions are even more
difficult to formulate and interpret for the smaller diagnostic groups.

In the epileptics, particularly those in the subgroup of genuine
epilepsy (which was diagnosed in 13 of our cases), there seemed to be a
genetic factor at work. In 11 out of our 29 cases, that is to say in somewhat
more than a third, there was a history of mental illness and/or epilepsy in
relatives of the first grade: for the group as a whole the comparable figure
was 30%.

A social history of aggressive and/or auto-aggressive and addictive behaviour was found in the families of 4 of the 29 cases, that is to say
in about a seventh: this was less than in the group as a whole, where the
figure was 23%. Not much weight can be attached to this finding.

Previous criminal record

In contrast to the lower rate of antisocial behaviour found in first-grade relatives of the epileptic offenders, there was one result which pointed nevertheless to a higher tendency for certain individuals in this diagnostic group to show aggressive forms of behaviour: almost three-quarters of the 29 epileptics (n = 19), as against a third of the group as a whole, had been guilty before the crime of some form of bodily harm. About half of the offenders (n = 13) had been charged previously with insulting, defamatory or threatening behaviour towards other people. Of 24 epileptic offenders who had a previous criminal history, 22 had committed these crimes during their illness, and two partly before and partly within the period of their illness.

There was, on the other hand, no instance of crime against life before the index crime. Only 5 of the 29 offenders had no history at all of previous crime, that is to say no form of crime against property, or indecent, defamatory, threatening or other delinquent behaviour. There was no real difference in this respect between those epileptics who suffered from defective intelligence and those who did not.

Items related to the illness

Examination of the duration of illness in the 29 epileptic violent offenders shows that more than half of them (n = 17) had been suffering from convulsions for ten or more years before the crime (Table 91). This is due to the fact that 13 offenders belonged to the aetiological subgroup of genuine epilepsy and 3 to the subgroup of residual epilepsy - forms of illness which mostly become manifest before the end of adolescence. The preponderance among the offenders of forms of epilepsy with a long history of convulsive attacks is also reflected in the number of cases with a history of at least one admission to a psychiatric hospital before the crime; this applied to 20 out of the 29

Table 91. *Duration of illness for 29 epileptic violent offenders*

Duration	No.
Up to 1 year	1
1-5 years	2
5-10 years	8
More than 10 years	17
Not known	1
Total	29

offenders, a proportion which is higher than that of the group as a whole,
50% of whom had received in-patient psychiatric treatment at least once before
the crime. A further finding was that most of the cases showing defects of
intelligence (10 out of the 16) fell within the group of offenders with a
long history of epilepsy (see Table 92): this group may be assumed to include
many patients with deteriorating intelligence, that is to say with processes
of dementia, as has already been mentioned above.

Epileptic twilight states were present at the time of the crime
in only 8 of these offenders, a number which from study of the literature we
would have expected to be higher. Delusions were likewise infrequent, being
documented in only about a fifth of the 29 cases. In this connection it may
be said that presumably an epileptic with psychotic symptoms is considerably
restricted in his capacity for goal-directed, planned action, including acts
of violence, and that he is recognised as severely disturbed and may be
admitted for in-patient treatment more quickly than epileptics who are not
psychotic.

Lastly it should be mentioned that 3 epileptic offenders had been
given a supplementary diagnosis of schizophrenia and 2 more a diagnosis of
exogenous psychosis following brain injury.

Table 92. *Twilight states and delusional psychoses in epileptic offenders
with and without defects of intelligence*

	All epileptic offenders (n = 29)	Epilepsy	
		with intellec- tual defects (n = 16)	without intellectual defects (n = 13)
Genuine epilepsy	13	7	6
Residual epilepsy	3	3	0
Symptomatic epilepsy	12	5	7
Epilepsy in cerebral atrophy	1	1	0
Twilight state at time of crime	8	2	6
Delusions present in illness	6	3	3

Behaviour during the six months preceding the crime

In view of the large proportion of epileptic offenders who had a previous criminal history of bodily harm, it seemed likely that, by analogy with the data from the group as a whole, there would also be numerous instances of aggressive behaviour in the six months preceding the crime. This was in fact the case: aggressive and threatening forms of behaviour on the part of the patient towards those around him were particularly frequent, such behaviour being recorded in more than three-quarters of the cases ($n = 21$), as against a half for all the 533 mentally ill offenders of all diagnostic groups. Epileptic violent offenders thus showed a warning phase of perceptible aggressiveness towards their intimate partners and those standing in secondary relationships to them; this phase was at least of several months' duration. The argument that such patients are liable to unaccountable explosions seems to apply in only a few cases.

Signs of considerable social isolation ($n = 7$) and suicidal tendencies (threats and attempts; $n = 3$) were on the other hand somewhat less frequent than in the group of offenders as a whole.

The crime and the victim

About a third ($n = 10$) of the epileptic offenders had killed at least one person (1 was responsible for three victims, and 2 for two victims). Attacks with fatal outcome were thus somewhat less frequent than in the group as a whole, where half of all the patients had killed one person. Nineteen epileptic offenders, almost three-quarters of this group, injured their victims without killing them (three had injured two persons each), a higher proportion than in the group as a whole where the figure was 53%.

As mentioned, 8 offenders committed their crimes while under the influence of an epileptic twilight state: 3 of these were also under the influence of alcohol, while alcoholic influence on its own was recorded in 7 cases.

Eight of the 29 offenders, i.e. somewhat more than a quarter, had planned the crime in advance: the corresponding ratio for the group as a whole was about 48%, that is to say about a half. More than a third (11 out of 29) acted with apparently no premeditation and with no quarrelling beforehand; about a third (10 out of 29) were involved in a dispute with the victim beforehand. These figures are somewhat higher than for the group as a whole where they amounted to about a quarter in each case.

Suicide associated with the crime was much less frequent than in all the other diagnoses, occurring in only 2 cases as against a quarter of the group as a whole. There was no instance of extended suicide.

The 29 epileptics killed in all 14 victims and injured 24. Most of the victims were adults (n = 23) and the numbers for men and for women were roughly the same. Seven epileptics attacked children, and here again there was no difference between the sexes. These figures are about the same as corresponding figures for the group of mentally abnormal offenders as a whole.

Here again it is significant that two-thirds of the epileptic offenders (n = 19) chose victims from the circle of family or other intimate relationships (the figure for the group as a whole was about 60%). In the case of the large number of unmarried offenders the victims were mostly parents or siblings. Only in 2 cases was the victim unknown to the offender. In 6 cases the victim was a casual acquaintance.

About half of the offenders (n = 14) perpetrated their attack from motives which were not delusional: in 4 cases the motive was delusional, while in somewhat more than a third of the cases (n = 11) there was no apparent motive.

9.2 Violent offenders with late-acquired brain damage and cerebral atrophy

As we have seen, the epileptic offenders represented a selection of almost exclusively male patients who had for a long time before the crime been conspicuous for their aggressive moods and for their tendency to use insulting and threatening behaviour: they also tended to have a previous criminal history of bodily injury, to show intellectual defects and to have very long histories of illness. Our findings thus seemed to support the views of previous investigators who believed that it is not the epileptic attacks themselves, and only to a small extent the epileptic psychoses such as the epileptic twilight state, which contribute to the risk of violence, but much more those phenomena which are directly or indirectly associated with the convulsive disorder (for example cerebral disintegration, intellectual impairment (dementia), personality change, effect of social relationships, and much else besides). A personality factor which is independent of the illness seems also to play a decisive part, as has already been shown in the group of mentally abnormal offenders as a whole.

By analogy with these findings and considerations it may be assumed that other forms of illness which can lead to brain damage will also show a marked incidence of violence, provided that: (1) there has been fairly severe cerebral deterioration and considerable damage to the structure of personality and character; (2) the premorbid personality has already shown evidence of antisocial, aggressive forms of behaviour.

In view of these and other general hypotheses we considered it useful to bring together the very heterogeneous group of 'brain-damaged patients' and to analyse it quantitatively. It was possible to divide it into

I. Those with *late-acquired brain damage* (due to traumatic, toxic or inflammatory processes and with no innate or early cerebral damage), $n = 43$.

II. Those with *cerebral atrophy* caused by presenile or senile processes or deterioration (dementias), $n = 40$.

According to reports in the literature, the rate of criminal violence in patients whose cerebral functioning is affected by senile and presenile involutional processes is lower than in persons who have suffered brain damage due to trauma or inflammatory processes (H.W. Müller & Hadamik; Bürger-Prinz & Lewerenz; Roth). In the case of elderly abnormal offenders it is not in Roth's view the normal phenomena of senile deterioration which can lead to serious acts of aggression but psychological accompaniments and complications such as, for example, chronic alcoholism or paranoid syndromes.

In what follows we shall as far as possible present groups I and II together. Only where clear differences can be demonstrated will we evaluate them separately. We shall again begin by presenting some important demographic data on the 43 violent offenders with late-acquired brain damage and on the 40 with cerebral atrophy.

Sex

As in the case of the epileptics, there is again a clear preponderance of male offenders: 40 out of the 43 with late-acquired brain damage were men, and 35 out of the 40 with cerebral atrophy.

Age

As is to be expected, the peak age for offenders in group I and particularly for those in group II was high (Table 93): for those with late-acquired brain damage it was between 40 and 60, while those with cerebral atrophy were, with one exception, aged 50 and over.

Marital status

The fairly high figure for married offenders is in keeping with the preponderance of higher age groups. This applied particularly to group II (28 married, 3 single), while the offenders in group I were to a relatively larger extent unmarried (21 married, 14 single). In both groups the proportion who were married was somewhat higher than in the group of abnormal violent offenders as a whole.

It is noteworthy that, as with the epileptics, there were more patients in these groups without work (out of work or incapable of work) than in the group of abnormal offenders as a whole (Table 94). This may be connected with the higher age of these offenders, particularly in group II; so far as group I is concerned it may also be connected with factors associated with the illness.

Table 93. *Age distribution of violent offenders with late-acquired brain damage (group I) and with cerebral atrophy (group II)*

Age	Group I	Group II
14-19	2	0
20-29	8	0
30-39	8	0
40-49	12	1
50-59	12	17
60 and over	1	22
Total	43	40

Table 94. *Distribution or occupations in violent offenders with late-acquired brain damage (I) and with cerebral atrophy (II)*

Occupation	Group I	Group II
Out of work/incapable of work	15	24
In training	2	0
Auxiliary worker and comparable occupations	10	3
Skilled worker and comparable occupations	12	8
Higher professions	2	0
Housewife	2	5
Total	43	40

Personality traits

More than a third (16 out of 43) of those with late-acquired brain damage and about half (18 out of 40) of those with cerebral atrophy had a documented defect of intelligence,[1] which in group II was naturally likely to reach a higher proportion.

Antisocial psychopathy was given as a subsidiary diagnosis in a quarter ($n \doteq 11$) of those with late-acquired damage, but only in an eighth ($n = 5$) of those with cerebral atrophy. (In the group as a whole, covering all diagnoses, it was recorded in about a fifth of the cases.)

The two groups differed considerably in regard to alcoholism and addiction: in group I almost half ($n = 21$) were chronic alcoholics, which is far more than in the group of all abnormal offenders as a whole, where the rate was about 1 in 7. Group II on the other hand, with 6 alcoholics, showed about the same rate as the group of abnormal offenders as a whole.

Heredity

There was no real difference between the two groups in regard to mental illness and socially conspicuous behaviour in first-grade relatives. The rates recorded for both these items, which fluctuated between a fifth and an eighth, were below the rates for the group as a whole (group I: history of mental illness in 6 cases, and of conspicuous behaviour in 9 cases; group II: history of mental illness in 5 and of conspicuous behaviour in 7 cases).

Table 95. *Previous crimes in violent offenders with late-acquired brain damage (I) and with cerebral atrophy (II)*

Previous crimes	Group I	Group II
No previous crime	8	21
Insulting, libellous, threatening behaviour	15	18
Bodily harm and rape	20	8
Crimes against life	3	1
Total	46[a]	48[a]

[a] The total differs from the number of cases because the cases were counted according to categories exhibited, and combinations were therefore counted more than once.

Previous criminal record

While the offenders in group I showed a higher rate of antisocial personality disturbances and chronic alcoholism than those in group II, the tendency of offenders with late-acquired brain damage to show aggressive forms of behaviour came very clearly to the fore when we looked at the history of previous crime (Table 95).

The patients affected by cerebral atrophy had, it is true, more often made themselves conspicuous by their threats and abuse of others, that is to say by troublesome, offensive or intimidating behaviour; but they committed distinctly fewer serious assaults involving bodily harm or danger to life than did the group of abnormal offenders as a whole, and fewer also than the offenders with late-acquired brain damage.

In both groups the majority of previous crimes fell within the period of the illness (group I, 24 cases; group II, 13 cases).

Items related to the illness

Taking first the duration of illness for the two groups, we again find differences (Table 96): the group with late-acquired brain damage shows a slightly higher proportion of offenders who had been ill for more than five years (25 out of 43 as against 15 out of 40 for the group with cerebral atrophy).

It is of interest here to consider how many offenders in both groups had at the time of the crime suffered from additional mental disturbances of any considerable degree, apart from their basic organic cerebral

Table 96. *Duration of illness in violent offenders with late-acquired brain damage (I) and cerebral atrophy (II)*

Duration of illness	Group I	Group II
Up to 1 month	2	0
Up to 6 months	3	4
Up to 1 year	2	3
1-5 years	10	16
5-10 years	6	10
10 years and over	19	5
Not known	1	2
Total	43	40

Table 97. *Delusions and accompanying psychoses in violent offenders
with late-acquired brain damage (I) and with cerebral atrophy (II)*

	Group I	Group II
Delusions present in the illness	21	23
Cases with accompanying psychosis:		
Total	21	26
Schizophrenia	6	2
Affective psychoses	3	2
Unclassifiable endogenous psychoses	2	2
Exogenous psychoses	10	20

disorders of late brain damage acquired through mechanical, inflammatory or
toxic processes or senile deterioration (Table 97).

It is worth noting that an accompanying psychosis, usually an
exogenous psychosis, was diagnosed in more than half of the offenders with
cerebral atrophy. This means that at the time of the crime the offender was
suffering not only from a deterioration in cerebral functioning but also from
a disturbance of consciousness which in these cases amounted to a loss of
conscious control over aggressive emotions that was of great significance and
was clearly more common than any similar occurrence in the twilight states
that affected the epileptic offenders. Moreover the productive psychotic
symptom of delusion was documented in about half the cases, including the
exogenous psychoses, in both groups of offenders suffering from cerebral
organic changes; this is roughly of the same order as was noted in offenders
with manic-depressive illness (about 56%) but decidedly less common than in
the case of the schizophrenic offenders, of whom about 90% exhibited
delusional symptoms.

In both groups there was a considerable proportion of patients
with functional (endogenous) psychoses.

Behaviour during the six months preceding the crime

Aggressive behaviour on the part of the offenders with cerebral-
organic changes was not less frequent during the six months preceding the
crime than among the 533 abnormal offenders in our group as a whole: in those
with late-acquired brain damage it was even slightly higher (Table 98). In
this respect they were, however, surpassed by the epileptics. But both groups
of cerebral-organic patients showed a more marked tendency to suicide,

Table 98. *Behaviour in the six months preceding the crime in violent*
offenders with late-acquired brain damage (I) and with cerebral atrophy (II)

Form of conspicuous behaviour	Group I	Group II
Aggressiveness (threats and/or violence)	28	20
Suicidal behaviour (threats and/or attempts)	14	17
Considerable social withdrawal (isolation, autism)	14	11
Total	56[a]	48[a]

[a] The total differs from the number of cases because the cases were counted
according to categories exhibited, and combinations were therefore counted
more than once.

particularly those with cerebral atrophy, and there was more reference in their
files to a tendency to withdraw from special relationships than was the case
with the epileptic patients.

The rate of suicidal behaviour is well above the average for all
diagnoses (10%), especially for offenders with cerebral atrophy, a finding
which is in accordance with the high incidence of successful suicide shown in
the Federal Statistics for the age group of 60 and over.

The crime and the victim

As in the case of the epileptic offenders, this group showed fewer
crimes with fatal outcome than attacks that did not end in death. Nineteen
offenders in group I killed at least one victim (in 2 cases there were three
killed); in group II the corresponding figure was 12. In 24 cases in group I
and 20 in group II the victims were only injured. In so far as these figures
can be used as a basis for prediction, they would seem to imply that the senile
patients are slightly less dangerous than those with a traumatic, toxic or
inflammatory cerebral disorder, who are on average younger.

In keeping with the high rate of chronic alcoholism among those
with late-acquired brain damage, there is also in this group a high record of
alcohol intake at the time of the crime: in more than a third ($n = 17$) of
these offenders the influence of alcohol was noted. This is well above the
figure for the cerebral atrophy group where the proportion of such cases
($n = 9$) was about a fifth, which is around the average for all male abnormal
offenders in the study.

The figure for premeditated crime in both groups was similar to the average for the group as a whole (group I: 24 offenders; group II: 17 offenders). Impulsive attacks not preceded by any quarrel or dispute with the victim were much less common than in the epileptic group, being found in between a sixth (group I: n = 7) and about a fifth (group II: n = 9) of the cases. In 9 cases in group I and 14 in group II the violence arose from a quarrel with the victim.

Suicidal behaviour associated with the crime was much more common than in the epileptic group and reached about the same proportions as in the group as a whole. There were 12 cases in each group. Five of these in each group involved extended suicide acts; only one patient, with cerebral atrophy, actually killed himself in an extended suicide act, the rest being registered as extended suicide attempts.

The 43 offenders with late-acquired brain damage killed a total of 24 victims and injured 30. The 40 with cerebral atrophy killed 14 and injured 27 victims. As with the epileptic group, most of the victims were adults

Table 99. *Choice of victim by violent offenders with late-acquired brain damage (I) and with cerebral atrophy (II)*

Type of victim	Group I	Group II
Adult		
Total	35	39
Male adults	14	15
Female adults	18	23
Both male and female adults	3	1
Children		
Total	10	2
Male children	7	1
Female children	1	1
Both male and female children	2	0
Victims from:		
Family/intimate circle	27	26
Circle of acquaintances	3	1
Persons in authority	1	4
Casual acquaintances	10	9
Strangers	2	0

(Counted in number of offenders.)

(group I: n = 35 cases; group II: n = 39 cases), and most were women. The two groups differed in that those with senile brain disorders almost exclusively attacked adults and also attacked comparatively more women than did those with late-acquired brain damage.

Table 99 shows that both groups of cerebral-organic offenders chose their victims mainly from the intimate circle. In keeping with the large number of married offenders, it was mainly the marriage partner who was attacked.

If we look finally at the ostensible motives for the crimes, we find that in contrast to the epileptic group delusional motives played a significant part: they were documented in more than half the cases of cerebral atrophy (n = 25) and in about half the cases of late-acquired brain damage (n = 20). These figures correspond roughly to the frequency with which delusions were recorded in the course of these brain-damaged patients' illnesses. Patients whose record contained no mention of motive were more frequent in the epileptic group (about a third) than in the cerebral-organic group (about an eighth of the cases). Sixteen offenders in group I and 11 in group II had committed their violent crime from motives that did not involve delusions.

9.3 Mentally abnormal violent offenders with chronic alcoholism

As already explained in Chapter 3, we admitted to our study only those mentally abnormal offenders who suffered from 'major mental disorders', meaning essentially persons who were psychotic, severely brain-damaged, epileptic or mentally defective. Psychopathic syndromes such as personality disorders (psychopathies), neuroses, perversions and addictions, including chronic alcoholism,[2] were recorded as subsidiary diagnoses.

The most common subsidiary diagnosis was alcoholism, which is a form of addiction that can lead to and affect the course of associated personality changes, or be accompanied by extensive disturbances. It therefore seemed worthwhile to assemble, in addition to the diagnostic groups already discussed, a separate group consisting of those offenders who in addition to severe psychological and behavioural disturbances such as schizophrenia or mental deficiency, suffered from chronic alcoholism. We have already presented some data on this subject in our paired comparison of violent and non-violent offenders (Chapter 3).

In all, 79 mentally abnormal violent offenders (14.8%) were given the subsidiary diagnosis of chronic alcoholism; in six cases the addiction was combined with other forms of addiction.

Table 100. *Age distribution of mentally*
abnormal violent offenders with a
subsidiary diagnosis of chronic
alcoholism

	n	%
14–19	3	4
20–29	23	29
30–39	22	28
40–49	15	19
50–59	12	15
60 and over	4	5
Total	79	100

Sex and age

The group consisted predominantly of male patients (n = 74). The
age distribution showed a small peak in the third and fourth decades (Table
100).

Marital status

About half of the offenders were unmarried (n = 39), more than a
third were married (n = 27), barely a seventh (n = 11) were separated or
divorced, and two were widowed.

Occupation

A good third of the cases were out of work or incapable of work at
the time of the crime (n = 29) or were in unskilled occupations such as
auxiliary worker, farm labourer, etc. (n = 30). Only 18 alcoholics were working in skilled or comparable occupations. There were none in the higher
professions. Two were documented as housewives.

Personality, previous criminal record, heredity

As might be expected, the violent alcoholic offenders were to a
large extent people with severe disturbances of personality. The subsidiary
diagnosis of 'antisocial psychopathy' was, for example, recorded in about
half the cases (n = 38). Far more than half of the chronic alcoholics had
already been guilty of violent acts against life and limb (n = 46) and there
were only 11 cases in which no mention was made of previous crimes.

More than half of the group were also recorded as being of low intelligence, ranging from slightly subnormal to mentally deficient ($n = 14$).[3]

In about a quarter of the cases ($n = 19$) there was a record of mental deficiency or mental illness among Grade I relatives; a social heredity of addictive, aggressive or auto-aggressive behaviour was documented in just under a third of the cases ($n = 24$).

Items related to the illness

It was of interest here to find out which main diagnoses and important psychopathological syndromes were associated with chronic alcoholism at the time of the crime (Table 101). Half of all the violent alcoholics ($n = 39$) had delusional symptoms. In far more than half of the cases ($n = 45$) the addiction was accompanied by a psychosis.

Behaviour in the six months preceding the crime

In view of the high rate of previous violent crimes and antisocial personality disturbances, the group of alcoholics might also be expected to show a high incidence of aggressive behaviour in the months preceding the crime. This was indeed the case: almost three-quarters of these offenders

Table 101. *Association of chronic alcoholism with other diagnoses in the whole group of mentally abnormal offenders*

Chronic alcoholism associated with:	n	%
Schizophrenia	22	24.2
Unclassifiable endogenous psychoses	5	5.5
Affective psychoses	3	3.3
Exogenous psychoses	15	16.5
Epilepsy	8	8.8
Late-acquired brain damage	19	20.8
Senile/presenile dementia (cerebral atrophy)	5	5.5
Mental deficiency	14	15.4
Total	91[a]	100.0

[a] Including multiple diagnoses, which is why there are 91 diagnoses for 79 cases.

(n = 58) had shown threatening behaviour, aggressive tensions or violence towards those around them, while suicidal behaviour had been noted in just under a quarter (n = 17). Considerable social isolation or autism was recorded in about a fifth (n = 16) of these offenders.

The crime and the victim

The number of crimes ending in death (n = 25, or 31.6%) was lower than in the group as a whole, where just under half of all the offenders had killed one victim. In 54 cases (68.4%) the victim suffered only bodily harm. In view of the variety of main diagnoses involved, it would be difficult and of little profit to analyse the victims by number and sex.

As might be expected, a very substantial proportion of these offenders were under the influence of alcohol at the time of the crime, namely 54, or 68.4%, which is considerably higher than the figure for the group of mentally abnormal offenders as a whole (17.1%).

The rate of premeditated crime (n = 34) was of the same order as that in the group as a whole. Suicidal behaviour after the crime (n = 13) was somewhat less frequent than in the group as a whole.

The alcoholic offenders again chose their victims to a large extent from the family or intimate circle (42 cases, or 53.2%). But the proportion of offenders who attacked acquaintances was higher here than in the group of all diagnoses (26 cases, or 32.9%, as against 23.4% for the group of all mentally abnormal offenders).

Crimes with no ostensible motive (n = 6) were much less common than in the control group. Just under half of the chronic alcoholic offenders (n = 36) acted from purely delusional motives, 11 from disappointed love and jealousy (including delusional jealousy), 37 from motives which were not associated with delusion. It was not possible, however, to define clearly to what extent the motivation was associated with the effects of alcoholism or with the effects of the mental illness recorded as the main diagnosis.

To sum up, one has the impression that chronic alcoholism as an additional complication of mental illness, mental deficiency and many syndromes of defect, implies a considerable increase in the risk of violence, which is reflected in the very high rate of previous violent crime and aggressive behaviour in the months preceding the actual crime. If chronic alcoholism is associated with antisocial personality traits, brain damage with personality change, or below-average intelligence or slight mental defect, and/or if there are delusional symptoms, then the risk of violence is perceptibly increased, particularly when the use of alcohol helps to precipitate the crime.

10. SUMMARY AND DISCUSSION

It is not our intention at this point merely to reproduce all the findings of the investigation in a comprehensive summary. Our aim is much more to review and clarify these findings on the basis of the discussions already set out in the individual chapters: this will, it is hoped, make it easier to place our study within the framework of current psychiatric knowledge and to derive from it some measures of prevention.

Our study has one considerable advantage over previous relevant investigations. It began with a relatively well defined and sufficiently large body of material which was capable of being more or less comprehensively surveyed. The base population (the legally responsible adult population of the GFR, numbering about 42.6 millions) and the risk period (10 years) are such that it can reasonably be claimed that the group investigated is representative and forms part of a whole on which comprehensive data are available.

The representativeness of our subgroups, for example that of mentally abnormal offenders who committed suicide after their crime and who fall particularly within the diagnoses of 'depression' and 'affective psychoses', must be viewed with somewhat more reserve. Nor can we claim that our findings would be fully valid for any other period. The decade covered by our study, 1955 to 1964, coincides with a relatively stable period of economic and social-political development in the GFR. Criminal rates were running on a more or less regular continuum and showed no real qualitative changes. Crimes committed by foreigners were still very few, as was the proportion of offenders who might have been influenced by different cultural factors. Our study was practically unaffected by violent crimes with a political background, or by crimes subject to extraordinary influences such as drug abuse, which increased from 1968 onwards and in which mentally abnormal offenders could possibly be under- or over-represented. We can therefore in the first place assume that our predictions apply only to 'normal' conditions governing the development of violence in the GFR and perhaps to other nations which are culturally comparable.

The advantage of this relatively solid methodological basis, which makes it possible for the first time to arrive at fairly reliable figures for violent crime committed by the mentally abnormal, has associated disadvantages. As we said at the outset, questions of overall crime rates for the mentally abnormal must remain unanswered, as must questions of overall crime rates for diagnostic categories other than those we studied, such as personality disturbances and neuroses. We included in our study those offenders who came within the diagnostic categories of 'mental deficiency, epilepsy, endogenous and exogenous psychoses, and degenerative syndromes (such as dementia), as well as psychological changes due to organic disturbances of cerebral functioning'. In so far as the crime was concerned, we based our study on an operational definition that took account of the reason for the crime and the content of the crime, content being essentially a serious attack on the life of another person.

This definition embraces one type of crime which occupies a special position, namely, attempts at extended suicide. Such a crime differs from most other types of crime mainly because of the special importance of suicidal intentions in motivating the act and determining its course. A different form of questionnaire might have placed extended suicide in the category of auto-aggressive violence, that is to say violence directed against the offender himself. But in our study it counted as an act of violence, on the same footing as any other act which led, or at least might have led, to the death of another person. Since we were concerned with the 'dangerousness' of the mentally abnormal, it followed that our operational terms must enable us to arrive at findings that would throw light on different types of dangerous crime, on their areas of motivation and on their relationships to different diagnostic categories.

Individual suicide, however, which injures only the offender himself, or perhaps by negligence also involves other people, remained outside the scope of our study. One reason for this decision was that to include such cases would have called for a new and very much extended investigation. Comprehensive surveys of completed and attempted suicide present one of the most difficult problems in psychiatric epidemiology, to which reliable solutions have not yet been found. The risk that mentally disturbed persons who commit suicide - apart from deliberate extended suicide - will constitute a danger to other people is quantitatively insignificant and did not seem to justify a wide-ranging expansion of our research programme.

All our findings - and this must again be emphasised in connection with our methodology - must be viewed in the context of our basic data and their validity and reliability at the time of the study. It should not be forgotten that our data were collected from secondary sources and could not yield more than the original documents contained. In testing various hypotheses, therefore, for example in the area of the influence of the offender's family and of his personality upon the risk of violence, we had to use indices which were probably characteristic only of a part of the qualities we wished to study. In selecting such indices from the data documented we had moreover to consider not only their reliability but also their availability, which preferably should be close on 100%: in other words, we wanted as low as possible a ratio of 'not knowns'. This explains also why we were often unable to use the indices which are customarily employed in psychiatry, criminology and sociology.

Where possible we tried to increase the general validity of the findings by testing the same hypothesis in correlation with different items of equal or similar significance. We adopted similar procedures when we did not have reliable or completely adequate relative numbers. Thus, for example, when making the vital comparison between rates of violence for the mentally abnormal and rates for the general population, we used figures drawn from different sources (police statistics of crime, court sentences, and statistics of the causes of death). By such pragmatic means we tried to decrease the margins of error in our results.

Probably the most important finding from our study is that the 533 mentally abnormal individuals investigated, who had committed a violent crime in the GFR between 1 January 1955 and 31 December 1964, represented about 3% of the total number of comparable violent offenders during this period. The number of victims killed was 293, which represents a roughly equivalent proportion, based on corrected estimates, of the deaths by violence shown in the official federal statistics of causes of death. Although we did not have available the requisite comparative figures, i.e. the frequency (incidence and prevalence) and age distribution of those suffering from illnesses in the same diagnostic categories in the general population (as no such epidemiological data are available for the GFR), we were able to draw upon estimated rates from fairly comparable investigations in other countries. The resulting conclusion is: the mentally abnormal in general are not more likely, and are in fact less likely, to commit violent crimes than are the mentally normal.

In this formulation, of course, the concept of 'mentally normal' implies no more than the absence of a mental illness falling within the category of a psychosis, a mental handicap (mental deficiency), an epileptic disorder, or any kind of psychological defect based on organic cerebral impairment. It leaves untouched the much-discussed question, that is often studied with inadequate means and that has not so far been answered, of what proportion of violent offenders suffer from 'minor psychiatric disorders', in particular personality disorders (psychopathy) and neuroses. Psychiatry certainly still has many research problems to solve in this area of criminology.

We have set forth in detail the facts and considerations which support our prediction. Two basic objections must, however, also be taken into account:

(1) *The influence of the dark figure could alter the proportion of violent offenders who are mentally abnormal.* Crimes of violence include an unknown number of undiscovered cases. It is, of course, not possible to include this dark figure as an unknown quantity in the estimation or calculation of the risk of crime. If it does not contain an equal distribution of mentally abnormal and other offenders, then it is more probable that the mentally abnormal offenders have less chance of concealing their crime and escaping detection than the mentally 'normal' and mentally less handicapped violent offenders. Assuming that the dark figure is higher for mentally 'normal' violent offenders, this means that the proportion of all violent offenders who are mentally abnormal would be lower than the figure of about 3% at which we arrived.

(2) *The more frequent loss of liberty suffered by the mentally abnormal might have led to an 'unreal' lowering of the risk of crime.* Mentally abnormal persons are, on account of their illness or handicap, admitted to hospital more frequently than the mentally normal and are thus prevented from committing crimes by their loss of freedom, which is presumably of longer than average duration. Against this hypothesis, however, it must be said that mentally normal violent offenders also have above-average rates of loss of liberty because of their previous convictions. It would therefore have been advisable to compare the average loss of freedom for these two groups before the crime. Unfortunately the requisite information, in the form of statistical data on previous convictions in violent offenders, was not available.

Our findings, however, provide an important and relevant pointer: about half of all the mentally abnormal offenders had not previously been in hospital. If we compare the duration of illness for those offenders who had and those who had not previously been admitted to hospital, we find there is no real difference between the two groups. This means that the effect of hospitalisation is unlikely to be considerable, since it would have to be apparent in a postponement of the crime, that is to say in an increase in duration of illness for those offenders who had been in hospital as compared with those who had had no previous admissions.

Finally we may make this objection more specific and hypothesise that mentally abnormal offenders have an advantage in regard to risk period, in that during acute phases or exacerbations of their illness they are restrained from possible crimes by their immediate admission to hospital. But this argument, too, is not very telling, since according to our findings - and this applied also to offenders with no previous hospital admissions - the crime was not very often associated with acute phases or exacerbations of the illness. Moreover about 40% of the offenders who had been in psychiatric hospitals committed their violent crime during the first six months after discharge. If loss of freedom, focused as it is on phases of the illness, had a delaying effect on the risk of crime, then this would probably continue to rise or even be over-compensated for during the subsequent risk period.

Consideration of these two objections thus gives no indication that our estimate of the proportion of violent offenders who are mentally abnormal is too low, or that the low rate is essentially governed by the intervention of such influences as admission to hospital and loss of liberty.

10.1 The 'dangerousness' of the mentally abnormal

If we define the dangerousness of the mentally abnormal as the relative probability of their committing a violent crime, then our findings show that this does not exceed the dangerousness of the legally responsible adult population as a whole. This finding puts a clear question mark against the assumption that mental illnesses are a principal cause of violence or are likely to make individuals liable to commit violent crimes.

One conclusion may be drawn from this, the practical implications of which should be rated very highly: it is not necessary or justifiable to treat a large proportion of the mentally abnormal under conditions of increased control because of an increased risk of violence. The general trend in psychiatry towards more open care of the mentally ill seems justified so far as the risk of violence is concerned.

At all events the mentally abnormal are not according to our findings more dangerous, in the defined sense of the word, than the legally responsible adult population as a whole. At the same time it is necessary and justifiable to apply measures of security and prevention to those patients for whom the risk is increased. We must therefore try to direct such measures as accurately as possible towards their target. To achieve this we need more precise knowledge of the groups with high risk and of the predictors of imminent violence.

10.2   Danger to the self and to others

The problem of the dangerousness of the mentally ill quickly leads to the problem of their dangerousness to themselves. Unfortunately we could not tackle this question empirically on the basis of an adequate comparison, because the analogous data on suicide are unreliable and above all incomplete. Starting as we did with the total number of deaths from violence, we could, as already explained, arrive at only an estimated figure. For the period of our investigation the annual average of such deaths was around 1000 cases. The annual average number of suicides recorded stood many times higher, at 10 000 cases. This takes no account of the fact that the dark figure for suicide is very high - it is estimated at twice or more the number of registered cases - presumably higher than that for deaths from violent crime. The proportion of suicides who are mentally disturbed is variously estimated to be between 5% and 20%;   exact figures are not known. The proportion of abnormal violent offenders who have killed their victim is around 3%.

Studies of the course of illness in cohorts of different composition have provided better information about the risk of suicide in individual groups of mentally ill patients. The findings are not entirely comparable; but the order of size can nevertheless be estimated. The proportion of patients with depressive psychoses or manic-depressive illnesses whose cause of death was suicide lies between about 9% (Kinkelin, 1959; Ciompi & Lai, 1969) and about 50% (Freming, 1951; Helgason, 1964). The last two of these studies, with findings of 50% (Freming, Bornholm) and 53% (Helgason, Iceland), deserve to be given special weight, in as much as they are based not only on former hospital patients but also on cohorts of analogous-risk groups in the general population.

For schizophrenia the corresponding figures are between about 6% (Helgason) and about 10% (Freming). The data published more recently on the basis of cumulative case registers are admittedly not comparable but confirm at least this order of size (cf. Gardner *et al.*, 1964).

If we compare these figures with the probability, based on the number of new cases, that the patient will kill another person (again this is not exact but represents only the possible order of size) then we see that the risk of suicide for schizophrenics is higher by a factor of 10^2, and for depressives by a factor of 10^3 to 10^4, than the risk of killing another person.

This comparison, imprecise as it is, still makes it clear that schizophrenics are a hundred times more in danger, and depressives a thousand times more in danger, of killing themselves than of killing other people. It is probably justifiable to predict that the danger to the patient himself is many, many times greater than the danger to other people, allowing for some variation in this respect in the other groups of the mentally ill in the narrower sense. The conclusion which can be drawn from this and which has implications for the orientation of psychiatric therapy and for the organisation of psychiatric services of treatment and care, is as follows: preventive, remedial and protective measures designed to keep the patient from endangering his own person should be in the foreground for a large majority of patients. Only a very small proportion of those patients who require care need measures of security or other arrangements to lessen their dangerousness towards other people. This is first and foremost a purely quantitative prediction, which should, however, be reflected in all laws relating to the committal of the mentally ill.

For the mentally defective, whose risk of suicide probably does not exceed their risk of violence to others to the same extent, we are unable to give an estimate because there are no suitable comparative data.

Finally it should be noted that about 23% of all the violent offenders in our study committed their crime either as a form of extended suicide and/or in association with suicide or attempted suicide. The largest subgroup of these offenders came typically within the category of the affective psychoses, the second largest within the category of the schizophrenias.

10.3 Risk of violence in individual groups of illnesses

We could arrive at only an approximate estimate of the illness-specific risk. For schizophrenics it was of the order of 5 per 10 000; for the mentally defective[1] and for those with affective psychoses it was about 6 per 100 000 new cases of illness. The estimate given for schizophrenics is probably rather high, as we have already explained in detail. For the affective psychoses the same source of error is certainly wiped out - in fact it may be over-compensated - by the fact that a proportion of the offenders who died in an extended suicide may have escaped our case-finding procedures, so that the risk may be assumed to be slightly higher than the figure at which we arrived.

We did not calculate risks for the other groups of illnesses, chiefly because the numbers of offenders were too low or the groups were heterogeneous. But it may be predicted, with some reservations, that none

of these groups of illnesses contained more violent offenders than one might
expect from a crude estimate of their share in the incidence of 'serious
psychiatric illnesses'.

Starting from the fact that we collected all the mentally abnormal
violent offenders in a population of about 42.6 millions (the legally
responsible adult population of the GFR), we may say that even these crude
predictions are of some significance. We may infer from them that there is no
support for the assumption that any form of mental illness or mental defect
is associated with an excessive tendency to violent crime. The risk of violence
in the mentally abnormal, which is close to the average for the adult population in general, is admittedly an average figure, which is slightly higher for
some specific diagnoses and slightly lower for others, but the diagnostic
variation in risk is relatively small.

10.4   General data on the crime and the victim

In the ten years between 1955 and 1964 the 533 mentally abnormal
offenders killed a total of 293 persons and seriously injured 362. Attacks on
one victim headed the list and, with the exception of the mentally defective
and to a less marked degree the chronic alcoholic, the victim usually was drawn
from the circle of close family relationships or intimate partnerships. The
crime was almost without exception committed by one offender alone, again with
the exception of the mentally defective offenders. The few offenders who
killed three or four people usually fell within the category of family suicide
and as a rule were also acting on their own.

Only two offenders killed or seriously injured more than four
people. One of the two, who attacked ten unknown passers-by on different days
with a hammer because his voices ordered him to do so, suffered from a
paranoid-hallucinatory schizophrenia. The other, the 'Volkhoven flamethrower',
had built himself a flamethrower and an iron lance, with which he attacked a
primary school. Eight children and two female teachers died, mostly of severe
burns, while 22 more were injured, some seriously. His motive seemed to be
delusional revenge for a long chain of failures and disappointments which he
laid at the door of various authorities and doctors. As he committed suicide
shortly after the event, the diagnosis of chronic paranoid schizophrenia was
made only on the basis of previous findings, though it was probably correct
(cf. Kiehne, 1965).

Comparable cases, such as that of the mass-murderer Wagner
described by Gaupp (1914), or the schizophrenic student who fired on strangers
from the tower of the University of Texas, are extraordinarily rare. Because

of the horror which such deeds inspire, however, they remain in the memory for a long time and thus constitute a kind of type of schizophrenic multiple murderer which can sometimes develop into or contribute to the development of a stereotype.

Looked at in the light of our findings, these men belong to the extreme end of a group of mentally abnormal offenders who have usually suffered for many years from a chronic delusional psychosis, without showing any deep change in personality, and who have committed their crimes in the end from delusional motives. The features which characterise this subgroup of schizophrenic offenders, together with some preliminary warning signs of impending violence, make preventive measures seem not altogether hopeless. We shall deal with this question further when we come to discuss schizophrenic offenders.

The crime

There are no particular features worth reproducing in regard to the manner in which the mentally abnormal offenders carried out their violent crimes. The preferred methods of the male offenders (blunt and sharp instruments: 65%) and of the female offenders (strangulation, poison or gas, and drowning: about 50%; and blunt and sharp instruments: 34%) show a sex difference which reflects general tendencies found in violent crime as a whole, as well as in some statistics on methods of suicide. Special brutality in executing the crime, such as extraordinarily cruel or perverse abuse of the living or dead victim, is very rare in mentally abnormal offenders. It is found more often in the violent crimes of 'normal' offenders and those with personality disorders (neurotic or psychopathic) than in crimes committed by the mentally ill or mentally defective in the narrower sense.

Influence of alcohol at the time of the crime

In the group as a whole the influence of alcohol at the time of the crime was evident to a certain extent though it did not play a major part. It was accepted as being present in 17% of all cases, almost exclusively those of the male offenders (21.5% as against 2.5% of the women). There were, however, great differences in respect of this item between the different diagnostic groups. Characteristic examples are the offenders with chronic alcoholism, about two-thirds of whom were under the influence of alcohol at the time of the crime; for the epileptics, for those with late-acquired brain damage and for the mentally defective the figure was about one-third, for the schizophrenics about 10% and for those with affective psychoses about 5%.

In just under 7% of the cases only, the offenders in question all
being male, was the crime associated with sexual activity, though this is
not to say that the motivation was then predominantly sexual. In this respect
the mentally defective offenders headed the list with 24%, being well in
front of the schizophrenics with about 5%, while the figure for the depressives
(affective psychoses) was 0%. This shows that the mentally ill patient in the
narrower sense does not contribute to any important extent to sexually motivated crimes - in so far as we arbitrarily interpret as sexually motivated only
those crimes which have frank sexual intent or accompaniments. Apart from
the small number of offenders in the mentally deficient group, it is clear
that it is offenders with personality disturbances or neurotic personalities
who chiefly account for the instinctual violent crimes that form part of
crimes of violence as a whole.

Violent crime and suicide

In 13.4% of all the cases the crime was committed as an extended
suicide, which is one of the characteristic forms of violence in the mentally
abnormal. If we add to this those offenders who committed or attempted
suicide in association with a crime perpetrated from other motives, then we
find that in 23% of the cases the crime was associated with suicidal acts.
For women this figure rises to 47% (17% for men), the high rate being
accounted for mainly by the massive over-representation of offenders with
affective psychoses, whose crime was in about 60% of cases classified as
extended suicide. If we bear in mind that our survey probably failed to
include some offenders who committed suicide in association with their crime,
then in all likelihood these percentages should be still further increased.

Offenders who repeat their crime

The mentally abnormal do not often repeat their homicidal crimes.
Only 8, or 1.2%, of the 533 offenders had previously killed someone, a
further 9 having made previous homicidal attempts. This means that 17 in all,
or 3.2% of the offenders, were guilty of a second crime that fell within the
same definition of a crime of violence. This low rate is probably partly due
to the fact that mentally abnormal offenders are easily apprehended after a
homicidal crime and are often then committed for a lengthy period of time.
This assumption is supported by the finding that less serious aggressive
acts, such as bodily injury, were recorded in the previous history of a third
of the offenders. Here again there were considerable diagnostic differences.

It follows from this that at least some small, fairly

circumscribed groups of mentally ill offenders present a not inconsiderable danger of repeated violent crime. In the language of psychiatry, this means that we have to reckon with small groups of patients with different diagnoses who have a special predisposition to violence. Clearly this dangerousness is not randomly or blindly distributed over the whole range of the mentally abnormal. We shall deal with the preventive implications of this when we come to discuss the risk factors and the warning signs or indicators of violence in individual groups of illnesses.

Choice of victim

The victims of the mentally abnormal offenders were drawn to a striking degree from the circle of close human relationships. About 60% of the victims belonged to the immediate families of the offenders - marriage partners, children, parents, siblings - or had intimate relationships with them. Only about 9% were strangers, unknown to the offenders, while about 7% had played some kind of authoritative role in their lives, being, for example, doctors, judges, police officers and so on. The remaining victims, about 23%, were friends or acquaintances of the offenders. It may be inferred from this that intimate human relationships play an important part in motivating violent crimes by the mentally abnormal.

Attacks on strangers, for example from motives of material gain or gratification of instincts, which form a large part of the 'normal' crimes of violence, are thus the exception so far as the mentally abnormal are concerned. It is not often the widow living alone, the bank messenger, or the woman going home alone at night, who is threatened by the potential violence of the mentally abnormal, though the mentally deficient are somewhat of an exception here. It is much more the closest relatives and most intimate partners of the patient who are in immediate danger. Sixty-two per cent of the female offenders - who were mostly suffering from endogenous depression and whose crime was extended suicide - chose their own children as victims.

This specific tendency in dangerousness provides us with an important pointer so far as prevention is concerned. We must watch above all for warning signs of impending violence and of danger to specific persons within the patient's most intimate circle. In doing so we must remember that intimate partners are often, because of their emotional ties with the patient, inadequately equipped to recognise their own danger. Children usually remain to the end free of any suspicion of their mothers who are planning their extended suicide.

The future offender not infrequently gives indications in the

form of threats and hints as to the person whom he might attack, often direct-
ing these immediately at the threatened individual. In order to be able to
assess the seriousness of the danger, it is necessary to look to some extent
objectively not only at the warning signs but also at the way in which the
patient experiences the relationship that is so fraught with danger. An
important way of achieving this difficult goal is to draw the partner who is
possibly at risk into the orbit of psychiatric advice. Sometimes this is
better done by a doctor other than the one who is treating the patient, though
working in close collaboration with him. It is often necessary to consult
further relatives or friends of the patient who have good contacts with him
and can help to make the situation and its observation more objective.

The most important source of information – at least for the
relatively large group of cases of delusional 'family violence' is the
offender himself. As the danger increases, a temporary or sometimes permanent
separation of the offender from his endangered partner becomes necessary;
when the risk is serious, and the partner is likely to be harmed or the
delusional homicidal motivation is likely to be shifted on to other partners,
precautionary hospitalisation is required.

The legal provisions for this are inadequate, and there are great
differences in legal practice in regard to the administration of precautionary
committals. The threat to the civil rights of non-dangerous patients, if such
measures are widely used, is easily recognisable. But this does not absolve us
from the duty of seeking better ways of protecting the endangered relatives
of that small group of the mentally ill who are liable to commit violent
crimes.

The above considerations apply only to a limited proportion of
the offenders studied and diagnostically concern mainly the chronic paranoid
schizophrenics, though they apply also in part to the epileptic offenders and
to those with late-acquired brain damage and cerebral atrophy, as well as to
some of the chronic alcoholic offenders. So far as the depressed female
offenders are concerned, attention must be paid to the serious risk of
extended suicide and to the danger this implies for those close to them,
particularly their own children: delusional fears of perishing must be studied
with particular care. The most important precautionary measure here is
probably in-patient treatment, which should continue as long as there is a
serious risk of suicide.

Adult relatives should be thoroughly briefed on the danger, the
direction it is likely to take and the warning signs that may appear: this
preventive step is to be recommended in such illnesses and is indispensable

where suicidal acts or threats, or desires to include others therein, give
warning of the danger that may accompany the next phase of the illness.

The tendency to choose victims from the intimate family circle -
'normal' violent offenders seem, on the other hand, to prefer victims from
outside the family - is not found in the mentally defective group and was
less common in the chronic alcoholics, who to a large extent were suffering
concurrently from another mental illness. The behaviour of the mentally
deficient in this respect was more like that of the 'normal' offenders: 25%
of their victims were strangers, about 40% acquaintances or friends, and
only about 30% members of their immediate family or intimate partners.

It might be argued that the preference of the mentally ill for
victims from their family circle is associated with the fact that they are
more often married and living in family surroundings than, for example, the
mentally defective offenders who are mostly unmarried: such an objection,
however, seemed to us of only limited importance. The epileptic offenders,
who were also to a large extent unmarried, also chose two-thirds of their
victims from the immediate family circle. Of 37 offenders with affective
psychoses, only two attacked someone who was not related to or intimately
associated with them, the other 35 choosing only members of the family as
victims. One of these two was suffering additionally from florid mania and
while in a beer-tent had struck someone sitting at the same table over the
head with the beer-measure - a crime with local colour that according to
our findings was extremely unusual for depressive offenders.

The prediction that choice of victim will tend to be associated
with the type of mental illness, or with personality factors, was borne out by
analysis of the content of motives, particularly for the two groups of
'endogenous depression' and 'chronic paranoid schizophrenia'.

Arguing on the hypothesis that marriage rates might affect the
choice of victim, we might presumably expect that absence of the married state
in the case of depressed patients would reduce the risk of violence to almost
nil. For mentally defective patients, on the other hand, the support of a
positive family setting would possibly decrease the risk of violence. For
patients with schizophrenia and some allied illnesses (particularly delusional
illnesses) - or, rather, for that small group of such patients who are liable
to be violent - close emotional ties represent a special risk factor. The
hypothesis that avoidance of close emotional ties would lessen the risk of
violent crime in delusional patients is not without foundation.

Since recent research in schizophrenia has shown (cf. Brown,
Monck, Carstairs, Wing, 1962) that close and intense relationships play a part

in causing relapses, we can hardly doubt that a parallel exists between the
two processes. Violent crimes on the part of such patients cannot, however,
be interpreted as the exact equivalent of a relapse into illness. The offenders in this group, who are mostly chronically ill, do not often show an
exacerbation of symptoms coinciding with the crime. One may point rather to a
general disturbance in their capacity for integration and for reality-based
control of deep emotions, such a disturbance being possibly a necessary part
of the specific vulnerability of schizophrenics who are in danger of
relapsing as well as of the pathological deviations and elaborations seen in
violent schizophrenic offenders.

Practical conclusions may at any rate be jointly inferred concerning patients of this type who are in danger of relapsing or who are liable
to aggressive violence. If close affective ties and emotional overstimulation
are significant trigger mechanisms, then their avoidance, and the maintenance
of a more remote attitude, even at the cost of more severe isolation at the
emotional level, is a real and sometimes essential measure of prevention. The
isolation can as a rule be partly overcome by strengthening clearly structured
and regulated social contacts at the level of secondary relationships. This
goal has to be approached by ways that have to be selected in the light of
individual potentialities. These range from an adequate maintenance dosage of
antipsychotic or neuroleptic drugs to measures of social therapy, such as
admission to a patients' club or to a sheltered hostel, and finally to a
regime of continuous advice given to the marriage partner and members of the
family. As already mentioned, these must go as far as separation from a partner or a family with whom a potentially violent patient is entangled
inextricably in a delusionally governed state of hostility.

The matter seems important enough for us to close this section
with a rule - to which there will be many exceptions - namely: the danger
inherent in those mentally ill, as opposed to mentally deficient, patients
who are inclined to be violent, is greatest in the area of their strongest
emotional relationships. These are often also the patient's most intimate and
tense relationships. It is only in depressive patients that such ties are not
mainly of a marital or other intimate kind: in depressives they are the very
close and by no means tense relationships between married mothers and their
own children.

Motives and planning of the crime

We have already shown in detail why the greatest reserve must be
used in evaluating direct data about motives. Nevertheless there is one

useful finding which contradicts the older psychiatric concepts, namely the low proportion (18.5%) of our mentally abnormal offenders for whom no motive could be ascertained. In fact this figure is probably too high, because in a case of clear and severe mental illness or mental defect the search for motives is usually accorded low priority. It is possible that some of the examining psychiatrists started by assuming that the crimes were chiefly senseless and out of keeping with the personality, and in addition there is a relatively small proportion of mentally abnormal patients whose inner world remains very inaccessible. The last-named factor may explain the disproportion-ately high number of hebephrenic or autistic schizophrenics with a clinically quiet symptomatology who are found among the apparently unmotivated offenders, in so far as other syndrome-specific reasons do not account for this finding.

Apart from this, the different groups of illnesses show a propor-tion of apparently unmotivated offenders which is close to the average of about 1 : 5. Only the chronic alcoholics - including all cases which were given another diagnosis as well, say of schizophrenia or mental deficiency - had a lower figure of 10%, while the epileptics showed the somewhat higher proportion of one-third.

So far as motives themselves are concerned, it was possible only to make a comparison of trends between our group and the group representing violent crime in general, in whom, at least according to all the records from the GFR, the motives that headed the list were gain and concealment of a punishable offence. This corresponded to the findings for the mental defec-tives in our study, of whom more than two-thirds came within these categories of motivation. In the other groups of illnesses this combination of motives occupied a much lower place, with figures of around 10%. Heading the list of motives in the schizophrenic group was that of revenge, usually based on close emotional relationships, frequently with delusional causes or compon-ents, which accounted for about 40% of the cases. Next came mainly delusional motives such as defence against a delusionally experienced threat (16%) and jealousy (15%). However many reservations there are regarding the reliability of these findings, it cannot be denied that they supplement to an adequate degree the statements which we encountered when we examined the content of offender-victim relationships in our schizophrenics. They also define some-what more precisely, in terms of the content of the relationships, the range of persons who are at risk.

So far as the chronic alcoholics are concerned, motives such as jealousy and disappointment in love were more to the fore. Depressed offend-ers again occupied a special position. In more than three-quarters of the cases the idea of finding release in death from some delusionally feared and inescapable evil was prominent in the list of motives. The conspicuous part played by delusional experience in the motivation of mentally ill, as opposed to mentally defective, violent offenders is confirmed by a few further data: more than 50% of those suffering from processes of cerebral disintegration, usually aged 60 and over, and about half of those with late-acquired brain damage, had delusional motives. In 68% of the schizophrenic cases the victim was delusionally involved before the crime. In so far as the content of the delusions was concerned, the offender most frequently felt himself injured or threatened. The general inference that can be drawn from this, and the most important one from the point of view of prevention, is as follows: if a person with whom such a patient has close emotional ties is involved in the patient's delusions, particularly if it is a question of delusional jealousy or erotic delusions, and if the delusional experience is associated with injury or a threat to life, then the risk of such a person being the victim of a violent crime exceeds that which is normal for the basic illness in question. This is based on the assumption that the patient is then not the average brain-injured or schizophrenic individual, but is a person who because of certain risk factors is liable to become violent.

Information about the proportion of crimes which are premeditated is even more questionable than data about motivation. Here presumably only the positive results have any predictive value. Impulsive acts appear to be most frequent in epileptic offenders and in the mentally defective, with a figure of around a third. For schizophrenics impulsive crimes were recorded in about a quarter of the cases, but in affective psychoses only in 20%. Usually the crime was planned in advance. Though women are often considered to be impulsive, 60% of all the mentally abnormal female offenders had planned their crime beforehand (as against 33% of the men). This again is connected with the marked over-representation of women in the depressive group who as a rule did not commit extended suicide impulsively, in a state of raptus melancholicus, but planned it carefully and usually over a long period of time. More than 70% of the offenders with affective psychoses had made plans for their crime. In the schizophrenic group about half of the crimes, and in the mentally defective group about two-fifths, were explicitly described as planned. The epileptic group, with 8 out of 29, showed a markedly lower proportion of planned crimes. This group of 'explosive' patients, who committed their crimes while under the influence of alcohol or twilight states, and a third of whom became violent after a quarrel or without any recognisable cause, showed the highest rate of unplanned or impulsive delinquency.

Planned crimes of violence naturally have a higher 'success rate'; they more frequently lead to the death of the victim. On the other hand, in so far as specific preventive measures have prospects of success, plans contemplated by offenders over a fairly long period of time are accessible to intervention. Impulsive behaviour, on the other hand, can be mitigated only by more general measures such as, for example, continuous anticonvulsive and sedative treatment of an epileptic patient who shows violent tendencies.

We were left with the impression that unaccountable, impulsive behaviour contributes to the violence of the mentally abnormal in a way that is related to diagnosis but that is on the whole only of minor significance. Much more common are the morbidly motivated crimes which are more or less carefully planned in advance and directed against a specific person whose relationship with the offender is close and often affected by delusions.

Causes and precipitating factors

Recent research has increasingly recognised the importance of precipitating factors which trigger off a psychotic episode, particularly in the schizophrenias and the affective psychoses (Brown & Birley, 1970). We therefore tried to investigate stress factors in the lives of our offenders which might be considered as causes of the crime. The relatively small number of violent crimes which were associated with relapse into illness, and the unexpectedly high number of crimes which were planned a long time beforehand, particularly in the case of mental illnesses in the narrower sense, show that there is a clear distinction between the triggering of a psychosis and the precipitating of a violent crime. Crimes planned in advance need no immediate cause - a 'favourable opportunity' or an exchange of words can at times suffice to set in motion the premeditated crime that has already been decided on or is smouldering under the surface. In other instances a violent quarrel, a deep humiliation, or a relaxation of inhibitions due to alcohol, can cause the patient to lose his self-control, which is already weakened by his illness (for example in the case of epileptic or mentally defective offenders), and thus act as the trigger or immediate occasion of the crime.

These examples show that the question of precipitating factors is more complicated where violence is concerned than it is in causing psychotic episodes. The answers, if indeed there are any, are to be found at very different levels, concerned with such factors as, for example, the strength of motivation, specific and non-specific emotional provocation, and decrease in self-control.

shift towards the older decades. This finding lends support to the hypothesis that age seems in general to have more influence than mental illness on the risk of violence. Looking at the evidence critically, all we can say at present is that membership of the male sex and of an age group with a high risk of violence constitutes a basis for the manifestation of violence, irrespective of whether this risk is heightened by mental illness or not. As mentioned, however, the affective psychoses are an exception to this rule.

The shift in age of the mentally abnormal offenders was a striking feature: with a mean of 34.6 years as against 26.4 for the mentally normal offenders, this amounted to about 8 years. We have discussed some of the possible explanations for this. One hypothesis, for example, might be that the illness does not affect the age of manifestation of violent crimes. It would then follow that the age shift is only a statistical artefact, caused by the higher average age of the mentally abnormal and its effect on the age distribution of our sample of violent offenders selected according to our criterion of mental illness. Although we could not test this hypothesis precisely, we were able to show that this is probably only a partial explana-tion of the age shift. For the offenders with degenerative cerebral dis-orders - a form of illness with maximal manifestation in the higher age groups - this age shift plays a decisive role. For the mentally defective offenders, whose average age was largely in line with that of the 'normal' violent offenders but who also shared with them numerous other characteristics, the age factor probably no longer counts, or may even work in the opposite direction because of the lower expectation of life.

The possibility that the age shift is caused by the event of illness, or by factors associated with the illness, is one that must be seriously considered. It finds support not least in the very long period of time that generally elapses between the onset of the illness and the committ-ing of the violent offence. We considered at one time that the illness might operate as a partial defence factor, by delaying the manifestation of violence in predisposed personalities. An argument against this is, however, that it would lead also to a perceptible fall in the incidence of violence, which is not the case, at least not in schizophrenics. On the other hand illness might restrict the danger of violence to a narrow area of risk, which would then be influenced by factors associated with the illness and would be affected temporally by the course of the illness. It seems highly likely that this is what happens in the case of the depressed offenders.

To account for the age shift in the largest group of mentally abnormal offenders, namely the schizophrenics, we prefer the hypothesis that

secondary processes, which are associated causally and temporally with the
illness, play an essential part. An example of this is the development of a
systematic paranoid delusion. In the course of the illness, which generally
lasts for years, the marriage partner is drawn into the delusion, marital
relationships slowly deteriorate, partly as a result of this, and tensions
mount, all of which may produce a growing risk of violence. A similar situation arises when epilepsy is complicated by a slowly progressive process of
cerebral deterioration which leads to a reduction in self-control and a
lowering of emotional balance, and thus to an increased risk of aggressive
outbursts. We cannot, of course, overlook the fact that there are other
factors that affect the age distribution or the age-dependent risk of
violence. For example, very few of the jealous offenders were unmarried.
Marriage, and the relatively long period of time it usually takes for
pathological or delusional jealousy to develop, raises the average age of
jealous murderers considerably, as Mowat (1966) has pointed out.

We have thus been able only to put forward some points of view
about the interpretation of this interesting finding: we cannot claim to
have explained it fully and reliably. There is also the complicated question
of the effect which withdrawal of liberty has on abnormal offenders, who are
admitted to hospital more frequently than the 'sane' offenders. This is
another factor which might contribute to the higher average age of the
abnormal offenders and has already been discussed in detail in connection
with a possible resultant fall in the incidence of violence: our provisional
conclusion was negative (see p.281).

Sixteen offenders committed their crimes while they were in a
psychiatric hospital or institution. They included, as might be expected, a
high proportion of long-stay patients, namely eight schizophrenic and five
mentally defective offenders.

Diagnosis

We have already shown the diagnostic distribution of our cohort
of mentally abnormal violent offenders (p.83). At the top of Fig. 3, and
considerably ahead of the rest, come the schizophrenics with 53.4%; next are
the mentally defective with 12.7%, followed by those with late-acquired brain
damage (8%), cerebral atrophy (presenile and senile deterioration of varied
genesis) with 7.5%, affective psychoses with 6.9%, unclassifiable endogenous
psychoses (climacteric and involutional psychoses, mixed psychoses, emotion
psychoses (*Emotionspsychosen*), puerperal psychoses with no clear symptoms of
schizophrenia or endogenous depression, etc.) with 6.4% and the epileptics

with 5.4%.

There were only three diagnostic groups - schizophrenia, mental
deficiency and affective psychoses - for which it was possible to calculate
the relative incidence compared with that in the general population. The
schizophrenics maintained their leading position. Even when possible sources
of error are taken into account this would still be the case, since the
estimated risk in the case of schizophrenia is about ten times higher than
that for the other two diagnostic groups.

It was impossible, for many reasons, to arrive at even a rough
indication of the risk for the other diagnostic groups, such as epilepsy,
late-acquired brain damage or degenerative cerebral processes. The absolute
figures for these groups nevertheless suggest that they are not grossly over-
or under-represented.

The chronic alcoholics formed a special group, since alcoholism
was associated with several diagnoses. According to our criteria of classification, these patients were assigned to main diagnoses such as late-
acquired brain damage, mental deficiency or epilepsy and they consequently
do not appear in our tabulation. They numbered in all 79, or about 15% of
the total group of mentally abnormal offenders. Quantitatively, therefore,
they came second in the list, after the schizophrenics. But because of the
lack of various essential data we could not make any estimate of the risk
factor involved. If, however, we disregard the fact that the diagnosis was
often a multiple one, we find that the number of alcoholics in our study
was roughly the same as might be expected from comparison with relevant rates
in the general population. This does not in any way affect the finding that
when a cerebral syndrome, be it mental defect, epilepsy or late-acquired brain
damage, is complicated by the presence of alcoholism, the risk of violence is
perceptibly increased.

10.6   The special case of 'cyclothymic mania'

It seems to us particularly significant that one diagnosis which
is often widely incriminated where violence is concerned, namely cyclothymic
mania, in fact occurred extremely rarely. Among our offenders with affective
psychoses, who suffered almost exclusively from depressions, there was only
one case of classical mania: this was the female patient who while in a beer
tent took a measuring jug and smashed it on her neighbour's head.

One single act of violence in ten years, and moreover one which
was an unpremeditated emotional outburst that could be classed as 'brawling',
suggests that in terms of our criteria manic patients are the reverse of

dangerous. This is presumably because bipolar affective psychoses are
generally accompanied by low aggressiveness or even by inhibition of
aggression which in mania is replaced by a superficial lack of control. In
depression this inhibition of aggressiveness is narrowly limited or dis-
appears when murderous and suicidal impulses are combined: such an assumption is in line with the views we expressed earlier (Häfner, 1962) and with
findings arrived at by V. Zerssen *et al.* (unpublished) in psychometric
studies of personality in bipolar affective psychoses.

In connection with the low incidence of serious violence
in cyclothymic mania we should mention here the case of a second
offender whom we could not include in the category of manic offenders
because of the existence of several concurrent illnesses. This case
is so complex that it was not possible to mention it specially in our
first publication, which gave only a summary of illness-dependent risks
(Häfner & Böker (1972) Geistesgestörte Gewalttäter in der Bundesrepublik: Eine epidemiologische Untersuchung. (Mentally abnormal
violent offenders in the Federal Republic: an epidemiological study.)
Nervenarzt, 43, 285-91.) But as the patient in question committed
at least one of his violent attacks while in a state of manic excitement, it is appropriate to report the case in detail here:

The patient was a former railway mechanic, whose mother
had committed suicide at the age of 60. The crime which brought him
on to our index was attempted murder, committed in 1962, when he
was 67, as a result of a quarrel.

The following diagnoses were made: (1) mental subnormality (IQ 77), (2) cerebral atrophy with incipient dementia,
(3) bipolar affective psychosis (cyclothymia).

At the age of 42 the patient had tried, while depressed,
to kill his two sons who were then 7 and 12 years old and had also cut
his own veins. The two boys sustained considerable head injuries but
recovered, as did the patient. The motivation and the circumstances
of the attempt were typical of extended suicide in endogenous
depression: the patient was mistakenly convinced that he and his
sons were suffering from an incurable disease.

He made two more suicide attempts, both within the framework of depression but involving himself only, at the age of 51,
while being assessed psychiatrically in connection with the first
offence.

After suffering only from depressions up to the age of

57, he then developed a paranoid delusion of being threatened and
influenced by his daughter-in-law, fought with his alleged enemy
and had again to be compulsorily detained in a psychiatric hospital.
On examination he was in a state of hypomanic excitement and showed
disturbances of thought and of orientation. An epileptic twilight
state was suspected and cerebral atrophy was assumed, though no air
encephalogram was carried out.

At the age of 62 he was again in trouble with the law.
In the course of a quarrel he broke his lodger's window with a spade
and then attacked him physically though without inflicting serious
injury.

It emerged that for a long time he and his wife had
been quarrelling a lot and had often had noisy altercations, at
times coming to blows. On several occasions the lodger had come to
the aid of the wife. Possibly because of this, the patient had
developed delusional ideas of jealousy and believed that the lodger
had had indecent relationships with his wife in the cellar.

He had also quarrelled with the neighbours, had threatened them and put broken glass in front of their door.

On examination he was again partially disorientated,
his mood was one of hypomanic excitement and he showed defects of
memory and of intellect.

The diagnosis read: 'Cerebral atrophy with cyclothymia'.
He was not prosecuted and was detained for only a short time.

When he was 65 he was again admitted because one of his
frequent quarrels had again led to violence. He had threatened his
wife with an axe, the lodger came to her aid and suffered head
injuries.
The clinical picture was unchanged.

At 67 he committed the index offence which has already
been mentioned. Again there was a quarrel and his wife went to the
lodger's room for help. The patient followed and struck the lodger
with an iron bar, causing a severe fracture of the skull and fracture
of the lower arm, as well as other injuries.

A week earlier the lodger had gone to the local police
station where he registered a complaint and emphasised the great
danger that threatened him and the patient's wife. He expressly asked
that the police should take action, but nothing was done.

On admission the patient was excited and restless,

showing a marked flight of ideas. There was again no prosecution and
he was discharged after a short stay.

In accordance with our criteria, we entered this patient
under the main diagnosis of affective psychosis. His first offence,
when he tried to kill his two sons, was typical in all respects of the
kind of violence that is found in endogenous depressives. It was,
however, difficult to view the later offences as associated solely
with manic phases of his illness.

There seems no doubt that a syndrome of hypomanic excitement, accompanied at times by flight of ideas, was present in fluctuating degree during the second half of this patient's life. But it is
also clear that his aggressiveness was not confined to these phases of
mood disorder and was not predominantly caused by them. The long
history of quarrelling with his wife and his lodger, which was
accompanied by jealous and other paranoid ideas including, for
example, the belief that the lodger was threatening to poison him
with gas, played a much more important part. Moreover his instability
was no doubt increased by the process of cerebral deterioration with
its accompanying lessening of control over aggressive impulses.

We consider, therefore, that multiple causal factors
were involved in this patient's second phase of aggressive misdemeanours and in the crime which ultimately led to his entering our
cohort at the age of 67. The cyclothymic-manic component, which
presumably existed, could not be regarded with sufficient certainty
as being the main cause. For these reasons we did not include him
as a straightforward second case of violence in cyclothymic mania.

10.7 Duration of illness before the crime

One of the most important and in some respects unexpected findings was the small number of offenders who committed a violent crime at the
beginning of their illness. Only 3.3% of all the mentally abnormal offenders,
and only 2.9% of the 284 schizophrenic offenders, committed a violent crime
within four weeks of the onset of their illness. In fact 83% of all the
abnormal offenders, and 84% of the schizophrenics, had been ill for more than
a year at the time of the crime, and 55% for more than five years. This
finding refutes at least quantitatively the view that violence is a prodromal
symptom of schizophrenia, a view which has found its way into psychiatric
doctrine and which is based on numerous case studies such as those cited at
the beginning of this book.

The low number of violent crimes committed in the initial phases
of illness is in keeping with the low ratio of impulsive as opposed to planned
acts and with the predominance of chronic illnesses. The very high average
duration of illness is noteworthy: excluding the mentally defective patients,
for whom the duration of illness equals their age at the time of the crime,
the average duration was more than five years. This casts some light on the
age difference between the mentally abnormal and the 'normal' violent offenders. Some of the reasons already advanced to account for that difference are
relevant also to the long duration of illness. The finding is moreover of
practical importance, since it gives grounds for hoping that as a rule there
may be sufficient time available to translate any knowledge gained into
preventive treatment.

To a certain extent the affective psychoses again represent an
exception. More than a tenth of this group committed a violent crime in the
first four weeks of their illness, and about a third of them within the
first six months. The reason for this is that in contrast to most other
groups of illness, this group shows a direct relationship between the crime
and an illness which, although recurrent, clearly follows an acute course.
The most frequent form of crime, namely extended suicide, is committed during
the depressive phase and its morbid motivation has its roots in that phase.
The high proportion of offenders (one-third) who commit a crime in their
first depressive phase is also worth noting. This may be influenced by the
inhibiting effect of increasing age in subsequent spells of illness. Another
reason why the likelihood of crime decreases with age during later depressive
phases is that children grow up and there is not the same symbiotic relationship between them and their parents – a relationship which is frequently found
in extended suicide by depressed mothers.

10.8 Previous treatment of mentally abnormal offenders

The proportion of mentally abnormal offenders who had had previous
psychiatric treatment proved to be unexpectedly low. The mental abnormal
non-offenders in the control group, who had been matched for age, sex and
diagnosis, had been treated more frequently and for longer periods as in-
patients in psychiatric hospitals, although the average duration of their
illness was less than that of the mentally abnormal offenders.

About a half of the mentally abnormal offenders had not been
treated in a psychiatric hospital before their crime. Since the offenders
and the controls differ in their need of hospital care and in the duration
of their illness, this finding cannot be clearly interpreted. Nevertheless,

in view of the generally long duration of illness, it would seem to indicate
a low level of treatment for those groups of illness which usually require
in-patient care, particularly by comparison with the mentally abnormal non-
offenders.

When we come to examine the main groups of illnesses, we find
that we can leave aside the mentally defective offenders, since in their case
the basic illness - if it is present with the degree of severity now under
discussion - does not as a rule call for in-patient treatment. About half of
the offenders with affective psychoses had had previous in-patient treatment:
in other words, there was no significant difference between them and their
control group of non-offenders. It is worth noting, however, that 41% of the
schizophrenic offenders had had no previous in-patient treatment, and this is
significantly different from the 27% of non-offenders. The position becomes
even clearer if we look at treatment in the six months preceding the crime.
Ninety per cent of the offenders had been ill for at least six months before
the crime. Only about 10% had received out-patient treatment and only 22%
in-patient treatment. Treatment by general practitioners because of the existing mental disturbance, or analogous care by social workers (whose numbers
have possibly since increased), did not play any significant part in the
cohort we studied. This means that about two-thirds (68%) had received no
treatment or care in the six months preceding their crime - a period which
must be regarded as one of increasing risk at least for a proportion of the
offenders. (It should be borne in mind, however, that these findings apply
only to the decade 1 January 1955 to 31 December 1964.)

In the group of schizophrenics, 91% of whom had shown symptoms
of illness six months before the crime, only about 30% had received in-
patient or out-patient psychiatric treatment or care during this period.
The findings in the control group were similar and there was no significant
difference between the two groups.

10.9 Period of risk after discharge from a psychiatric hospital

The most spectacular finding in our study, and at the same time
the most significant from a practical point of view, is that discharge or
abscondment from in-patient treatment is followed by a marked period of risk
of violence. This finding does not, of course, apply to all psychiatric in-
patients, but only to the very small proportion who are predisposed to
violence. Moreover, since we did not start with a sample of discharged
psychiatric patients, but with a cohort of violent offenders, we do not

know what is the incidence of violence in the first six months for discharged patients as a whole. In the absence of control figures for the decade in question, let us assume that 60 000 to 80 000 patients with analogous diagnoses are discharged annually from psychiatric hospitals and institutions in the GFR:[3] relating this figure to the 10 or so patients per year who committed a violent crime within six months of their discharge, we arrive at some idea of the relevant proportions.

Out of 248 offenders discharged from psychiatric hospitals, 99, or 39%, committed a violent crime within six months of leaving hospital: 29, or 12%, of them had left the hospital against medical advice or had absconded. Some became violent within a few days of leaving. In the control group of non-violent patients, only 2% were recorded as absconding or discharging themselves against medical advice within the same period of time. Although the numbers are small, one may with some caution conclude that the offenders tend to be more active in their rejection of treatment and their refusal to have their liberty curtailed. Non-offenders tend to be more co-operative in so far as in-patient treatment is concerned.

The associated finding that hospital psychiatrists were able to form a fairly reliable judgement of the general increased risk in a proportion of the potentially violent offenders is of great practical importance. On the other hand, however, a large majority of the patients (88%) who committed violent crimes within six months of leaving hospital had been discharged with medical consent. In these cases there are clearly no reliable indicators of risk, unless we assume that some of the patients were less thoroughly examined or were discharged for other reasons, perhaps because of pressure on the part of relatives, against the doctor's judgement but with his consent.

We examined in detail the possible reasons for the period of risk that follows discharge from hospital. The most obvious assumption, namely that it is chiefly a question of relapses brought on by professional or personal difficulties in adjusting to life outside the hospital, is not borne out in the majority of cases. It may apply to some offenders, but it was not possible to reach a quantitative assessment on this point. It could not, however, apply to more than one-third of the offenders, since only approximately a third of them showed signs of deterioration during the period in question. Among the non-violent patients, who showed significantly fewer readmissions in this period (23% as compared with 39% of the offenders), symptoms of deterioration were recorded in almost half of the cases.

These two trends - namely for the non-offending patients frequent worsening of the patient's condition with a slightly higher readmission rate in the first six months after discharge, and for the violent offenders less frequent deterioration with a marked increase in the rate of violence during the same period - reflect a partial distinction between factors that are related to the illness and factors that are related to violence.

This finding, which suggests that the chief factors affecting the increased risk of violence do not have their origin directly in the illness, again does not hold good for the depressed offenders where the opposite seems to apply. Here we find on the one hand a frequent association between the crime and a deterioration in the patient's state after discharge, while on the other hand the incidence of violence within six months of leaving hospital was extremely high (11 out of 18 discharged patients). The offence was usually committed in the first three months.

We therefore concluded, and this was confirmed by our analysis of the content of case records, that these depressed patients usually committed their violent acts, which in most cases involved extended suicide, in the same phase of illness as that for which they had been receiving treatment in hospital. The risk of violence in such patients can be treated to a large extent in the same way as their risk of suicide. Studies by Stengel & Cook (1958) showed that in psychotic depression the peak suicide rate does not coincide with the peak severity of clinical symptoms. It tends rather to be higher in the second stage of the illness, when the defence mechanisms of depressive inhibition and delusion have reduced the level of pathological dynamics and have themselves considerably receded. Patients often go through this risk period without the help of hospital or out-patient treatment. One reason for this is that the patients or their families may insist on early discharge. It is noteworthy that almost all the depressed patients who became violent within six months of discharge had left hospital with medical consent.

It is possible also that confrontation with the outside world and its tasks, and with those persons who are involved in the patient's fears of calamity, can reactivate the depressive symptoms. Depressed patients who are in danger of committing extended suicide - and this probably applies also to the risk of suicide by depressed patients in general - are clearly most at risk and most dangerous in the second stage of an illness of this kind. Admittedly at this stage clinical symptoms have passed their peak and the patient's ability to communicate with the outside world has been restored. Depressive delusions are usually less intense but their content is still present and unchanged. In certain circumstances these can be translated into action via the accompanying dynamics of depressive rage against the patient

himself or against those most dear to him, or in a desperate longing for
release in death. In individual cases we certainly had the impression that
the motive, although the patient might at first deny it, was a plan already
conceived in hospital to press by every means for a speedy discharge and then
to pursue at home the fatal sequence leading to extended suicide.

We assume that these risk factors, formulated in the first
instance for affective psychoses, apply also to a large extent to offenders
with psychotic-depressive syndromes based on other illnesses, for example
severe depressive syndromes occurring in schizophrenia. We would recall here
that 13.4% of the offenders (38% of all the female but only 6.2% of all the
male abnormal violent offenders) had committed or attempted extended suicide.
Looked at from the point of view of level of motivation, the schizophrenic
offenders, who apart from the unclassifiable endogenous psychoses came next
to the depressive psychoses, showed in 9.3% of cases an analogous motive of
'release from dreaded suffering'.

It seems to us highly important from the practical point of view
to regard the syndrome-specific risk of extended suicide (it is also illness-
specific for polar and bipolar endogenous depressions) as occupying a special
position, quite separate from all other categories, and as calling for
specific measures of treatment.

Of the 23 mentally defective offenders discharged from hospitals
or similar institutions, 7 became violent in the first, and 5 in the second
six months after discharge. In this group of offenders there was very often
a history of aggressive behaviour and of crimes such as bodily harm. It must
therefore be assumed that being in a hospital or institution prevents at
least a proportion of them from committing violent crimes, such acts being
committed after discharge in some cases as if 'making up for lost time'.

The increased risk following discharge is even more marked in
schizophrenic offenders. In this group 59, or 37%, of the 160 discharged
patients became violent offenders within six months, as against 26% of the
schizophrenic non-offenders who were readmitted to hospital. In the second
six months after discharge the figure for the two groups was nearly the
same at around 15%.

We have already discussed possible explanations. There is not
much support for the argument that difficulties in social rehabilitation,
which are often invoked as reasons for relapse, play a dominant part. The
problems seem to lie much more in the area of intimate human relationships.
We have already drawn attention to the parallel case of intense emotional

relationships which according to recent studies significantly increase the relapse rate in schizophrenics.

It may be assumed that a fairly long absence from those intimate partners with whom the patient has a tense and often delusional involvement may have the effect not only of releasing tension but also in some cases of increasing the schizophrenic's difficulties. A delusional patient may, for example, temporarily lose the ability to control his ideas of jealousy or harm and these may become considerably stronger. Moreover the intimate partner may have been involved in the committal of the patient to hospital against his will and this initiative is again delusionally misinterpreted by the patient. Finally, the stay in hospital and the reaction of the outside world may be experienced by the patient as a severe insult. Such assumptions receive support from the observation that the offenders are emotionally and socially more active and at the same time have more numerous and more intense family relationships than the patients in the control group.

The possible effect of the hospital milieu on the risk of violence must remain an open question, as our study provided no data on which we can base an answer. It is possible that some patients who suffer from delusional fears of injury or destruction may experience their loss of liberty and the actual hospital situation as a further impetus to fight and seek revenge, but this has not been demonstrated. In individual cases, for instance of offenders whose violent crimes were committed inside the hospital, the motive recorded was one of revenge for real or delusional injury. But it can hardly be claimed that the majority of these offenders experienced while in hospital an increase in their aggressiveness which then manifested itself in violence after their discharge.

10.10   Implications for prevention and treatment

What can be done? Any answer to this question must take account not only of the risk period just mentioned but of the entire life history of the small group of potential violent offenders. The first requirement is better knowledge which will enable us to identify those patients in whom the risk of violence is great. Several pointers have been given in this direction. The second requirement is a closely woven net of specialist medical care, particularly in the transitional period from hospital to family life or partnership. When it comes to translating these requirements into therapeutic reality, however, scientific considerations give way to practical problems. A large proportion of these sufferers are among the psychiatrist's most difficult patients. We may for the present leave aside those depressives who

deny their intentions and who, even though they have taken their firm decision
to commit suicide, are to outward appearance undergoing a sudden remission of
their depressive psychosis.

It is difficult to persuade chronic schizophrenics, particularly
those who are paranoid, quarrelsome and suspicious but whose social adaptation is adequate, that they are mentally ill and should seek psychiatric help.
The involvement of relatives, who may themselves share the same hereditary
tendency to illness or may be more or less overtly ill, also plays an important part. Close and often subjectively involved associates moreover find it
easier to recognise as illnesses those mental changes which are of acute onset than those which are insidious and progressive, particularly if they are
accompanied by real tensions between patient and observer. The answer to
this question of early detection and early treatment can only be the
unsatisfactory one that we must have more enlightenment in the field of
mental health. Such enlightenment should in particular make family members
and associates who are not themselves pathologically involved with the
patient aware of his illness and motivated to seek help and intervention.

The next difficulty lies in the continuous medical care of withdrawn hebephrenics who make little contact. The group at risk among these
patients, who nurse considerable suppressed hostility, tend to deny their
illness, to discontinue the necessary medication and to break off contact
with those treating them.

So far as medication is concerned, the possibilities of
controlled long-term therapy have in the meantime improved considerably,
thanks to the introduction of depot-neuroleptics. The other difficulties
remain unchanged. It is necessary to review them closely in each individual
case and to plan one's therapeutic strategy accordingly. It is usually
helpful to apportion therapeutic and rehabilitation functions so that, for
example, a social worker collaborating closely with the doctor will undertake
the task of advising members of the family. This serves to remove the doctor
from the all too powerful role of sole therapeutic adviser, a role which may
sometimes provoke paranoid reactions. The same purpose may be served by
advice or helpful intervention by a discreet and realistic member of the
family or by a friend of the patient who is not involved in his pathology.

With regard to the question of avoiding a period of risk after
discharge from hospital, the answer is that at least a proportion of these
patients continue to require hospital treatment. In every case, however,
careful consideration should be given to the possibility that partial
hospitalisation or some other alternative to in-patient care might offer

better prospects of success. If the patient has been compulsorily admitted to hospital, the possible discharge must be carefully planned and prepared, especially in the case of paranoid and jealous schizophrenics. On his admission and during his stay persistent and firm efforts should be made to establish the patient's co-operation in his treatment. This is of course no easy matter with patients whose trust and confidence have been badly shaken and a frank, consistent attitude is called for in all one's dealings with them. This can be achieved only if the psychiatrist has a good insight into his own behaviour and responsibilities and if the hospital conditions and personnel are favourable.

However much we try to improve prevention and treatment, there will certainly still remain a hard core of patients who have to have compulsory long-term detention because they constitute such a high risk. These are the very ones who are likely to abscond or to offer a serious risk if they are given an early discharge. Discharge and resettlement in the community must therefore be planned and prepared with the greatest care, if indeed they are considered to be at all justifiable. Controlled maintenance of neuroleptic therapy, trial periods of discharge and continuous care and supervision must be assured. A further indispensable step so far as estimating the risk is concerned is to try to establish any special area of danger, such as a tension-laden, delusional relationship with the marital partner. In this and other areas in which warning signs might be expected to show themselves, the indications of future conduct must be just as carefully examined as the observed symptoms of illness.

It must finally be remembered that the recurrence rate for aggressive crimes is particularly high in the small group of mentally defective offenders with behavioural disorders. Most of these patients are at the present time inaccessible to any form of treatment in the narrow sense. It is doubtful whether the methods of applied behaviour or learning therapy can bring about a long-term modification of behaviour in some cases. In the small group of mentally defective offenders whose violence is of sexual, instinctive origin, consideration should be given to anti-androgen therapy or to voluntary sterilisation.

A large proportion of the mentally defective violent offenders probably require long term management or control, the extent of which has to be judged individually in each case. In some ways these patients are particularly difficult and if they are committed to psychiatric hospitals they make high demands on the staff and on their fellow-patients. From a long-term point of view they should therefore be sent to special institutions for disturbed mental defectives where there are specially trained personnel and special occupational facilities. Drug therapy often helps to reduce their aggressive tendencies: in childhood this can be done, surprisingly, with stimulant drugs, but later a maintenance dosage of neuroleptics is usually required.

These few pointers to treatment and prevention must of course be regarded as very generalised. We have looked at a large cohort of mentally abnormal offenders, made up of widely varying subgroups. In many cases circumstances were much more complicated than our research procedures could handle. If we have demonstrated only a few typical problems and principles, this is chiefly due to the fact that our study was an epidemiological one and not an enquiry into the success and practicability of treatment programmes and other methods of dealing with mentally abnormal violent offenders.

10.11 Factors relating to family and personality

On the basis of our material it was of course possible to make only a partial assessment of the part played by hereditary and familial factors in producing a tendency to violence in the mentally abnormal. We nevertheless tried when possible to examine in our group of mentally abnormal offenders the predictors of criminal behaviour, such as disorganised or broken families, antisocial behaviour, alcoholism, parental crime, etc., which have been found to apply in studies of normal groups (S. & E. Glueck; Guze, Goodwin & Crane; Robins & Lewis, etc.).

The data we were able to collect showed hardly any significant differences between the mentally abnormal offenders and the control group of abnormal non-offenders so far as familial loading with mental illness was concerned. This was in line with our expectation. Significant differences were, however, evident in regard to suicide, alcoholism and criminality in the parental family: taking these three loadings together we found them in 23% of the abnormal offenders as compared with 9% of the abnormal non-offenders. When the main diagnostic groups were examined separately, very different findings emerged. The mentally defective offenders easily headed the list, with about 50% whose parental families showed at least one of the three loading factors: parental criminality was the most frequent factor present, the second most common being alcoholism. In the affective psychoses suicide was the most common factor found, criminality and alcoholism being of very little significance. For the schizophrenic offenders, suicide, alcoholism and criminality were all present, though to a lesser degree.

Broken homes were found in about a quarter of both the abnormal offenders and the non-offenders. Contrary to our expectation, this seemed to be of little real significance so far as the tendency to criminal violence was concerned. It was only in the mentally defective offenders that the rate rose to 54%. Comparison with the non-offenders was of little value here, since in the control group, which was drawn from psychiatric admissions, there was probably an over-representation of mentally defective patients with behaviour disorders and inadequate family care.

It is probable that broken homes are to some extent relevant so far as the risk of violence in the mentally defective is concerned. It was not possible for us to determine, however, whether this worked directly, by disturbing the process of socialisation, or indirectly through a lack of support and supervision of subjects who are at risk because of low self-control. The same applies basically to the antisocial behaviour of parents: the studies of Robins & Lewis have shown a high measure of consistency in this respect over generations and we do not yet know to what extent this is brought about by genetic transmission or by learning processes. It is more-over probable that the high rate of antisocial behaviour found in the parents of mentally defective offenders has an effect on the frequency of broken homes.

There is an association between the behavioural characteristics of the parents and many of the personality traits found in the group of offenders.

About three-quarters of the mentally defective offenders, namely 48 out of 65, showed features of an antisocial personality. The main character-istics included in this category were habitual signs of easily aroused, frankly aggressive, quarrelsome, or repeatedly criminal (usually fraudulent) behaviour. We would also recall in this connection the high incidence of chronic alcoholism among the defective offenders. The defectives were similar to the offenders with late-acquired brain damage in that about a quarter of them showed antisocial personality and about half were alcoholics. The patients with affective psychoses again represented a complete contrast, in that only one of them, who was atypical in other respects also, showed signs of an antisocial personality. The large group of schizophrenic offenders contained 8% with antisocial personalities, which was considerably less than the average, though distinctly more than the schizophrenic non-offenders with 3%. Antisocial personality was rare in the epileptic group (about one in seven) and in the much older group of offenders with cerebral deterioration.

These data again show the different significance attached to antisocial personality traits in the various diagnostic groups. The overall figure of 20%, which significantly distinguishes the abnormal offenders from the abnormal non-offenders, thus reflects only a global tendency.

Looking at the results as a whole, and remembering the high concordance with the relevant behavioural characteristics in the parents and with broken homes, we must ask ourselves whether for mentally defective offenders and for those with late-acquired brain damage the antisocial personality disorder is in fact the primary disorder from which the tendency to violence springs. A tendency to violence would then be a personality trait which in these cases was correlated with other traits coming into the category of 'antisocial personality'. Criminal violence in the mentally defective would thus be in line with 'normal' violent delinquency, which it resembles in many respects such as age, sex distribution, motives, choice of victim, etc. The combination of violence and other antisocial personality traits is characteristic of a large group of 'normal' violent offenders.

Looked at in this way, mental defect would be a complication of the personality disorder that carries with it a tendency towards violence, the risk of violence being increased by a weakness of self-control and by a lower capacity for adjustment and regulation. Alcohol and late brain damage can to a limited extent be regarded as similar complicating factors which in an antisocial personality inclined to frank aggressiveness can carry the risk of violence beyond the threshold.

Such an interpretation is of course a simplification which would apply presumably only to a proportion of cases. It ignores the fact that mental defect, late brain damage and to some extent also chronic alcoholism may be associated with cerebral changes which in turn are accompanied by abnormalities of affect or personality. In such cases, which may for example be characterised by a high degree of excitability, one may assume that the illness has a more specific influence on the risk of violence.

A limited proportion of antisocial personality disorders with a more or less marked tendency to violence seemed to be distributed, though unevenly, over the other diagnostic categories, contributing as part of a multifactorial aetiology to the higher risk of violence in these categories. The only exception is found in offenders with depressive psychoses, in whom this combination is practically unknown. In this disorder personality factors, which we have already discussed in another context, are not involved in the same way in a tendency to violence. If a previous history of aggressive crimes is taken as a presumably more specific indicator of a violent disposition than antisocial personality, then the associations become even plainer: 33.6% of the mentally abnormal offenders, as against only 4% of the control group, had committed crimes against life and limb, usually bodily harm (29% of the offenders): the difference is highly significant. It is clear from this that the small group of mentally abnormal persons who commit violent crimes are at least characterised by a strong habitual tendency and not only by occasional and totally unpredictable outbursts.

The rates for the different diagnostic groups correspond only partly to the relevant rates for antisocial personality. No depressive offender had a record of bodily harm or similar overt aggressive behaviour. As already mentioned, there were only three cases in which there had been an earlier attempt at extended suicide. This confirms the view that this group shows above-average control of general aggressiveness and an extremely specific risk of extended suicide.

In contrast to the findings in regard to their antisocial personality, the schizophrenics show a high incidence of previous bodily harm (33.6% of the offenders). In 42% of the cases there was a history of crimes involving threats against the person. There is thus no doubt that for the majority of the schizophrenic offenders there was inherently a much more specific danger of violence than for the mentally defective offenders with their general antisocial personalities. It was only in a small proportion of the schizophrenic offenders that this risk seemed to stem from an antisocial personality. It is our firm opinion that the same difference is reflected in the association between violence and tense relationships which was found in the schizophrenic offenders and which is seen also in their distinctive motives and in their choice of victims. In the mentally defective offenders, on the other hand, there is no specific association between symptoms of illness and violent crime: nor are these offenders very specific in their motives and choice of victim.

The highest record of previous criminal aggression was found in a group containing few antisocial personalities, namely, the patients with convulsive disorders. More than two-thirds of these offenders had been guilty of bodily harm or a similar offence; less than a fifth of them had no record of aggressive offences. This group also covered patients with alcoholism, dementia and organic psychoses (twilight states), and their crimes - unlike those of the schizophrenic and depressed offenders - were very often impulsive or arose from a quarrel. The risk here would therefore seem to be also specific to the illness, though somewhat different in nature. It is presumably associated with a pathological aggressiveness or excitability on the one hand, and with a lack of inhibition or loss of control brought about by the illness and by secondary factors on the other (alcohol was involved in about a third of the crimes). The mentally defective offenders, and those with late-acquired brain damage, showed similar tendencies: more than half of them

had a previous history of crimes against life and limb. One may adduce in
both groups a combination of low powers of self-control and a personality that
predisposed the individual to aggressiveness and antisocial behaviour. The
effect of this combination on behaviour may be judged by the fact that in
these two groups only about a fifth of the offenders had no previous history
of criminal aggression (including insulting and threatening behaviour, etc.).
If we disregard the main diagnosis we find the same activating combination
clearly present in patients with chronic alcoholism. Here again about half
of the offenders had a previous history of crimes against life and limb and
only a quarter had no previous history of aggressive offences. To complete
the picture we would mention that the corresponding findings for offenders
suffering from cerebral deterioration were about a quarter and a half
respectively.

10.12   Intelligence, education, marital and occupational status

The group of mentally abnormal offenders contained a higher
proportion of high-grade defectives (IQ 70-89) than did the control group
(23% as against 13%), but there was no significant difference in regard to
the number of low-grade defectives (IQ less than 70) found among the remaining diagnoses. Though this finding may be affected by the more thorough testing carried out on the group of offenders as compared with the control group,
it is nevertheless of some practical importance. It may well be that a less
severe degree of defect increases to some extent the risk of violence in
individual groups of offenders. A considerable degree of defect has, however,
the opposite effect. Taking mentally defective offenders as a whole, the
risk of violence is relatively low and mental defect is not a factor that
can be expected to increase such a risk.

In so far as educational and occupational levels were concerned,
there were no significant differences between the violent and the non-
violent mentally abnormal. This means that professional status, and probably
also social class, have no demonstrable influence on the risk of violence in
the mentally abnormal. As it happened, both the offenders and the control
group were drawn predominantly from the lower and middle classes, which may
reflect on the one hand the higher prevalence of those with below-average
intelligence and on the other the downward drift in social class that is
frequently found in those epileptic and schizophrenic patients who become
ill at an early age or who are socially handicapped even before the onset
of their illness. The patients with affective psychoses showed no over-

representation of lower social class or lesser intelligence, which was in keeping with the distribution found in previous prevalence studies.

The differences in family and social relationships are illuminating. Considerably more offenders than non-offenders were married (45% as against 36%, taking age into account). About 70% of the two groups were living with their families at the time of the crime or of admission to hospital. As mentioned, it was only in the mentally defective that lack of family relationships seemed to represent a risk factor of some importance. For some of the schizophrenic and many of the depressed offenders, however, family relationships represented an area of definite risk. In fact disturbances in this area were considerably more frequent among the offenders, the depressed group again forming an exception. Conflict and tension with the marital partner were the most frequent features found (46% as against 21% in the control group).

A congruent finding was that in the offenders social contacts were more often tense or at least were more often inclined to cause tension. More non-offenders were socially isolated (28% as against 16% of the offenders). More non-offenders were also unemployed, but the difference was not significant.

These social data emphasise the trends already revealed by the study of personality traits: few of the mentally disturbed violent offenders seem to be socially isolated or passive. This applies to the schizophrenic offenders in particular. Most of them are more active than the control group and surpass them so far as external hallmarks of adjustment are concerned, such as family status and extent of social contacts. In the quality of their relationships, however, the offenders are clearly more tense and quarrelsome, and more frequently show overt hostility and aggressiveness. Their behaviour is more often regarded clinically as 'excited' or 'moody' and less often as apathetic or autistic.

Again, as might be expected, the depressed offenders form an exception. Their previous history differs clearly from that of the non-offenders, by virtue of the burden of auto-aggressive acts and suicide attempts.

Summing up the indications provided by family history, personality and social situation, we may say that the following factors may point to an increased risk of violence:

1. *A history of criminality, alcoholism and suicide in the parental family:* in particular crime and alcoholism in the mentally defective, and suicide in the depressives.

2. *Broken home:* this applies only to mentally defective offenders.

3. *Antisocial personality traits:* this applies particularly to the mentally defective and chronic alcoholics; to a lesser extent to those with late-acquired brain damage and to schizophrenics; to a slight extent to those with cerebral atrophy and to epileptics; and not at all to depressives.

4. *Overt aggressiveness, particularly a previous history of criminal aggression:* this applies particularly to epileptics, mental defectives, those with late-acquired brain damage and chronic alcoholism; it also applies to schizophrenics and to offenders with cerebral deterioration. Apart from attempts at extended suicide, it does not apply to depressive offenders.

5. *Previous history of attempted suicide:* significant only for depressive offenders.

6. *Tense and conflicting relationships with marital or other intimate partners:* applies particularly to schizophrenics, but also to alcoholics, epileptics and those with late-acquired brain damage and cerebral deterioration. Probably of no significance in depressives. Does not apply to mentally defective offenders who generally are neither married nor involved in this way.

7. *Systematic paranoid delusion, or more rarely delusional jealousy, accompanied by the conviction of being harmed, deceived or destroyed by someone, particularly if the partner in a close, tense, emotional marital or other intimate relationship is involved in this delusion:* this is most marked in chronic schizophrenics, but applies partly also to chronic alcoholics and to those with late-acquired brain damage. Does not apply to the mentally defective or to those with affective psychoses. (In depressives this is replaced by delusional fears of unavoidable evil threatening the patient and his family and by fantasies of release and thoughts of suicide.)

8. *Increased tension and conflict in social relationships outside the family:* this applies in varying degree to all diagnostic groups except the affective psychoses.

9. *Alcoholism (and alcohol consumption at the time of the crime):* applies particularly to epileptics and to all forms of brain damage including mental defect (quantitatively this is of lower significance and is not very specific). (There is more distinct association with illness factors.)

10.13 Warning signs

For methodological reasons we examined this important question by looking for any forms of behaviour during the six months before the crime which might possibly count as warning signs. It was found that a 'deterioration' in clinical state played an important part only in the case of depressive offenders.

If we disregard the complications often caused by exogenous psychoses in cerebral organic and epileptic syndromes, we find that clinical deterioration occurred considerably less often in the other groups of offenders than in the control group. This finding reflects the predominance of chronic illnesses in the offenders and the relative infrequency of a direct association between the illness and the crime. It does not relieve us, however, of the need to examine closely the course of illness in patients who are highly at risk.

The clearest indications to be found in the overt behaviour of the potential offender are, of course, aggressive utterances such as threats against the person of those who are in danger (48% of the offenders) and not infrequently aggressive crimes (15% of the offenders as against 2.3% of the control group). Such signs are particularly important when they are associated with a paranoid delusion and are directed against a close partner who is delusionally regarded as threatening or harmful. This means that a good estimate of the risk involved cannot be made solely on the basis of warnings conveyed by overt behaviour. These must be supplemented by psychiatric findings, by observation of the danger areas - for example, a tense marital situation - and by the way in which the warning signs are reflected in the morbid and normal experiences of the patient.

Aggressive behaviour, which was also not infrequently observed in the wider circles of the patient's life, is nevertheless an extremely important indicator, since it can alert the lay public to the dangerousness of the situation. It may thus be more effective than many other warning signs in bringing about serious medical attention for patients who have no insight into their illness and do not wish to be treated for it.

Social isolation, autism and passive disengagement do not usually provide an indication of increased risk, since they are found much more frequently in non-violent patients. There is, however, a small group of predominantly schizophrenic offenders who develop such symptoms before their crime.

A decline in social status or extremely unfavourable social circumstances, such as particularly loss of employment or lack of family or comparable relationships, seem on the whole to provide no good indication of the risk of violence, as we have mentioned in another connection. They are, however, fairly frequent in epileptic, mentally defective, alcoholic and some brain-damaged offenders, and may play some part there as risk factors. But they are not indicators in the narrower sense, since their incidence is not markedly higher in the six months before the crime.

Altogether our study shows that general warning signs are found only in a limited proportion of all or at least most diagnostic groups. Such warning signs as are characteristic and possess high predictive value exist mainly in association with a developing crisis that culminates in the crime. In so far as the illness is directly or indirectly involved in this development, they are therefore more specific to the illness than are earlier forms of behaviour. In the review which now follows of the characteristics of violent behaviour in various diagnostic groups, we shall return to this question.

10.14 Typology of violent offenders in various diagnostic groups

It is not proposed to go into detail in this concluding section Our intention is rather to summarise individual characteristics into constellations which are to some extent typical and which may serve as points of orientation for proposals and practical intervention.

Schizophrenic psychoses

Violent schizophrenic offenders are mostly male and belong to the younger or middle age groups. Most of them (60%) are single, though this status is found even more frequently among the schizophrenic non-offenders. A small group suffers concurrently from mental defect (15 *Pfropfschizophrenien*) or intellectual retardation and are of a considerably lower educational level. On average the offenders are professionally and socially no less well adapted than non-violent schizophrenics in the control group.

Schizophrenic offenders show predominantly a chronic, productive symptomatology with systematic paranoid delusions. Only a small proportion of them are clinically quiet, with such symptoms as flatness of affect and autism. The illness is usually of several years' duration: violent offences in the first four weeks of the illness are extremely rare (about 3%). In about 40% of cases there is a deterioration in clinical symptoms in the six months preceding the crime: this is less than the corresponding deterioration in non-violent schizophrenics before admission to hospital. It should never

be forgotten that the decision to carry out a planned crime may release the
offender from tensions, much as the decision to commit suicide brings relaxation to depressives. This often results in a facade of improvement and shortly
before the crime the patient may seem less disturbed, less hostile or less
deluded. This observation applies only to a small number of patients.

In spite of the long duration of their illness, a large proportion of the schizophrenics (41%) had never received psychiatric treatment.
Schizophrenics headed the list of offenders who had absconded from a
psychiatric hospital or left against medical advice (14.5%), thus demonstrating their tendency to refuse specialist or clinical treatment. This is in
keeping with the lack of insight and the suspiciousness of the paranoid
patient and with his fears of being deprived of liberty and power. On the
other hand the high quotas of untreated schizophrenics is no doubt also
partly due to the generally slow progression of the illness which makes it
escape the notice of those around the patient and also makes it easier for
his immediate family to deny the illness than would be the case with attacks
of acute onset. This is probably reflected also in the relatively high quota
of untreated cases among the hebephrenic offenders with low symptomatology.

The patients' most intimate partners are often closely involved
in their delusions, so that they deny overtly pathological behaviour and
clear symptoms of illness or participate in dangerous unrealities. In some
of the cases studied this undoubtedly facilitated the crime.

At the same time it must be remembered that schizophrenics in
general tend to come from disturbed families or to have relatives who suffer
from various mental illnesses (Häfner, 1971). In marital and other partnerships the schizophrenics' selective choice of partner leads to an over-
representation of those who are mentally disturbed. Any efforts at early
detection and adequate and continuous therapy for such patients must take
account of this fact.

Married schizophrenics often live in very tense relationships
with their spouses. If such marital or extramarital partners are drawn into
the paranoid delusion and regarded as 'enemies', they are particularly at
risk. Schizophrenic offenders tend to choose as victims the partners of
their most intimate relationships. The predominant motives for their crimes
are delusionally based revenge, self-defence and jealousy.

There is another, less frequent constellation of attributes
which differs in several respects from the above, so that it is possible to
speak of two types of schizophrenic offender: Type A is more common and
therefore to some extent shows more clearly the characteristic features of

the group as a whole. It consists mainly of married male schizophrenics in the middle age group whose illnesses are chronic paranoid or paranoid-hallucinatory. They suffer from systematic delusions of persecution and believe that they are threatened in life and limb. This experience of threat is often associated with bodily hallucinations or delusions of bodily harm. The patient's personality remains to a large extent unimpaired: he can dissociate himself from his morbid experiences and is usually fairly well adjusted professionally and socially, though he is frequently at odds with those around him.

In contrast to this active, bellicose type A, there is the much more passive type B. These are younger, mostly unmarried offenders, whose illness is on average of shorter duration. Usually withdrawn, often described as autistic, these patients suffer more frequently from unproductive symptoms more akin to hebephrenia or schizophrenia simplex. Delusions are not so common but the patient more often hears imperative voices which at times order him to commit violent acts. Some of these patients are socially fairly well adjusted but passive, autistic behaviour is common, as well as some eccentric or even aggressive conduct. Others in this group show serious signs of personality disintegration. The motives are more difficult to determine than in type A and it is not so easy to say who is in danger of falling victim to violent acts, which seem more often to be committed impulsively.

The different constellations of risk factors in these two types of schizophrenic offender show clearly that any estimate of risk and any measures of prevention must take account of a great variety of characteristics in many areas of behaviour.

This review of schizophrenic offenders cannot be concluded without referring to the two somewhat atypical multiple murderers in our cohort who belonged to this diagnostic category. Unlike the majority of these offenders in their choice of victim, their attacks were made upon strangers. In both cases the underlying motivation was probably partly delusional errors, pathological hatred or desire for revenge, in one case accompanied by imperative voices. The question whether such extreme violent crimes are characteristic of schizophrenics cannot be answered quantitatively. Two multiple murderers in ten years with a diagnosis of schizophrenia is a result which falls within the limits of chance, particularly as more than half of our cohort belonged to the schizophrenic category. It is only the similarity in motivation between this and other reports published from time to time of comparable multiple murders by schizophrenics that suggests that this might be a question of extremely rare crimes which are nevertheless characteristic of the criminally violent personality of schizophrenics. When we look at multiple murderers as a whole, however, it should again be repeated that quantitatively they appear to play only a small part.

We may summarise briefly some of the chief risk factors for the two types of schizophrenic violent offenders as follows:

Type A

1. Mainly married men of middle age with chronic psychoses of a paranoid or paranoid-hallucinatory type, whose illness is of several years' duration.

2. Systematic, usually 'paraphrenic' delusions in individuals of well maintained personality and good professional and social adjustment, who have from time to time shown 'bellicose' forms of behaviour.

3. Contentious and tense relationships with marital or other intimate partners.

4. Involvement of the partner in conflict as a 'dangerous enemy' or object of jealousy in delusional threats or delusional jealousy.

5. Periods of greatly increased risk in the first few months after absconding from a psychiatric hospital, or significantly increased risk after discharge from hospital (possibly only if the period in hospital has involved a considerable loss of liberty).

6. Warning signs in the form of threats and violence.

Type B

1. Usually single men in younger age groups suffering from a predominantly 'unproductive' hebephrenia or very rarely from catatonic schizophrenia.

2. Frequent imperative voices, more rarely systematic delusions in individuals whose personality and social adjustment is to some extent unimpaired, and predominantly autistic, withdrawn behaviour, or severe disintegration of personality and long-term institutional stay.

3. Crimes of violence that seem to be less planned and more impulsive. Some preference for close partners as victims, but this is less marked than with type A.

4. Risk periods after absconding or discharge as in type A. Crime may also occur in the psychiatric hospital

5. Warning signs in the form of threats and violence, often also outside the family.

Affective psychoses

Offenders with affective psychoses are almost exclusively married women aged between 30 and 40 with children under legal age. They come from intact parental families, sometimes with a family history of depression and suicide. Of normal intelligence, they belong mainly to the middle classes. They are usually housewives, whose marriage is at least to outward appearances free from conflict. They are socially well adjusted and show hardly any anti-social or habitually aggressive personality traits.

The illness is almost exclusively characterised by a severe 'endogenous' depression with delusional fears of unavoidable harm or threatening disaster. Manic syndromes are of little importance so far as the risk of violence is concerned.

The violence of depressive offenders is nearly always associated with suicide or attempted suicide and the intention is generally to commit extended suicide. The victims, who are usually involved in the patient's nihilistic delusions, are generally their own children. The motive is a delusionally based idea of obtaining release. In all other areas of overt aggressive behaviour, and probably also of crime in general, the depressive patients seem to be well under-represented.

Warning signs of violence are suicide attempts or suicidal thoughts rather than overt aggressive behaviour. Suicidal intent must be regarded as the most important warning sign, though it is not always present. Talk of extended suicide must be taken very seriously indeed.

The crime rarely occurs at the beginning of a depressive phase, but usually in the second stage when depressive inhibition has decreased and delusions have somewhat receded into the background. This may explain why almost two-thirds of the offenders discharged from psychiatric treatment - with medical consent - became violent within the next six months.

The number of depressive offenders is small but if we consider the relatively high number of victims they constitute a very dangerous group. Their violent acts are delusionally motivated and carefully and realistically planned, their victims are unsuspecting and defenceless and they themselves are to outward appearance relatively harmless. After reaching their decision they behave outwardly, as do many schizophrenic offenders, as though they had suddenly recovered from their illness, as though depression, fear and oppressive worry had vanished. An apparently complete remission of this kind, which may often take place overnight, should be viewed with alarm.

The victims came almost exclusively from the immediate family.

Such patients, who are usually anything but hedonistic, have little interest in alcohol, nor do instinctual desires or sexual considerations enter into the picture.

The risk of violence in these depressed patients is certainly very difficult to recognise: they are usually reserved and able to behave in a well adjusted manner, and there are no striking and characteristic signs. The fact that there are promising therapeutic possibilities, and that the risk of violence coincides both qualitatively and temporally with the simple risk of suicide, would seem to make it necessary to extend the appropriate preventive measures to all patients who show these symptoms. This is also justifiable in that treating the risk of suicide and the risk of violence do not in any way conflict with the basic therapeutic requirements of the illness.

The most important risk factors may be summarised as follows:
1. Married housewives in the middle age group (30-40), who are suffering from a severe endogenous depression.
2. Delusional fears of unavoidable harm, associated with delusional ideas of release involving the family and in particular the patient's own young children.
3. Previous suicide attempts and talk of suicidal intent, particularly if this concerns extended suicide.
4. Period of greatly increased risk immediately after discharge from a psychiatric hospital.

Unclassifiable endogenous psychoses

We did not set up this group of patients as a separate entity. The reasons for this were purely methodological. We could not hope for reliable results, for example in regard to risk factors or illness-specific forms of violence, if the groups studied were not diagnostically as homogeneous as we could possibly make them. We therefore used relatively strict diagnostic criteria, such as had proved suitable, for example, in epidemiological studies of twins (Kringlen, 1967). This probably enabled us to detect a substantial number of significant and useful differences between the various diagnostic groups. Between affective psychoses and schizophrenia such differences would, for example, have been considerably reduced, sometimes to the level of chance, if we had, in spite of the uncertainties of classification, apportioned the unclassifiable endogenous psychoses between these two categories.

As it turned out, our findings in this group justified the methods used. In several respects the unclassifiable endogenous psychoses occupied an intermediate position. They included some violent offenders who corresponded to those with affective psychoses in regard to sex, motivation and choice of victim, and others who resembled type A schizophrenic offenders. There was a small group of female offenders whose psychotic illnesses were mainly depressive but also schizophrenic-depressive and puerperal and who seemed to fall into a special category. Their victims were newborn babies or infants and their violent acts were associated with attempted suicide: in these respects and in their motivation they corresponded more or less entirely to the typical constellation that characterises cyclothymic-depressive female offenders. It can with justification be argued that the characteristics and risk factors set out above for schizophrenics and for patients with straight-forward affective psychoses apply also to patients with 'unclassifiable' endogenous psychoses. The predominant syndrome, a severe delusional nihil-istic depression within the framework of schizophrenia, or a severe delusion of jealousy within the framework of an involutional psychosis, seems to play a more important part, so far as the specific risk of violence and the choice of victim are concerned, than allocation to a particular category of illness. Because of the small number of offenders whose syndrome and illness could be unambiguously categorised, however, we were unable to carry out a reliable test of this hypothesis.

One important consequence of these observations must still be mentioned: if we add to our schizophrenic and depressive groups those offenders who possibly belong diagnostically to one or the other group, the risk of violence both in schizophrenia and in the affective psychoses becomes greater. This applies particularly to offenders with affective psychoses. Their number could be increased by about 30 to 60% if we included those offenders from the group of unclassifiable endogenous psychoses whose illnesses might be 'presumed' to count as affective psychoses. We have moreover already mentioned that the number of depressive offenders is reduced by the fact that when the person committing the crime has died - and the combination of suicide and violence in depressives considerably increases the likelihood of this happening - the act is more likely to go unrecorded than if the offender survives.

We would therefore once more emphasise that the risk rate of 6 violent offenders per 100 000 new cases of affective psychosis is pitched too low. Taking the two main sources of error into consideration, we would estimate that this rate should be multiplied by 2 or 3, giving a figure that would still be relatively low compared with, say, schizophrenia.

The risk rate for schizophrenia would only be slightly raised by adding doubtful cases from the category of unclassifiable endogenous psychoses.

Apart from the fact that considerably less than 50% of those with unclassifiable endogenous psychoses showed a clinical resemblance to schizophrenia,
the increase would still be in the region of 5-10% when set against the total
number of schizophrenic offenders. It would not therefore materially affect
our estimate of a risk of around 5 per 10 000 new cases of schizophrenia.

Mental deficiency

Compared with the other diagnoses, the mentally defective group
contained a high proportion of male offenders (sex ratio 6 : 1 as against
3 .5 : 1 for the cohort as a whole). The unusually low risk of violence in
female defectives is noteworthy. The explanation may lie in the sex differences found in the behaviour of defectives of disturbed and particularly of
antisocial personality. The offenders were mostly between 20 and 30 years old,
which is less than the average age for mentally abnormal offenders as a
whole, but in line with the maximum age for normal offenders.

Unlike all the other groups of mentally abnormal offenders they
came frequently from broken homes. They had a family history of mental
defect and mental illness and particularly of criminality and alcoholism.

They belonged almost exclusively to the lower social classes and
were nearly all unmarried; family ties were usually loose and about half of
them were not living with relatives. Their record in regard to employment
and social adjustment was usually bad and there was generally a history of
conflict with the environment.

A large majority of them showed an antisocial disturbance of
personality. Overt aggressive behaviour and, in contrast to all the other
diagnostic groups, sexual offences were marked and frequent features in their
previous history. Mentally defective violent offenders include a high
proportion of individuals whose behaviour is consistently characterised by
overt aggressive deviations and who are in considerable danger of committing
repeated violent crimes.

This group of offenders did not include individuals with average
or uncomplicated mental retardation - such a population shows no real risk of
violence - but consisted of defectives who were behaviourally disturbed; to
put it more specifically, they were antisocial personalities, with a bad
family history, whose behaviour patterns were largely aggressive and to some
extent instinctual, who suffered from a mild to average degree of mental
defect and who at the same time lacked family support. This is not to say
that family support would have kept these offenders from becoming violent:
it is just as likely that most of them were incapable of forming ties and
would scarcely have integrated into any family.

Severe grades of mental defect are as a rule incompatible with
dangerous violence. There are, however, exceptions. For example an imbecile
naively wanted to take a 3-year-old child for a walk in the woods; he did this
and then abandoned the child there, freezing and crying, until in the end he
died of cold and exhaustion. He did not harm the boy in any way but was just
unable because of his severe intellectual defect to foresee the consequences
of his behaviour.

There is of course no deterioration in the degree of defect before
the crime. Nor do abnormal reactions play any particular part, if we except
the consumption of alcohol which featured in almost a quarter of the cases.
Warning signs are in particular threats or violent behaviour.

Motives for the most part resemble those of 'normal' criminals.
Gain, concealment of other crimes and instinctual motives head the list,
while pathological motivation such as delusional self-defence, extended
suicide, etc., hardly ever enter into the picture. Where the motivation
included negative emotions, as in acts of revenge, there were always real
injuries or other causes to account for it. The victims at risk were therefore less frequently family members or partners in a close emotional relationship but rather, for example, outsiders who were associated with the offender's gainful or instinctual interests. The crime is more likely to be preceded by quarrels or to be committed on impulse than to be planned long in
advance. The proportion of crimes with fatal outcome is therefore lower
than average.

The mentally defective offenders thus differ in many respects
from the other mentally abnormal violent offenders. Though not entirely
comparable, they are more like normal violent offenders, at least in their
choice of victim, in their motivation and partly also in their personality
traits.

Mental defect would itself seem to be not so much a specific
causal factor as a complicating factor, acting through lower self-control or
higher excitability or instinctive drive. It is probable that an antisocial
personality disturbance, such as was evident in a majority of the mentally
defective offenders, predisposes them to aggressive behaviour and constitutes
a more specific factor in increasing the risk of violence.

On the basis of our material it was not possible to examine the
question of whether and how far the actual defect is involved in this personality disturbance and in the resultant severe disturbance of the individual's
capacity for social adjustment, perhaps by way of a general cerebral organic
tendency or a low capacity for socialisation.

To sum up, the most important risk factors are as follows:

1. Broken home, family history of criminality and alcoholism.
2. Antisocial personality disturbance, tendency towards overt aggressive behaviour, inadequate occupational, social and family adjustment.
3. Previous history of bodily harm and sexual offences.
4. Chronic alcoholism and alcohol consumption at the time of the crime.
5. The chief warning signs are excitable mood disorders, and aggressive and instinctual deviations of behaviour amounting at times to violence.

The following diagnostic groups were too small to be subjected to statistical tests. The opinions given, which are based on a quantitative analysis of the data, cannot therefore be generalised without due care.

Convulsive disorders (epilepsies)

Offenders with convulsive disorders (epilepsies) are almost exclusively male, generally between 20 and 30 years old, single, and living alone. Their family history is often relatively tainted. Their occupational and social situation is usually unfavourable. They tend to come from the lower social classes and the early onset of their disorder often hinders their educational and occupational progress or causes early invalidism.

Their behaviour is governed by mood disorders and excitability, and by a tendency to aggressive reactions and deviations. They show an abnormality of character which is at least partly connected with their cerebral disorder, though it is probably rooted also to a varying degree in factors of primary personality and temperament. The previous history therefore very often contains instances of overt and serious aggressiveness, such as bodily harm. Violence and threats are the main warning signs and no other diagnostic group shows such a high incidence of these forms of behaviour during the six months preceding the crime.

It is thus clear that epileptic patients include a very small number whose personalities are such that they fairly consistently behave aggressively and are therefore liable to commit violent offences: the risk of their repeating these crimes is relatively high. They seem to be fairly easy to distinguish from the general run of patients with convulsive disorders who are not dangerous.

When this group of offenders is divided into diagnostic subgroups, genuine and traumatic epilepsies are almost equally prominent. Residual and

other symptomatic epilepsies are rare. In nearly all cases the convulsive disorder is complicated by either an intellectual handicap (mental defect or
dementia), a change in personality, twilight states or the consumption of
alcohol. More than a quarter of the 29 epileptic offenders committed their
crime while in a twilight state.

At the time of the crime the illness is usually of more than five
years' duration. Clinical deterioration, such as the onset of a twilight state,
plays a certain part. The act is often impulsive, and preceded by excitement
or triggered by a quarrel. Victims are usually drawn from the immediate
environment of the patient, for example parents or siblings. Motives are only
to a small extent influenced by delusional ideas. The seriousness of the
crime, as measured by the rate of fatal outcome, is usually below average.
The victim seldom dies, particularly when the patient's consciousness is
considerably disturbed or he is intellectually impaired. One result of this
is that excited twilight states, which are notoriously considered to be
dangerous, have less serious consequences when consciousness is more
severely disturbed.

One may therefore say of the epilepsies too that they carry a
fairly high risk of violence only when they are combined with other unfavourable factors and when the individual's character structure disposes him
specifically to aggressive forms of behaviour.

Late-acquired brain damage
Offenders with late-acquired brain damage are mostly married men
in the middle to higher age groups. Their brain damage is frequently caused
by trauma. With them also, serious complications are well to the fore. One in
three showed a definite intellectual decline, and alcoholism played a
prominent part: two in every five offenders committed their crime while under
the influence of alcohol. There was a markedly high incidence of disturbed
consciousness (exogenous psychoses) at the time of the crime; this applied to
10 out of 43 cases and underlines the decisive importance of this complication in increasing the risk of violence. Personal disposition nevertheless
also plays an important part, as the relatively high proportion of antisocial
personality disturbances shows. Bodily harm, violent behaviour and threats
are frequently present in the previous history: together with disturbances of
consciousness, they may be regarded as the main warning signs of impending risk.

As might be expected from the high incidence of psychotic
complications, delusional symptoms and quarrels are prominent features of the
motivation of the crime. Victims are in the main intimate partners, usually
the spouse. Suicidal acts are much more frequently associated with the crime

than in the case, for example, of mentally defective offenders.

Here again we may with due reservation say that patients with late-acquired brain damage include a small number who are disposed to act violently. This group also tends fairly consistently to behave with overt aggression. The cause can hardly be the late brain damage alone. It is much more likely that the risk is multifactorial in origin and that it may, for example, involve an antisocial excitable personality, traumatic dementia with a decrease in self-control, and an exogenous psychosis accompanied by delusions and disturbances of consciousness.

Cerebral deterioration (presenile and senile dementia)

Offenders with syndromes of cerebral deterioration are usually married men suffering from processes of presenile and senile atrophy who therefore are as a rule more than 50 years old. Symptoms of less serious dementia are frequent, being limited in a small number of cases to personality changes and to the organic psychosyndrome. There were no offenders with more severe dementia in our cohort, confirming the view that has often been expressed, namely that with the transition to severe mental disintegration the risk of violence subsides again to nil.

Personality disturbances such as antisocial and habitually aggressive behaviour play a relevant though comparatively small part, as does the consumption of alcohol. On the other hand, the insidious nature of the process is reflected in a certain increase in overtly aggressive behaviour during the six months before the crime. The most striking finding is the high incidence of exogenous psychoses at the time of the crime: with a figure of 20 out of 40 cases, this clearly exceeds the corresponding rate for brain-damaged offenders. Delusions similarly play an important part in motivating the crime. Victims thus again come from the family circle – again mainly the marital partner. Offenders in this group are more likely than those in the other brain-damaged groups (mental defect, epilepsy, late-acquired brain damage) to commit suicidal acts before or in association with the crime. In depressively inclined patients of this group acts of extended suicide play a definite if subordinate part. Actively bellicose and overtly aggressive behaviour is not so prominent. The crime is not infrequently preceded by passive behaviour and a withdrawal from social relationships, this being associated as a rule with depressed affect.

In summary it may be said that offenders with cerebral deterioration belong to the higher age groups and that, as in the case of late-acquired brain damage, the risk of violence is multifactorial in origin. The

complications of cerebral deterioration, in particular exogenous psychosis
with delusions and disturbances of consciousness, are of more importance here,
while somewhat less significance is attached to antisocial and aggressive
personality trends. So far as behaviour, motivation and form of crime are
concerned, this group of offenders is somewhat less homogeneous and therefore harder to define. Depressive syndromes in particular, which represent a
frequent complication of cerebral deterioration, exercise a modifying effect,
bringing into play the features which characterise a tendency to violence in
endogenous depressives. This makes it more difficult to establish general
criteria of risk and it is necessary to weigh up the various risk factors in
each individual case.

Alcoholism and alcohol consumption at the time of the crime

Misuse of alcohol in the form of chronic alcoholism is a common
complication of other mental disturbances. It is very rarely found in
depression and in the processes of senile deterioration that are sometimes
accompanied by depressive syndromes. It also occurs relatively rarely in
schizophrenic offenders, but is very often found in the organic syndromes
of the middle and younger age groups which at their onset are accompanied by
a loss of control: this applies particularly to late-acquired brain damage,
mental defect and epilepsy. Underlying this there is a disposition to misuse
alcohol which varies in degree and which is presumably strengthened by
several other factors. There is, for example, a high incidence among
alcoholics of antisocial personality disturbance and of family taints.

All that can be said with certainty from our study, however, is
that chronic alcoholism raises the risk of violent crime, particularly when
it is combined with brain damage, which leads to impaired self-control, and
when it is associated with antisocial personality disturbances. The chronic
consequences of alcohol misuse, such as personality disintegration and
delusions of jealousy, play some part in this, as do the acute effects of
alcohol in stimulating aggressive forms of behaviour and relaxing inhibitions that might control them. Old age, which encourages abstinence, has an
incalculable effect, as has the influence of depressive syndromes, and this
frees relevant patients from one of the risk factors. Taking mentally abnormal
offenders as a whole, alcohol is only of minor significance, and in the
decade examined this applied even more plainly to all other addictions. Its
effect is lowest when the illness itself has a very strong influence on the
motivation and risk of violence. It is greater when the violence resembles
'normal' violence in regard to motivation and form of crime and when self-
control is weak or already impaired.

10.15 Conclusion

However comprehensive the enquiries may seem which we instituted into violence in the mentally abnormal, and however cautiously one interprets the conclusions drawn from our findings, in both these aspects our study is of necessity one-sided and condensed. We tried at the outset to state clearly the limits imposed by our methodology. As the study continued, the limits imposed by our material became increasingly evident. On the basis of our data we could only make quantitative statements and indicate global associations. Detailed and penetrating questions, such as what governs the psychological process that begins with an intimate partnership and ends with a fatal blow, must perforce remain unanswered. In many respects, therefore, our findings need to be supplemented by direct investigations using sociological, psychological and psychopathological methods: this is particularly true where motivation is concerned, or the part played by morbid psychological processes. Such investigations might be possible within the framework of a prospective study of cohorts that are particularly at risk.

In spite of the inadequacies of our study and although it leaves many questions open, we still believe that it represents a new epoch in research into violence in the mentally abnormal: it is a quantitative investigation of the risks of violence and of the risk factors operating in the main diagnostic categories, using the methods of epidemiology and making the best possible use of a large volume of documented material and secondary records. We believe that we have thus taken an important step towards our real goal, which is the establishment of reliable estimates of risk as a preliminary stage in the setting up of effective preventive measures. At the same time we have succeeded in demonstrating that the mentally ill and the mentally handicapped as a whole, while they admittedly sometimes constitute a higher risk to themselves, do not represent an increased risk so far as violence towards those around them is concerned. If we could identify the 'dangerous ones' more reliably, then even such risk as exists would be further decreased.

Reflections on the problem of the legal responsibility of the mentally abnormal

These final considerations lead away from our theme into the area of judging the legal responsibility of those mentally abnormal individuals who are guilty of crimes of violence. Our comments are intended to contribute to the discussion of such problems and perhaps to provide a forward-looking view of possible developments.

The largest group of mentally abnormal violent offenders, namely the schizophrenics, have till now usually been regarded as not being responsible for their actions: this view has followed a principle of 'agnosticism' such as was advanced in particular by Schneider, Gruhle and more recently also by Haddenbrock. If, however, the risk of violence is no greater, or only slightly greater, in the mentally abnormal as compared with the normal population, and if factors of personality and situation frequently outweigh the importance of the illness in governing the criminal act, then one must ask whether the practice hitherto followed is fully justified. Schematic exculpation, based solely on diagnosis, takes no account, for example, of the fact that a chronically deluded patient may still preserve considerable portions of his personality intact. The delusional motivation of a violent crime does not mean that the person committing it had at the time no insight into the culpability of his delusionally motivated act and was incapable of behaving in accordance with that insight. It is quite conceivable that even when the patient has no insight into the morbid nature of his delusions, insight and self-control are still maintained so far as his criminal and aggressive desires are concerned.

We found that several mentally abnormal violent offenders admitted responsibility for their crime and would have preferred severe punishment to internment in a psychiatric hospital. This observation is of course of no scientific value. In some circumstances it could arise from the resentment felt by offenders who are detained in mental hospitals for years with no foreseeable end to their internment. Nevertheless the fact that they have this feeling suggests that its content should at least be subjected to examination.

We are at any rate of the opinion that a differential approach to the psychiatric assessment of responsibility is required. This should make a clearer distinction between diagnostic groups than has for a long time usually been the case. There is no doubt that certain illnesses are associated with an inclination to commit certain acts which have their direct origin in the dynamics of the illness. The classical example of this is extended suicide in depressives. This would in many cases seem to be carried out, without or even against the patient's insight, with a forcefulness equal to that with which the illness itself governs the patient's behaviour. But only a small number of illnesses and of offenders can be judged in this way, namely on the grounds that the violence is governed by the course of the illness. There are on the other hand illnesses which affect only part of the personality and which possibly do not affect crucial areas of insight - we do not mean insight into the morbid nature of delusions but insight into the heinousness of killing a person because of delusional jealousy or revenge - and which possibly do not affect self-control. Some factors associated with the illness, such as delusional jealousy, are sometimes very close in nature to the motives of 'normal' offenders. They increase the risk of violence in that they provide motives and dynamics for the crime. But there are other characteristics shared with normal offenders who are, however, partly judged by different standards. It should seriously be considered whether in such cases an automatic exculpation should not be replaced by a careful and balanced assessment of these factors.

In this global review of the subject there is, finally, a third group of illnesses which deserve mention and which bring in their train a loss or decrease in the capacity for insight or self-control. These include chiefly the exogenous psychoses that occur in various cerebral disorders, in epilepsy and also in mental deficiency. Psychiatric specialists have always taken it for granted - and this gives cause for reflection - that in these cases one should estimate the extent of the impairment and use this as a basis for judging the degree of responsibility or the absence of responsibility involved. In practice it is no more easy to assess responsibility in many cases in this group than it is, for example, to weigh up the different factors involved in the responsibility or otherwise of an offender with a paranoid psychosis. The difference, which presumably has contributed to the different principles on which the two groups are judged, lies in the fact that objective and measurable findings are available for one group, namely those with organic syndromes.

It must be admitted that our views run counter to a current trend which, without seriously considering the capacity for insight and self-control, seeks to remove from legal responsibility all offenders whose motivation is abnormal. We make no apology for expressing our doubt as to whether this facile exculpation, which is applied now to increasingly trivial mental illnesses, is really humanitarian. We would again draw attention to the fact that many abnormal offenders do not by any means share that view.

Society must impose sanctions on those of its members who take the life of another person or seriously endanger it. When the offender is judged to be fully responsible for his act, the principle of relativity is followed and the possibility of rehabilitation considered, provided he has atoned for his offence and there is no real risk of its being repeated. The same possibility, and the possibility of treatment if this holds promise of success, should be offered to abnormal offenders, whether they were responsible

for their acts or not, and regardless of whether they were committed to
hospital because of their illness or sentenced to ordinary imprisonment. The
question of responsibility will then return to the level on which it really
is based, even by those who make the laws: a balanced judgement of guilt
according to the force with which the offender is driven to commit his crime
and his capacity for insight and self-control. If these requirements are met,
it will mean the rejection of the principles of wholesale exculpation of the
mentally abnormal and there will be no alternative to establishing a differential way of judging the origins of violent crime and the personality of
violent offenders according to the dimensions we have mentioned.

APPENDIX : DATA SHEETS

Name	Serial number
	1 2 3
	Sex
	4

Age at time of crime

First name(s)
                          5 6

Marital status
1 = unmarried; 2 = married;
3 = separated, living;
4 = divorced; 5 = widowed;
9 = not known

                           7

Maiden name

Religion
0 = no denomination;
1 = Evangelical; 2 = Catholic;
3 = Other denomination;
9 = not known

                           8

Date of birth

Number of own children
0 = none;
1 = one; 2 = two; 3 = three;
4 = four; 5 = five; 6 = six;
7 = seven; 8 = 8 and over;
9 = not known

                           9

Place of residence at time
of study

Education
0 = did not attend school;
1 = remedial or special school;
2 = primary school, not completed;
3 = primary school, completed;
4 = middle school completed;
5   upper school, not completed;
5 = upper school completed (*Abitur*);
6 = higher studies, not completed;
7 = higher studies, completed
    (Diploma, Certificate);
8 = other;
9 = not known

Names and addresses of
relatives

                         10

Prosecuting office

Court

File reference

Intelligence
 1 = mental deficiency (IQ under 50);
 2 = feebleminded (IQ 50-69);
 3 = subnormality (IQ 70-89); 4 = normal (IQ 90-110);
 5 = gifted (IQ more than 110); 9 = not known

11

Occupational attainment
 0 = not applicable, never gainfully employed;
 1 = below average throughout; 2 = fluctuating; 3 = normal;
 4 = above normal; 5 = many changes of job, good performance;
 6 = many changes of job, fluctuating or bad performance;
 9 = not known

12

Occupation (at time of crime)
 0 = out of work; 1 = incapable of work, or invalid;
 2 = still being educated; 3 = auxiliary worker or agricultural
     labourer;
 4 = technician, small farmer, low grade employee, low- and
     middle-grade civil servant;
 5 = master tradesman, farmer, employee or civil servant in
     middle grade;
 6 = high-grade employee or civil servant, self-employed with
     good income;
 7 = housewife; 8 = position uncertain; 9 = not known

13

Social class of the offender
 1 = lower class; 2 = middle class; 3 = upper middle class;
 4 = upper class; 9 = not known

14

Life events, environmental influences
 0 = none; 1 = occupational and material stress;
 2 = loss or threatened loss of intimate partner;
 3 = occupational and material stress + loss or threatened loss
     of intimate partner;
 4 = other personal stress;
 5 = occupational and material stress + other personal stress;
 6 = loss or threatened loss of intimate partner + other personal
     stress;
 7 = occupational and material stress + loss or threatened loss of
     intimate partner + other personal stress;
 8 = other; 9 = not known

15

Pattern of social behaviour
 0 = passive, poor initiative; 1 = shy and inhibited;
 2 = normally active; 3 = robust and successful;
 4 = overactive but not successful; 8 = other; 9 = not known

16

Pattern of emotional behaviour
  0 = cold affect (very few emotions); 1 = soft, labile;
  2 = even-tempered; 3 = over-sensitive; 4 = excitable, at times
      aggressive;
  5 = severe aggressiveness; 6 = cold affect + over-sensitivity
      (schizoid);
  8 = other; 9 = not known

17

Premorbid personality
  0 = normal childhood; 1 = previous history of neuroticism;
  2 = history of neuroticism with perversions and addictions;
  3 = history of neuroticism with homosexuality;
  4 = antisocial psychopathic traits;
  5 = antisocial psychopathic traits + perversions and addictions;
  6 = psychopathic history with homosexuality;
  8 = other special features; 9 = not known

18

===================================== FAMILY HISTORY =====================================

HEREDITY (GRADE I RELATIVES ONLY)
(a) Mental illnesses
O = none; 1 = endogenous psychosis (1 case);
2 = mental deficiency, epilepsy and other organic defects (1 case each);
3 = mental deficiency and endogenous psychosis (1 case each);
4 = more than 1 case of psychosis; 5 = more than 1 case of mental
deficiency or epilepsy or other organic defect;
6 = more than 1 case of endogenous psychosis and mental deficiency;
7 = one or more cases of death in mental hospital with uncertain
diagnosis;
8 = uncertain diagnoses only; 9 = not known

19

(b) Anomalies of behaviour
O = none; 1 = suicide; 2 = criminal record; 3 = suicide + criminal
record;
4 = alcoholism, addictions; 5 = alcoholism, addictions + suicide;
6 = alcoholism, addictions + criminal record;
7 = alcoholism, addictions + suicide + criminal record;
8 = other; 9 = not known

20

STRUCTURE OF PRIMARY FAMILY
(a) Up to the offender's sixth year
O = no parents (illegitimate);
1 = no parents (brought up in homes); 2 = broken home;
3 = disturbed family; 4 = antisocial parents, family outwardly intact;
5 = antisocial parents, disturbed family; 6 = antisocial parents and
broken home;
7 = normal parental family; 8 = other; 9 = not known

21

(b) After the offender's sixth year
O = no parents (illegitimate);
1 = no parents (brought up in homes); 2 = broken home;
3 = disturbed family; 4 = antisocial parents, family outwardly intact;
5 = antisocial parents, disturbed family; 6 = antisocial parents and
broken home;
7 = normal parental family; 8 = other; 9 = not known

22

===================================== ILLNESS OF THE OFFENDER =====================================

SYMPTOMS
(a) Delusions
O = no delusional phenomena; 1 = sensitive delusions of reference, no
vital threat;
2 = sensitive delusions of reference with vital threat;
3 = expansive delusions of persecution, no vital threat;
4 = expansive delusions of persecution, with vital threat;
5 = mixed form of delusion, no vital threat;
6 = mixed form of delusions, with vital threat; 8 = other;
9 = not known

23

(b) Dominant delusional theme
0 = none; 1 = delusions of interpretation, reference and injury;
2 = hypochondriacal delusions; 3 = delusions of grandeur and secular
   delusions of occupation;
4 = religious delusions; 5 = delusions of love;
6 = delusions of jealousy; 7 = delusions of guilt and nihilistic
   delusions;
8 = other/several themes, none dominant; 9 = not known

                                                                    24

(c) Hallucinations: visual and bodily
0 = none; 1 = visual; 2 = neutral/positive haptic; 3 = negative
   haptic; 4 = neutral/positive + negative haptic;
5 = visual + neutral/positive haptic; 6 = visual + negative haptic;
7 = visual + neutral/positive + negative haptic; 8 = other;
9 = not known

                                                                    25

(d) Auditory hallucinations
0 = none; 1 = acoasma; 2 = predominantly neutral voices;
3 = predominantly denigrating and abusive voices;
4 = predominantly imperative voices; 5 = positively experienced voices;
8 = other; 9 = not known

                                                                    26

(e) Thought disorders
0 = none; 1 = thought inhibition; emptiness and poor concentration;
2 = subjective thought disorders (thoughts spoken aloud, thought
   withdrawal, etc.);
3 = thought inhibition and subjective thought disorders;
4 = objective thought disorders (incoherence, fragmentation);
5 = objective thought disorders and thought inhibition;
6 = objective + subjective thought disorders; 7 = objective +
   subjective thought disorders + thought inhibition;
8 = other; 9 = not known

                                                                    27

(f) Predominant affect in illness
0 = no morbid affect or change from period before illness;
1 = mostly apathetic, dull; 2 = cold, callous; 3 = suspicious;
4 = morose, irritable; explosive; 5 = mostly sad; 6 = mostly hypomanic;
7 = labile; 8 = manic; 9 = not known.

                                                                    28

(g) Special, episodic mood changes
0 = no episodic mood changes; 1 = hypomanic, impulsive, excited
   episodes;
2 = depressive and anxious episodes; 3 = depressive/anxious episodes
   alternating with hypomanic, impulsive, excited episodes;
4 = ecstatic episodes; 5 = ecstatic episodes alternating with
   hypomanic, impulsive, excited episodes;
6 = ecstatic episodes alternating with depressive/anxious episodes;
8 = other; 9 = not known

                                                                    29

———

———————————————————————— DIAGNOSIS ————————————————

A. NON-PSYCHOTIC DISTURBANCES

1. CEREBRAL ORGANIC DISTURBANCES
0 = none; 1 = oligophrenias and innate or early-acquired defects
   of personality;
2 = late-acquired brain damage (trauma, inflammation, intoxication);
3 = senile and presenile dementia; 4 = epilepsy without demonstrable
   cause (genuine epilepsy);
5 = epilepsy with oligophrenia (residual epilepsy); 6 = epilepsy with
   acquired brain damage (symptomatic epilepsy);
7 = epilepsy with atrophy; 8 = other; 9 = not known

30

2. NON-ORGANIC DISTURBANCES
ALCOHOLISM, ADDICTIONS AND PERVERSIONS
0 = none; 1 = alcoholism; 2 = addictions, not incl. alcoholism;
3 = addictions + alcoholism; 4 = perversions; 5 = perversions +
   alcoholism;
6 = perversions + addictions not incl. alcoholism;
7 = perversions + alcoholism + other addictions;
8 = other; 9 = not known

31

NEUROTIC-PSYCHOPATHIC SYNDROMES
0 = none; 1 = neuroses (excl. obsessional neuroses);
2 = antisocial psychopathy or character neuroses; 3 = antisocial
   psychopathy/character neurosis + other neuroses;
4 = abnormal development + abnormal reactions;
5 = abnormal development + neuroses; 6 = abnormal development +
   psychopathies;
7 = neurotic obsessional illness; 8 = obsessional illness +
   psychopathy; 9 = not known

32

B. PSYCHOTIC DISTURBANCES

GROUP OF PSYCHOSES
0 = no psychosis; 1 = schizophrenia; 2 = unclassifiable endogenous
   psychosis;
3 = endogenous depressions; 4 = mania and cyclothymia;
5 = reactive depressions; 6 = twilight states; 7 = other exogenous
   psychoses;
8 = other; 9 = not known

33

BIOLOGICAL STAGE AT FIRST ATTACK
0 = not applicable, no psychosis present; 1 = no specific stage;
2 = puberty and adolescence; 3 = pregnancy; 4 = childbirth;
5 = climacterium; 6 = post-climacteric; 7 = old age;
8 = other; 9 = not known

34

PSYCHOPATHOLOGICAL PICTURE OF PSYCHOSIS
0 = not applicable, no psychosis present; 1 = no typical symptoms;
2 = clinically quiet; 3 = delusional-hallucinatory processes;
4 = motor-catatonic processes; 5 = rational-symptomatic-delusional
    processes;
6 = delirium, delusions; 7 = other organic pictures (e.g. Korsakoff);
8 = other; 9 = not known

35

—————————— COURSE OF ILLNESS UP TO TIME OF CRIME ——————————

Duration of illness
0 = no duration of illness; 1 = 1 to 7 days; 2 = up to 1 month;
3 = up to 6 months; 4 = up to 1 year; 5 = 1 to 5 years;
6 = 5 to 10 years; 7 = 10 years and more; 9 = not known

36

Course of illness
0 = no illness before the crime; 1 = phasic, with improvement;
2 = phasic, stationary or slightly progressive;
3 = phasic, acute deterioration before the crime;
4 = chronic course, with improvement; 5 = chronic course,
    stationary or slightly progressive;
6 = chronic course, acute deterioration before the crime;
8 = other; 9 = not known

37

Diagnostic control
0 = none; 2 = diagnosis confirmed; 3 = diagnosis revised,
    other mental illness;
4 = diagnosis revised, no mental illness; 5 = diagnosis uncertain;
8 = other; 9 = not known

38

================================ TREATMENT ================================

Timing and continuity of psychiatric treatment (during 6 months before
the crime)
0 = did not receive treatment; 1 = occasional treatment;
2 = continuously in treatment; 3 = occasional treatment, broken off;
4 = continuous treatment, broken off; 5 = occasional treatment,
    completed;
6 = continuous treatment, completed; 8 = other; 9 = not known

39

Social and non-specialist medical care (during 6 months before the crime)
0 = no form of care; 1 = social care because of other illness or
    disturbance;
2 = social care incl. care because of psychiatric illness;
3 = medical (not neuropsychiatric) treatment because of other illness;
4 = medical (not neuropsychiatric) treatment incl. treatment of
    psychiatric illness;
5 = social care and medical attention for non-psychiatric illness only;
6 = social care and medical attention incl. that given for psychiatric
    illness;
7 = in-patient treatment in non-psychiatric institution for non-psychiatric
    illness only;
8 = in-patient treatment in non-psychiatric institution incl. treatment
    of psychiatric illness;
9 = not known

                                                                            40

Duration of in-patient treatment before the crime
0 = no in-patient treatment; 1 = in hospital for less than 1 year;
2 = up to 2 years in hospital; 3 = up to 3 years in hospital;
4 = up to 4 years in hospital; 5 = up to 5 years in hospital;
6 = up to 6 years in hospital; 7 = up to 7 years in hospital;
8 = 8 years or more in hospital; 9 = not known

                                                                            41

Number of psychiatric admissions before the crime
0 = never received in-patient treatment; 1 = once; 2 = twice;
3 = 3 times; 4 = 4 times or more; 9 = not known

                                                                            42

Form of discharge (after last admission)
0 = never an in-patient; 1 = regular discharge, no aftercare;
2 = regular discharge, with social but no medical aftercare;
3 = regular discharge, continued medical care (at least once every
    2 weeks);
4 = regular discharge, occasional medical aftercare (less than once
    every 2 weeks);
5 = not discharged, on temporary leave with supervision;
6 = not discharged, on temporary leave without supervision;
7 = not discharged, absconded;
8 = not discharged, crime committed while in hospital; 9 = not known

                                                                            43

Outcome of psychiatric treatment
0 = never treated; 1 = condition unchanged; 2 = marked improvement;
3 = social remission; 4 = recovered; 5 = deteriorated; 8 = other;
9 = not known

                                                                            44

Interval between discharge, granting of leave, or absconding,
and crime
0 = not applicable, never in hospital, no leave or absconding;
1 = less than 1 day; 2 = 1 to 7 days; 3 = up to 1 month;
4 = up to 6 months; 5 = up to 1 year; 6 = 1 to 5 years;
7 = 5 to 10 years; 8 = 10 years and over; 9 = not known

                                                                            45

=========== SOCIAL BEHAVIOUR DURING SIX MONTHS BEFORE THE CRIME ===========

Aggressiveness
0 = nothing conspicuous before the crime; 1 = conspicuous because
of abnormal but not aggressive behaviour towards intimate partner;
2 = conspicuous also socially because of abnormal but not aggressive
behaviour;
3 = conspicuous because of threats or aggressive tension towards
intimate partner;
4 = conspicuous also socially because of threats or aggressive tension;
5 = serious violence towards intimate partner;
6 = serious violence also against other persons; 8 = other; 9 = not
known

46

Suicidal behaviour
0 = none; 1 = suicidal remarks; 2 = suicide attempt;
8 = other; 9 = not known

47

Signs of social isolation
0 = none; 1 = slightly withdrawn (withdrawal from society, etc.)
with suspicion, hostility;
2 = slightly withdrawn, depressive, inhibited, passive;
3 = considerable social isolation/suspicion, hostility;
4 = considerable social isolation/depressive, inhibited, passive;
5 = autism (considerable isolation from all partners) + suspicion,
hostility;
6 = autism (considerable isolation from all partners) +
depressive, passive, inhibited;
8 = other; 9 = not known

48

Sexual behaviour
0 = no anomalies in sexual behaviour; 1 = sexual activity much
reduced; 2 = sexual activity considerably heightened but not
abnormal in direction;
3 = abnormal sexual activity towards intimate partner;
4 = abnormal sexual activity towards others; 5 = instinctual
behaviour not overtly sexual in nature; 8 = other; 9 = not known

49

Living arrangements
0 = living in family; 1 = living alone, no fixed residence;
2 = living alone, fixed residence, independent;
3 = living with friends; 4 = living with close relatives;
5 = living in quasi-marital situation with person of opposite sex;
6 = living in quasi-marital situation with homosexual partner;
7 = living in institution; 8 = living in homes, camps, etc.
9 = not known

50

Contacts with primary family
0 = no primary family; 1 = not living with parents but good
   relationship with them;
2 = not living together, bad relationship; 3 = living together,
   good relationship;
4 = living together, conflicts present but outward appearances
   maintained;
5 = living together, conflicts present, outward appearances not
   maintained;
9 = not known

51

Contacts with marital or other intimate partner
0 = not married; 1 = living apart, has left partner; 2 = living
   apart, deserted by partner;
3 = living apart, separation mutually agreed, or situation uncertain;
4 = living together, good relationship; 5 = living together,
   bad relationship but outward appearances maintained;
6 = living together, bad relationship, outward appearances not
   maintained;
9 = not known

52

Contacts with own children
0 = no children; 1 = not living together, relationship bad;
2 = not living together, relationship good;
3 = living together, relationship good;
4 = living together, relationship bad but no maltreatment;
5 = living together, relationship bad, maltreatment; 9 = not known

53

Secondary social relationships (outside intimate circle)
0 = none; 1 = few, little conflict; 2 = few, much conflict;
3 = normal in number, little conflict; 4 = normal in number,
   much conflict;
5 = above normal in number, little conflict;
6 = above normal in number, much conflict
9 = not known

54

========================= PREVIOUS CRIMINAL HISTORY =========================

Previous crimes and illness
0 = never delinquent, never ill; 1 = never delinquent, has been ill;
2 = delinquent, but never ill; 3 = delinquent and has been ill, all
   crimes fell within the period of the illness;
4 = delinquent and has been ill, all crimes fell before the period
   of the illness;
5 = delinquent and has been ill, crimes occurred partly before
   partly within the period of the illness;
6 = delinquent and has been ill; crimes mentioned but no information
   about relationship to the illness;
8 = other; 9 = no details of crimes available

55

NATURE OF CRIMES
(a) Crimes against life and limb
0 = no violent crimes; 1 = bodily harm, outcome not fatal, once only;
2 = bodily harm, outcome not fatal, repeated; 3 = rape and/or
   other sexual violent crime, once;
4 = rape and/or other sexual violent crime, repeated;
5 = crime endangering life, once; 8 = one crime endangering life
   + bodily harm or rape;
9 = no details available

56

(b) Other crimes
0 = no other crimes; 1 = indecency, without use of violence;
2 = crime against property; 3 = indecency + crime against property;
4 = insulting, defamatory, threatening behaviour, etc;
5 = indecency + insulting, defamatory threatening behaviour;
6 = crime against property + insulting, defamatory, threatening
   behaviour;
7 = indecency + crime against property + insulting, defamatory,
   threatening behaviour;
8 = other; 9 = not known

57

DETAILS OF THE CRIME

Place of crime
0 = Baden-Württemberg; 1 = Bayern; 2 = Berlin; 3 = Hamburg or Bremen;
4 = Hessen; 5 = Niedersachsen; 6 = Nordrhein-Westfalen;
7 = Rheinland-Pfalz; 8 = Saargebiet; 9 = Schleswig-Holstein

58

Calendar year of crime

59   60

THE CRIME ITSELF
(a) Nature
0 = bodily harm, committed alone; 2 = bodily harm, with fatal
   outcome, committed alone;
3 = attempted homicide (murder or manslaughter), committed alone;
4 = murder or manslaughter, committed alone;
5 = bodily harm, with accomplice;
6 = bodily harm, with fatal outcome, with accomplice;
7 = attempted homicide (murder or manslaughter), with accomplice;
8 = murder or manslaughter, with accomplice;
9 = uncertain

61

(b) Method employed
0 = brachial pressure; 1 = strangulation or choking;
2 = blunt and sharp instruments; 3 = fire-arm; 4 = poison or gas;
5 = drowning; 6 = starvation, denial of care;
7 = combination of two or more of these methods;
8 = other methods; 9 = not known

62

Particularly savage features of crime, in single or multiple offenders
0 = single offender, no particular savageness, no sexual
    accompaniments;
1 = single offender, no particular savageness, with sexual accompani-
    ments;
2 = single offender, savage features, no sexual accompaniments;
3 = single offender, savage features, with sexual accompaniments;
4 = multiple offenders, no particular savageness, no sexual
    accompaniments;
5 = multiple offenders, no particular savageness, with sexual
    accompaniments;
6 = multiple offenders, savage features, no sexual accompaniments;
7 = multiple offenders, savage features, with sexual accompaniments;
8 = other; 9 = not known

63

Impulsive or planned aggression
0 = unpremeditated (no quarrelling); 1 = crime committed after
    quarrel;
2 = planned aggression, without intent to kill; 3 = planned killing;
8 = other; 9 = not known

64

Suicide or attempted suicide of the offender after the crime
0 = no suicide by offender; 1 = attempted suicide after the crime;
2 = suicide after the crime; 3 = extended suicide attempt;
4 = extended suicide (completed); 8 = other; 9 = not known

65

Clouding of consciousness
0 = no clouding of consciousness; 1 = intoxication with alcohol;
2 = intoxication with drugs; 3 = disorientation in cerebral disorder;
4 = crime committed in epileptic twilight state;
5 = alcohol + twilight state; 6 = alcohol + other factor;
8 = other; 9 = not known

66

=================================== THE VICTIM ===================================

Number of dead
0 = 0; 1 = 1; 2 = 2; 3 = 3; 4 = 4; 5 = 5; 6 = 6; 7 = 7;
8 = 8 and over; 9 = not known

67

Number of injured
0 = 0; 1 = 1; 2 = 2; 3 = 3; 4 = 4; 5 = 5; 6 = 6; 7 = 7;
8 = 8 and over; 9 = not known

68

AGE AND SEX
(a) Children
0 = no children; 1 = 1 child, female; 2 = 1 child, male;
3 = more than 1 child, female; 4 = more than 1 child, male;
5 = children of both sexes; 9 = not known

69

(b) Adults
O = no adults; 1 = 1 adult, female; 2 = 1 adult, male;
3 = more than 1 adult, female; 4 = more than 1 adult, male;
5 = adults of both sexes; 9 = not known   70

Objective relationship between offender and victim
O = none (total stranger); 1 = casual acquaintance;
2 = specific role (superior, judge, doctor, policeman, etc.);
3 = no specific professional role (e.g. colleague at work);
4 = parents, parents-in-law; 5 = children, stepchildren,
   grandchildren, adopted children, etc;
6 = other relations (incl. siblings);
7 = marriage partner; 8 = other intimate partner; 9 = not known

71

Delusional relationship to the victim
O = no delusional relationship to victim; 1 = only imperative
   voices ordering the crime; 2 = delusional association
   (victims are also being persecuted), voices ordering the crime;
3 = delusional association (victims are also being persecuted),
   crime not commanded by voices;
4 = delusional enemy (persecutor), crime commanded by voices;
5 = delusional enemy (persecutor) crime not commanded by voices;
6 = other delusional relationship, crime commanded by voices;
7 = other delusional relationship, crime not commanded by voices;
8 = other; 9 = not known

72

Motivation of the crime
O = no recognisable motive; 1 = delusional self-defence;
2 = revenge or retaliation for delusional suffering;
3 = revenge or retaliation for real suffering;
4 = disappointed love, jealousy (incl. delusional jealousy);
5 = abnormal or delusional methods of upbringing;
6 = release of victim from feared suffering or illness;
7 = other delusional motives (religious, ecstatic, etc.);
8 = other non-delusional motives (gain, removal of burdensome
   persons, concealment of punishable offence, etc.);
9 = not known

73

──────────── COMMITTAL OF OFFENDER AFTER CRIME OR AFTER CONVICTION ────────────

O = none, still at liberty; 1 = prison or detention; 2 = prison
   or detention, then institution (still detained or died in
   institution);
3 = prison or detention, then institution, now at liberty, no
   aftercare;
4 = prison, then institution, now at liberty, with aftercare;
5 = immediate committal to institution (still detained or died
   in institution);
6 = committal to institution (now at liberty, no aftercare);
7 = committal to institution (now at liberty, with aftercare);
8 = other forms of care or control; 9 = not known

74

———————————————— COURSE OF ILLNESS AFTER THE CRIME ————————

O = has not been ill; 1 = unchanged; 2 = deteriorated; 3 = improved;
4 = recovered; 5 = died by suicide in association with the crime;
6 = died later, no recovery; 7 = died after recovery; 8 = other;
9 = not known

                                                              75

———————————————————— FORM OF ENQUIRY ————————————————

1 = files only; 2 = personal examination only;
3 = files and personal examination; 4 = background investigation
    only;
5 = files and background investigation;
6 = personal and background investigation;
7 = files, personal and background investigation;
8 = other

                                                              76

Interval between investigation and crime (in years)

                                                    77   78

Form completed by
1 = Häfner; 2 = Böker; 3 = Schmitt

                                                              79

BIBLIOGRAPHY

Adelstein, A.M., Downham, D.Y., Stein, Z., Susser, W.M. (1968). The epidemiology of mental illness in an English city. *Soc. Psychiatry* *3*, 47-59.

Aichhorn, A. (1951). *Verwahrloste Jugend. Die Psychoanalyse in der Fürsorgeerziehung*, 3rd edn. Bern: Huber.

Alexander, R. (1926). Das verbrecherische Verhalten des Geisteskranken. Diss. *Hamburger Schriften zur gesamten Strafrechtswissenschaft 9*.

Alexander, R. & Nyssen, J. (1929). *J. Neurol. 29.* Cited in Langelüddeke, A. (1959). *Gerichtliche Psychiatrie*, 2nd edn. Berlin: de Gruyter.

Alström, C.H. (1950). A study of epilepsy in its clinical, social and genetic aspects. *Acta Psychiatr. Neurol. Suppl. 63.*

Alter (1913). Ein Fall von Selbstbeschuldigung. *Z. Neurol. 15,* 470-81.

Amelunxen, C. (1966). Ursachen und Delikte der Alterskriminalität. *Fortschr. Med. 84*(2), 41-2.

Aschaffenburg, G. (1912). *Die Sicherung der Gesellschaft gegen gemeingefährliche Geisteskranke.* Berlin: J. Guttenberg.

Bader, K.S. (1949). *Soziologie der deutschen Nachkriegskriminalität.* Tübingen.

Belknap, J. (1956). *Human Problems of a State Mental Hospital.* New York: McGraw-Hill.

Binder, H. (1952). *Die Geisteskrankheit im Recht.* Zurich: Schulthess.

Birley, J.L. & Brown, G.W. (1970). Crises and life changes preceding the onset of relapse of acute schizophrenia : clinical aspects. *Br. J. Psychiatr. 116,* 327-33.

Birnbaum, K. (1926). *Die psychopathischen Verbrecher*, 2nd edn. Leipzig.

Birnbaum, K. (1931). *Kriminalpsychopathologie und psychobiologische Verbrecherkunde,* 2nd edn. Berlin.

Bleuler, E. (1969). *Lehrbuch der Psychiatrie*, 11'th edn. Berlin, Heidelberg, New York: Springer.

Bochnik, H.J. (1961). The methodological problem involved in the delimitation of depressive syndromes in European psychiatry. *Acta Psychiatr. Scand. 37, Suppl. 162,* 210-27.

Bochnik, H.J., Legewie, H., Otto, P. & Wuster, G. (1965). Tat, Täter, Zurechnungsfähigkeit. *Multifaktorielle Analysen psychiatrisch-kriminologische Erfahrungen.* Stuttgart: Enke.

Bond, E.D. & Braceland, F.Y. (1937). Prognosis in mental disease. *Am. J. Psychiatr. 14,* 263–74.

Boor, W. de (1959). *Über motivisch unklare Delikte. Ein Beitrag zur Strafrechtsreform.* Berlin, Göttingen, Heidelberg: Springer.

Brack, E. (1957). Die Kriminalität der Schizophrenen. *Arch. Kriminol. 119,* 17–19.

Brack-Kletzhändler, E. (1954). Zum Problem der Kriminalität der Schizophrenen. *Monatsschr. Psychiatr. Neurol. 128,* 129–52.

Brandt, B. (1948). Über wahnkranke Mörder. Diss. Frankfurt.

Bremer, J. (1951). A social psychiatric investigation of a small community in Northern Norway. *Acta Psychiatr. Neurol. Suppl. 62,* 1–166.

Bromberg, W. (1961). *The Mold of Murder. A Psychiatric Study of Homicide.* New York: Grune & Stratton.

Brown, G.W. & Birley, J.T.L. (1970). Social precipitants of severe psychiatric disorders. In *Psychiatric Epidemiology,* ed. E.H. Hare & J.K. Wing. London: Oxford University Press.

Brown, G.W., Monck, E.M., Carstairs, G.M. & Wing, J.K. (1962). Influence of family life on the course of schizophrenic illness. *Br. J. Prev. Soc. Med. 16,* 55–68.

Brückner, G. (1961). *Zur Kriminologie des Mordes.* Hamburg.

Bumke, O. (1912). Gerichtliche Psychiatrie. In *Handbuch der Psychiatrie,* ed. G. Aschaffenburg. Leipzig, Vienna.

Bumke, O. (ed.) (1928–39). *Handbuch der Geisteskrankheiten.* Berlin: Springer.

Bundesamt für Statistik (1955-8). *Die Abgeurteilten und Verurteilten. Ergebnisse der Straferforschungsstatistik.* Wiesbaden.

Bundesamt für Statistik (1959-64). *Reihe 9 Rechtspflege: Bevölkerung und Kultur.* Mainz, Stuttgart: Kohlhammer-Verlag.

Bürger-Prinz, H. (1939). Schizophrenie und Mord. Eine kritische Auseinander-setzung mit dem gleichnamigen Buch von N. Schipkowensky. *Monatsschr. Kriminol. 30,* 29.

Bürger-Prinz, H. (1940-1). Schizophrenie und Mord. I and II. *Monatsschr. Kriminol. 31,* 125; *32,* 149–61.

Bürger-Prinz, H. (1950). *Motiv und Motivation.* Hamburg: Carl Holler Verlag.

Bürger-Prinz, H. & Lewerenz, H. (1961). *Die Alterskriminalität. Forum der Psychiatrie 3.* Stuttgart: Enke Verlag.

Campbell, D. (1912). Über Geistesstörungen bei Epilepsie mit Berücksichtigung ihrer forensischen Bedeutung. *Arch. Kriminal-Anthrop. Kriminalstat. 50,* 115.

Caudill, W. (1958). *The Psychiatric Hospital as a Small Society.* Cambridge, Mass: Harvard University Press.

Christiansen, K.O. (1968). Threshold of tolerance in various population groups illustrated by results from Danish criminological twin study. In *The Mentally Abnormal Offender. Ciba Foundation Symposium 1967.* London: Churchill.

Ciompi, L. & Lai, G.P. (1969). *Dépression et vieillesse: études catamnestiques sur le vieillissement et la mortalité de 555 anciens patients dépressifs.* Bern, Stuttgart: Huber Verlag.

Ciompi, L. & Müller, C. (1969). Katamneztische Untersuchungen zur Altersentwicklung psychischer Krankheiten. *Nervenarzt 40,* 349-55.

Claude, H. (1932). *Psychiatrie médico-légale:* Paris. Cited in Schipkowensky, N. (1938). *Schizophrenie und Mord. Monographien aus dem Gesamtgebiet der Neurologie und Psychiatrie 63.* Berlin, Springer.

Conrad, K. (1958). *Die beginnende Schizophrenie. Versuch einer Gestaltanalyse des Wahns. Sammlung psychiatrischer und neurologischer Einzeldarstellungen.* Stuttgart: Thieme.

Cramer, A. (1908). *Gerichtliche Psychiatrie.* Jena.

Cumming, E. & Cumming, J. (1957). *Closed Ranks. An Experiment in Mental Health Education.* Cambridge, Mass.: Harvard University Press.

Diagnostic and Statistical Manual of Mental Disorders, 2nd edn. (1968). Washington, DC: American Psychiatric Association.

Diamond, B. (1968). Diskussionsbemerkung zu J.Kloek: Schizophrenia and delinquency. In *The Mentally Abnormal Offender. Ciba Symposium 1967.* London: Churchill.

Dohrenwend, B.P. & Dohrenwend, D.S. (1965). The problem of validity in field studies of psychological disorder. *J. Abnorm. Psychol. 70,* 52-69.

Dohrenwend, B.P. & Dohrenwend, D.S. (1969). Social status and psychological disorder. A causal inquiry. New York: Wiley-Interscience.

Dolenc, M. (1913). Vierfache Kindesabschlachtung einer Mutter infolge Raptus melancholicus. *Arch. Kriminol 51,* 48.

Dollard, J. *et al.* (1939). *Frustration and Aggression.* New Haven, Conn.

Dukor, B. (1949). Die Erkennung von Geistesstörungen in der Haft. Schweiz. Verein f. Straf-, Gefängniswesen und Schutzaufsicht. Berufsausbildung der Angestellten in Straf- und Verwahrungsanstalten III. Sonderheft 1949.

Duncan, G.M. & Frazier, S.H. *et al.* (1958). Etiological factors in first-degree murder. *JAMA 168*(13), 1755-8.

East, N. (1936). *Medical Aspects of Crime.* London: Churchill.

Elsässer, G. (1939), Zur Frage des Familien- und Selbstmordes. *Z. Psychiatr. Grenzgeb.* 110, 207.

Ernst, K. (1938). *Über Gewalttätigkeitsverbrecher und ihre Nachkommen. Monographien aus dem Gesamtgebiet der Neurologie und Psychiatrie 65.* Berlin: Springer.

Esquirol, E. (1831). *Bemerkungen über die Mordmonomanie. Aus dem Französischen von Dr Bluff.* Nuremberg.

Esquirol, E. (1838). *Die Geistskrankheiten in Beziehung zur Medizin und Staatsarzneikunde,* vols. 1 and 2. Berlin.

Feuerbach, A. von (1849). *Aktenmässige Darstellung merkwürdiger Verbrechen,* 3rd edn. Frankfurt: Heyer.

Fodéré (1832). Essai médico-légale. Cited in Schipkowensky, N. (1938). *Schizophrenie und Mord. Monographien aus dem Gesamtgebiet der Neurologie und Psychiatrie 63.* Berlin: Springer.

Folkard, S. (1944). Aggressive behaviour in relation to open wards in a mental hospital. *Ment. Hyg. 44,* 155-61.

Folkard, S. (1956). A sociological contribution to the understanding of aggression and its treatment. *Proc. R. Soc. Med. 49,* 1030-4.

Freming, K.-H. (1947). *Morbidity Risk of Mental Diseases in an Average Danish Population.* Copenhagen. (English edn 1951.)

Gardner, E.A., Bahn, A.K. & Mack, M. (1964). Suicide and psychiatric care in the ageing. *Arch. Gen. Psychiatr. 10,* 547-60.

Gast, P. (1930). *Die Mörder. Kriminalistische Abhandlung 11.* Leipzig: E. Wiegandt.

Gaupp, R. (1914). Zur Psychologie und Massenmords; Hauptlehrer Wagner von Degerloch. Eine kriminalpsychologische und psychiatrische Studie. In *Verbrechertypen,* vol. 1, part 3, ed. H.W. Gruhle & A. Wetzel. Berlin.

Gaupp, R. (1938). Krankheit und Tod des paranoischen Massenmörders Hauptlehrer Wagner, eine Epikrise. *Zentralbl. Neurol. 163,* 48-82.

Genert, P.J. (1966). *A 20 Year Comparison of Releases and Recidivists.* Harrisburg: Pennsylvania Board of Parole.

Gibbens, T.C.N. (1958). Sane and insane homicide. *J. Crim. Law, Criminol. Police Sci.* Cited in West, D.J. (1965). *Murder followed by Suicide.* London: Heinemann.

Glaser, J. (1934). Tötungsdelikt als Symptom von beginnender oder schleichend verlaufender Schizophrenie. *Z. Neurol. 150,* 1-41.

Glueck, S. & Glueck, E. (1950). *Unraveling Juvenile Delinquency. Harvard Law School Studies in Criminology.* Cambridge, Mass.: Harvard University Press. (3rd edn 1957).

Goffman, E. (1961). *Asylums.* New York: Anchor Books.

Göppinger, H. (1971) *Kriminologie. Eine Einführung.* Munich: C.H.Beck'sche.

Greger, J. & Hoffmeyer, O. (1969). Tötung eigener Kinder durch schizophrene Mütter. *Psychiatr. Clin. 2,* 14-24.

Gross, K. (1936). Über paranoische Mörder. *Jahrb. Psychiatr. Neurol. 53,* 85.

Gruhle, H.W. (1933). Geisteskranke Verbrecher und verbrecherische Geisteskranken. In *Handwörterbuch der Kriminologie,* ed. A. Eister & H. Lingemann. Berlin & Leipzig: de Gruyter. (Reprinted in Gruhle, H.W. (1953). *Verstehen und Einfühlen. Gesammelte Schriften.* Berlin : Springer.)

Gruhle, H.W. (1940). *Selbstmord.* Leipzig: Thieme.

Gruhle, H.W. (1951). Über den Wahn. *Nervenarzt 22*, 125. (Reprinted in Gruhle, H.W. (1963). *Verstehen und Einfühlen. Gesammelte Schriften.* Berlin: Springer.)

Gulevich, G.D. & Bourne, P.G. (1970). Mental illness and violence. In *Violence and the Struggle for Existence.* Boston: Little, Brown.

Gunn, J. & Bonn, J. (1970). Criminality and violence in epileptic prisoners. *Br. J. Psychiatr. 117*, 450.

Gurin, G., Veroff, J. & Feld, S. (1960). *Americans View their Mental Health. Joint Commission on Mental Illness and Health. Monograph Series 4.* New York: Basic Books.

Guze, S.B., Tuason, V.B., Gatfield, P.D. et al. (1962). Psychiatric illness and crime with particular reference to alcoholism: a study of 223 criminals. *J. Nerv. Ment. Dis. 134*, 512-21.

Guze, S.B., Goodwin, D.W. & Crane, J.B. (1969). Criminality and psychiatric disorders. *Arch. Gen. Psychiatr. 20*, 583-91.

Haddenbrock, S. (1955). Zur Frage eines theoretischen oder pragmatischen Krankheitsbegriffs bei der Beurteilung der Zurechnungsfähigkeit. Monatsschr. Kriminol. 38.

Haddenbrock, S. (1967). Zur Frage der Verantwortungsfähigkeit auch 'schwerer' Psychopathen. *Nervenarzt 38*, 466-8.

Haffter, C. (1948). *Kinder aus geschiedenen Ehen.* Bern, Stuttgart: Huber.

Häfner, H. (1959). Von der 'moral insanity' zur daseinsanalytischen Gewissenspsychopathologie. *Confin. Psychiatr. 2*, 214-42.

Häfner, H. (1961). *Psychopathen. Daseinsanalytische Untersuchungen.* Berlin, Gottingen, Heidelberg: Springer.

Häfner, H. (1962). Struktur und Verlaufsgestalt manischer Verstimmungsphasen. *Jahrb. Psychol. Psychother. Med. Anthropol. 9*, 196-217.

Häfner, H. (1967). Situation und Entwicklungstendenzen der Sozialpsychiatrie. In *Die Verantwortung der Gesellschaft für ihre psychisch Kranken. Schriften des deutschen Vereins für öffentliche und private Fürsorge 235.*

Häfner, H. (1968). Rehabilitation bei Schizophrenen. *Nervenarzt 39*, 385-95.

Häfner, H. (1970). *Seelische Gesundheit in der Gemeinde. Aufgaben und Wege einer modernen Psychiatrie. Jahrbuch der Deutschen Caritas-Verbandes.* Freiburg.

Häfner, H. (1971). Der Einfluss von Umweltfaktoren auf das Erkrankungsrisiko für Schizophrenie. *Nervenarzt 42*, 557-68.

Häfner, H., Cesarino, A.C. & Cesarino-Krantz, M. (1967). Konstanz und Variabilität klinisch psychiatrischer Diagnosen über sechs Jahrzehnte. *Soc. Psychiatry 2*, 14-25.

Häfner, H. & Reimann, H. (1970). Zur Ökologie seelischer Erkrankungen. In *Neuroleptische Dauer- und Depottherapie in der Psychiatrie,* ed. K. Heinrich. Konstanz: Schnetztor.

Häfner, H., Reimann, H., Immich, H. & Martini, H. (1969). Incidenz seelischer Erkrankungen in Mannheim 1965. *Soc. Psychiatry 4*, 126-35.

Helgason, T. (1964). Epidemiology of mental disorders in Iceland : a psychiatric and demographic investigation. *Acta Psychiatr. Scand. 40, Suppl. 173.*

Hemprich, R.D. & Kisker, K.P. (1968). 'Die Herren der Klinik' und die Patienten. Erfahrungen aus der teilnehmend-verdeckten Beobachtung einer psychiatrischen Station. *Nervenarzt 39,* 433-41.

Hentig, H. von (1948). *The Criminal and his Victim.* New Haven: Yale University Press.

Hentig, H. von (1956). *Zur Psychologie der Einzeldelikte. II. Der Mord.* Tübingen: J.C.B. Mohr (Paul Siebeck).

Hill, D. & Pond, D.A. (1952). Reflections on one hundred capital cases submitted to electroencephalography. *J. Ment. Sci. 410,* 23-43.

Hillbom, E. (1960). *Acta Psychiatr. Neurol. Scand. 35, Suppl. 142,* 1-195. Cited in Roth, M. (1968). Cerebral diseases and mental disorders of old age as causes of antisocial behaviour. In *The Mentally Abnormal Offender. Ciba Foundation Symposium 1967.* London: Churchill.

Hoche, A. (1934). *Handbuch der gerichtlichen Psychiatrie,* 3rd edn. Berlin: Springer.

Hoel, P.G. (1962). *Introduction to Mathematical Statistics.* New York: Wiley.

Hoenig, J. & Hamilton, M.W. (1967). The burden on the household in an extramural psychiatric service. In *New Aspects of the Mental Health Services,* ed. H. Freeman & J. Farndale. New York: Pergamon.

Hopwood, J.S. (1927). Child murder and insanity. *J. Ment. Sci. 73,* 95-108.

Hübner, A.H. (1914). *Lehrbuch der forensischen Psychiatrie.* Bonn.

Iberg, G. (1905-6). Über Lustmord und Lustmörder. *Monatsschr. Kriminol. 2,* 596.

Ichiba, K. (1966). Homicide in the prodromal stage of schizophrenia. A type of psychogenic reaction. *Acta Criminol. Med. Leg. Jap. 32,* 12-13.

Jacobi, E. (1928). Zur Psychopathologie des Familienmordes. *Arch. Psychiatr. Nervenkr. 83,* 501-32.

Jaeckel, M. & Wieser, S. (1967). Studien zur 'unsichtbaren Schranke' bei psychisch Kranken. *Soc. Psychiatry 2,* 100-6.

Janz, D. (1969). *Die Epilepsien. Spezielle Pathologie und Therapie.* Stuttgart: Thieme.

Janzarik, W. (1956). Zur Beurteilung geordneter Wahnkranker bei zwangsweiser Unterbringung in einer geschlossen Anstalt. *Dtsch. Med. Wochenschr. 2,* 61-6.

Jaspers, K. (1965). *Allgemeine Psychopathologie,* 8th edn. Berlin, Heidelberg, New York: Springer.

Jossmann (1931). *Allg. Z. Psychiatr. 95,* 231. Cited in Langelüddeke, A. (1959). *Lehrbuch der gerichtlichen Psychiatrie.* Berlin: de Gruyter.

Juel-Nielsen, N. & Strömgren, E. (1962). Psykiatriske lidelser i almen laegepraksis. *Ugeskr. Laeg. 124,* 1103.

Karuth (1845). Über die Gemeingefährlichkeit der Seelengestörten. *Allg. Z. Psychiatr 2*, 74-86.

Kiehne, K. (1965). Das Flammenwerferattentat in Köln-Volkhoven. *Arch. Kriminol. 136*, 61-75.

Kielholz, P. (1965). *Diagnose und Therapie der Depressionen für den Praktiker.* Munich: J.F. Lehmanns (2nd edn, 1967).

Kinkelin, M. (1954). Verlauf und Prognose des manisch-depressiven Irreseins. *Schweiz. Arch. Neurol. Psychiatr. 73*, 100-46.

Klee, G.D., Spiro, E., Bahn, A.K. & Gorwitz, K. (1967). An ecological analysis of diagnosed mental illness in Baltimore. In *Psychiatric Epidemiology and Mental Health Planning*, ed. R.P.Monroe, G.D. Klee & E.B. Brody. *Psychiatric Reports of the American Psychiatric Association 22.* Washington.

Kloek, J. (1964). Schizophrenia and criminal behaviour. *Psychiatr. Neurol. Neurochir. 67*, 176-81.

Kloek, J. (1968). Schizophrenia and delinquency. The inadequacy of our conceptual framework. In *The Mentally Abnormal Offender. Ciba Foundation Symposium 1967.* London: Churchill.

Kögler, A. (1940). Über einen Fall von Kindesmord. Ein forensisch-psychiatrischer Beitrag zur Paranoiafrage. *Monatsschr. Kriminol. 30*, 162-77.

Kosyra, H. (1963). Beeinträchtigungswahn als Brandstiftungs- und Mordmotiv. *Arch. Kriminol. 135*, 163-6.

Krafft-Ebing, R. von (1892). *Lehrbuch der gerichtlichen Psychopathologie.* Stuttgart: Enke.

Kramer, M. (1969). Cross-national study of diagnosis of the mental disorders: origin of the problem. *Am. J. Psychiatr. 125*, 1-11.

Kreitman, N. (1969). The reliability of psychiatric diagnosis. *J. Ment. Sci. 107*, 876-86.

Kreitman, N., Sainbury, P., Morrissey, J., Towers, J. & Scrivener, J. (1969). The reliability of psychiatric assessment. An analysis. *J. Ment. Sci. 107*, 887-908.

Kretschmer, E. (1921) *Körperbau und Charakter.* Berlin, Göttingen, Heidelberg: Springer (23rd and 24th edns, 1961).

Kretschmer, E. & Enke, W. (1936). *Die Persönlichkeit der Athletiker.* Leipzig: Thieme.

Kringelin, E. (1967). *Heredity and Environment in the Functional Psychoses.* Oslo: Universitetsforlaget.

Lancaster, H.O. (1969). *The Chi-square Distribution.* New York: Wiley.

Lange, E. (1964). *Der misslungene erweiterte Suicid.* Jena: Fischer.

Lange, J. (1934). Manisch-depressiver Formenkreis. In *Handbuch der gerichtlichen Psychiatrie,* 3rd edn. Berlin: Springer.

Lange, J. & Boeters, H. (1936). Fall von Encephalitis epidemica mit aggressiven und andersartigen Drangzustände. *Monatsschr. Kriminol. 27,* 55.

Langelüddeke, A. (1940). Zur Motivierung des Kindesmordes. *Allg. Z. Psychiatr. 115,* 356-61.

Langelüddeke, A. (1959). *Gerichtliche Psychiatrie,* 2nd edn. Berlin: de Gruyter.

Lanzkron, J. (1963). Murder and insanity. A survey. *Am. J. Psychiatr. 119,* 754-8.

Leff, P.J. (1973). Trials of preventive medication. In *Tools for Evaluation. An Epidemiological Basis for Planning Psychiatric Services,* ed. J.K. Wing & H. Häfner. London: Oxford University Press.

Leighton, D.C., Hardin, J.S., Macklin, D.B., Macmillan, A.M. & Leighton, A.H. (1963). *The Character of Danger. Psychiatric Symptoms in Selected Communities. The Stirling County Study of Psychiatric Disorder and Sociocultural Environment.* New York: Basic Books.

Lennox, W.G. (1943). *Am. J. Psychiatr. 99,* 732-43. Cited in Roth, M. (1968). Cerebral disease and mental disorders of old age as causes of antisocial behaviour. In *The Mentally Abnormal Offender. Ciba Foundation Symposium 1967.* London: Churchill.

Leppien, R. (1963). Das open-door-system in Nottingham England, seine Voraussetzungen und Auswirkungen. *Nervenarzt 34,* 215-19.

Levy, L. & Rowitz, L. (1970). The spatial distribution of treated mental disorders in Chicago. *Soc. Psychiatry 5,* 1-11.

Lidz, T., Cornelison, A. & Fleck, S. (1965). *Schizophrenia and the family, Monograph Series on Schizophrenia 7.* New York: International Universities Press.

Lidz, T., Cornelison, A., Fleck, S. & Terry, D. (1957). The intrafamilial environment of the schizophrenic patient. I. The father. *Psychiatry 20,* 329-42.

Lidz, T. *et al.* (1959). Zur Familienumwelt der Schizophrenen. *Psyche 13,* parts 5 and 6.

Lindenberg, W. (1954). Hirnverletzte Berserker. *Ärztl. Wochenschr. 9,* 802-10.

Lombroso, C. (1887-90). *Der Verbrecher* (2 vols.). Hamburg: J. Richter.

Lorentz, W. (1932). *Die Totschläger. Kriminalistische Abhandlungen 18.* Leipzig: E. Wiegandt.

Lumpp (1913). *Bl. Gef. Kde 47.* Cited in Wilmanns, K. (1940). Über Morde im Prodromalstadium der Schizophrenie. *Z. Neurol. 170,* 583-662.

Lundquist, G. (1945). Prognosis and course in manic-depressive psychoses. A follow-up study of 319 first admissions. *Acta Psychiatr. Scand. Suppl.* 35.

Macdonald, J.M. (1963). The threat to kill. *Am. J. Psychiatr. 120,* 125-30.

Macdonald, J.M. (1967). Homicidal threats. *Am. J. Psychiatr. 124,* 475-82.

Maier, H.W. (1931). Psychopathologie und Strafrecht. *Abh. Psychiatr. Neurol. 61,* 93-117.

Mandelbrote, B. & Folkard, S. (1960). Some factors related to outcome and social adjustment in schizophrenia. *Acta Psychiatr. Scand. 37,* 223.

Mauz, F. (1937). *Die Veranlagung zu Krampfanfällen.* Leipzig: Thieme.

Mechanic, D. (1970). Problems and prospects in psychiatric epidemiology. In *Psychiatric Epidemiology,* ed. E.H.Hare & J.K. Wing. London: Oxford University Press.

Menninger, K. (1938). *Man Against Himself.* New York: Harcourt, Brace and World.

Menninger, K. (1968). *Das Leben als Balance, Seelische Gesundheit und Krankheit im Lebensprozess.* Munich: R. Piper.

Mikorey, M. & Mezger, E. (1936). Symptomarme Geisteskrankheit und schweres Verbrechen. *Monatsschr. Kriminol. 2,* 97-105.

Mishler, E. & Waxler, N. (1966). Family interaction process and schizophrenia. *Int. J. Psychiatr. 2,* 375-415.

Moeli, C. (1888). *Über irre Verbrecher.* Berlin: H. Kornfeld.

Mohr, P. (1938). Psychologische Grundlagen zum Delikt des Mordes und des Totschlags. *Schweiz Arch. Psychiatr. Neurol. 41,* 135.

Moravcsik, E.E. (1907-8). Gegen Menschenleben wiederholt begangenes Verbrechen eines Paranoikers. *Monatsschr. Kriminol. 4,* 40.

Mowat, R.R. (1966). *Morbid Jealousy and Murder.* London: Tavistock.

Müller, Ch. (1967). *Alterpsychiatrie.* Stuttgart: Thieme.

Müller, H.W. & Hadamik, W. (1966). Die Unterbringung psychisch abnormer Rechtsbrecher. *Abt. Gesundheitspflege.* Landschaftsverband Rheinland, Koln. *Nervenarzt 37,* 67-79.

Müller, H.W., Scheuerle, G. & Engels, G. (1970). Zur Hospitalisierung psychisch Kranker im Rheinland in den Jahren 1962-5. *Nervenarzt 41,* 234-46.

Munro, A.E. (1965). *Br. J. Prev. Soc. Med. 19,* 69.

Muralt, L. von (1906). Über Familienmord. *Monatsschr. Kriminol. 2,* 88-109.

Näcke, P. (1908). *Familienmord bei Geisteskranken.* Halle.

Nunnally, J.C. Jr (1961). *Popular Conceptions of Mental Health.* New York: Holt, Rinehart & Winston.

Pauleikhoff, B. (1957). *Atypische Psychosen*. Basel: Karger.

Peters, U.H. (1968). Dämmerattacken als Träger kriminellen Verhaltens.
  Psychiatr. Clin. 1, 375.

Pighini, G. (1927). Kriminalität und Dementia praecox. *Monatsschr. Kriminol.
  18*, 193.

Pinto de Toledo (1934). *Zentralbl. Neurol. 77*, 99. Cited in Wilmanns, K.
  (1940). Über Morde im Prodromalstadium der Schizophrenie. *Zentralbl.
  Neurol. 170*, 583-662.

Pitaval, G. de (1739-50). *Causes célèbres et intéressantes*. Paris: Theodore
  le Gras.

Podolsky, E. (1958). The psychodynamics of filicide and matricide. *Dis.
  Nerv. Syst. 19*, 475.

Podolsky, E. (1966). The psychodynamics of criminal behaviour. *Int. J.
  Neuropsychiatr. 2*, 166-74.

Pokorny, A.D. (1964). Suicide rates in various psychiatric disorders.
  J. Nerv. Ment. Dis. 139, 499-506.

Pöldinger, W. (1968). *Die Abschätzung der Suicidalität. Eine medizinisch-
  psychologische Studie*. Bern, Stuttgart: Huber.

Polizeiliche Kriminalstatistik der Bundesrepublik Deutschland (1955-64).
  Ed. Bundeskriminalamt, Wiesbaden.

Popella, E. (1964). Über den erweiterten Suicid. *Arch. Psychiatr. Nervenkr.
  205*, 615-24.

Prichard, I.C. (1835). *A Treatise on Insanity and Other Disorders Affecting
  the Mind*. London: Sherwood, Gilbert & Piper.

Prince, R. (1966). *An Ecological Study of Social Pathology in Central
  Montreal. Urban Social Redevelopment Project*. Montreal.

Rangol, A. (1959, 1963). *Mordstatistik*, ed. Statistisches Bundesamt,
  Wiesbaden.

Rangol, A. (1971). Rechtverletzungen Unzurechnungsfähiger. *Wirtschaft Stat.
  12*, 741.

Rangol, A. (1972). *Die Gewaltkriminalität im Spiegel der Zahlen*. Arbeitstagung
  1972 der Deutschen Kriminologischen Gesellschaft. Statistisches
  Bundesamt Wiesbaden VII-A.

Rappeport, J.R. & Lassen, G. (1965). Dangerousness. Arrest rate comparisons
  of discharged patients and the general population. *Am. J. Psychiatr.
  121*, 776-83.

Rappeport, J.R. & Lassen, G. (1966). The dangerousness of female patients.
  A comparison of the arrest rate of discharged psychiatric patients
  and the general population. *Am. J. Psychiatr. 123*, 413.

Rasch, W. (1964). *Totung des Intimpartners. Beiträge zur Sexualforschung 31.* Stuttgart: Enke.

Rasch, W. & Petersen, U. (1965). Kriminalität innerhalb endogen-phasischer Depression. *Monatsschr. Kriminol. 48,* 187-97.

Reid, D.D. (1966). Epidemiologische Methoden in der psychiatrischen Forschung. In *Sammlung psychiatrischer und neurologischer Einzeldarstellungen.* Stuttgart: Thieme.

Reimann, H. (1969). Die Gesellschaft und der Geisteskranke. *Soc. Psychiatry 4,* 87-94.

Reimann, H. & Häfner, H. (1972). Psychische Erkrankungen alter Menschen in Mannheim : eine Untersuchung der Konsultations-Inzidenz. *Soc. Psychiatr. 7,* 53-69.

Resnick, P.J. (1969). Child murder by parents:a psychiatric review of filicide. *Am. J. Psychiatr. 126,* 325-34.

Richmond. The criminal feebleminded. Cited by Werner, A. (1945), Die Rolle des Schwachsinns in der Kriminalität. *Monatsschr. Psychiatr. Neurol. 110,* 1-46.

Richter, H.E. (1967). *Eltern, Kindern und Neurose,* Stuttgart: Klett.

Richter, H.E. (1970). *Patient-Familie. Entstehung, Struktur und Therapie von Konflikten in Ehe und Familie.* Hamburg: Rowohlt.

Ringel, E. (1969). *Selbstmordverhütung.* Bern, Stuttgart, Vienna: Huber.

Rixen, P. (1921). *Die gemeingefährlichen Geisteskranken im Strafrecht, Strafvollzug und in der Irrenpflege. Monographien aus dem Gesamtgebiet der Psychiatrie und Neurologie 24.* Springer: Berlin.

Robins, L.N. (1966). *Deviant Children Grown Up.* Baltimore: Williams & Wilkins.

Robins, L.N. & Lewis, R.G. (1966). The role of the antisocial family in school completion and delinquency: a three generation study. *Sociol. Q. 7,* 500-14.

Robins, L.N. (1970). Follow up studies investigating childhood disorders. In *Psychiatric Epidemiology,* ed. E.H. Hare & J.K. Wing. London: Oxford University Press.

Roesner, E. (1936). Der Mord, seine Täter, Motive und Opfer nebst einer Bibliographie zum Problem des Mordes. *Z. gesamte Strafrechtswiss. 56,* 327.

Roesner, E. (1938). Mörder und ihre Opfer. *Monatsschr. Kriminol. 29,* 161-209.

Rosenberg, S.D. (1970). The disculturation hypothesis and the chronic patient syndrome. *Soc. Psychiatry 5,* 155-65.

Roth, M. (1968). Cerebral disease and mental disorders of old age as causes of antisocial behaviour. In *The Mentally Abnormal Offender. Ciba Foundation Symposium 1967.* London: Churchill.

Roth M. & Kay, D.W. (1956). Affective disorders arising in the senium. *J. Ment. Sci. 102,* 141-50.

Rüdin, H. (1909). *Über die klinischen Formen der Seelenstörungen bei zu lebenslänglicher Zuchthausstrafe Verurteilten.* Munich.

Rutter, M. (1966). *Children of Sick Parents: An Environmental and Psychiatric Study.* London and New York: Oxford University Press.

Schipkowensky, N. (1938). *Schizophrenie und Mord. Ein Beitrag zur Psychopathologie des Mordes. Monographien aus dem Gesamtgebiet der Neurologie und Psychiatrie 63.* Berlin: Springer.

Schipkowensky, N. (1958). Manie und Mord. *Wiener Z. Nervenheilk. 14*(2-3), 212-27.

Schipkowensky, N. (1963). Mitgehen und Mitnehmen in den Tod. *Psychiatr. Neurol. Med. Psychol. 15,* 226-34.

Schipkowensky, N. (1968). Affective disorders; cyclophrenia and murder. In *The Mentally Abnormal Offender. Ciba Foundation Symposium 1967.* London: Churchill.

Schneider, K. (1949). Die Untergrunddepression. *Fortschr. Neurol. 17,* 429.

Schneider, K. (1956). *Die Beurteilung der Zurechnungsfähigkeit,* 3rd edn. Stuttgart: Thieme.

Schneider, K. (1950). *Klinische Psychopathologie.* Stuttgart: Thieme.

Schröder, J. (1952). Zur Psychologie der Delikte gegen das Leben. *Schweiz. Arch. Neurol. Psychiatr. 69,* 287.

Schulte, P.W. (1970). Einige Ergebnisse der Basisdokumentation der psychiatrischen Landeskrankenhäuser in Baden-Württemberg. Lecture before the Committee for Youth, Family and Health in the German Federal Republic, 8 October 1970.

Schulte, W. & Mende, W. (1969), Forensische Psychiatrie in der Bundes-republik Deutschland. In *Lehrbuch der Psychiatrie* by Bleuler, M. Berlin, Heidelberg, New York: Springer.

Sellin, T. (1938). *Culture, Conflict and Crime.* New York: Social Science Research Council. Cited in Christiansen, K.O. (1968). Threshold of tolerance in various population groups. In *The Mentally Abnormal Offender. Ciba Foundation Symposium 1967.* London: Churchill.

Shapiro, A. (1968). Delinquent and disturbed behaviour within the field of mental deficiency. In *The Mentally Abnormal Offender. Ciba Foundation Symposium 1967.* London: Churchill.

Sharp, V.H., Glasner, S., Lederman, I.I. & Wolfe, S. (1964). Sociopaths and schizophrenics. A comparison of family interactions. *Psychiatry 27,* 127-34.

Shoor, H. & Speed, M.H. (1963). Delinquency as a manifestation of the mourning process. *Psychiatr. Q. 37,* 540-58.

Siciliano, S. (1961). Risultati preliminari de un' indagine sull' omicidio in Danimarca. *Sci. Positiva (Milano),* 718-29.

Slater, E. (1938). Zur Periodik des manisch-depressiven Irreseins. *Z. Neurol. Psychiatr. 162,* 794-801.

Spangenberg, H. (1932). Familienmord und erweiterter Selbstmord. Diss. Düsseldorf.

Spitz, R.A. (1946). Anaclitic depression. In *The Psychoanalytic Study of the Child*, ed. A. Freud *et al.*, vol. 2.

Srole, L., Langner, T.S., Michael, S.T., Opler, M.K. & Rennie, T.A.C. (1962). *Mental Health in the Metropolis: The Midtown Manhattan Study*. New York: McGraw-Hill.

Stabenau, J.R., Turpin, J., Werner, M. & Pollin, W. (1965). A comparative study of families of schizophrenics, delinquents and normals. *Psychiatry 28*, 1.

Star, S.A. (1955). *The Public's Ideas about Mental Illness*. Chicago: National Opinion Research Center, University of Chicago.

Statistisches Bundesamt Wiesbaden (1955-8). *Die Abgeurteilten und Verurteilten. Ergebnisse der Straferforschungsstatistik*. Mainz, Stuttgart: W. Kohlhammer.

Statistisches Bundesamt Wiesbaden (1959-65). *Bevölkerung und Kultur 9:* Rechtspflege. Mainz, Stuttgart: W. Kohlhammer.

Statistisches Jahrbuch (1970). *Statistisches Jahrbuch für die Bundesrepublik Deutschland*. Mainz, Stuttgart: W. Kohlhammer.

Steigleder, E. (1968). *Mörder und Totschläger. Die forensisch-medizinische Beurteilung von nicht geisteskranken Tätern als psychopathologisches Problem*. Stuttgart: Enke.

Stengel, E. & Cook, N.G. (1958). *Attempted Suicide. Maudsley Monograph 4*. London: Chapman & Hall.

Stertz, G. (1931). Encephalitische Wesensveränderung und Mordgutachten über die Zurechnungsfähigkeit. *Monatsschr. Kriminol. 22*, 320.

Stevens, B.C. (1973). Evaluation for rehabilitation of psychotic patients in the community. In *Roots of Evaluation. An Epidemiological Basis for Planning Psychiatric Services*, ed. J.K. Wing & H. Häfner. London: Oxford University Press.

Stierlin, H. (1956). *Der gewalttätige Patient. Eine Untersuchung über die von Geisteskranken an Ärzten und Pflegepersonen verübten Angriffe. Bibl. Psychiatrie und Neurologie*. Basel: Karger.

Stransky, E. (1904-5). Mordversuch eines Paranoikers (induziertes Irresein) an einem vermeintlichen Verfolger. *Monatsschr. Kriminol. 1*, 427-8.

Strassmann, F. (1916). Neue Erfahrungen über Familienmord. *Monatsschr. gerichtl. Med. offentl. San. Wesen 51*, 54-68.

Strohmeyer, W. (1928). Über angeborene und im frühen Kindesalter erworbene Schwachsinnszustände. In *Handbuch der Geisteskrankheiten*, by O. Bumke, vol. 6, pp. 1-192. Berlin: Springer.

Stumpfl, F. (1935). *Erbanlage und Verbrechen. Charaktereologische und psychiatrische Sippenuntersuchungen. Monographien aus dem Gesamtgebiet Neurologie und Psychiatrie 61.* Berlin: Springer.

Tanay, E. (1969). Psychiatric study of homicide. *Am. J. Psychiatr. 125,* 1252-8.

Többen, H. (1908). Die gerichtsärztliche Bedeutung der epileptischen Dämmerzustände. *Viertelj.-Schr. gerichtl. Med. III F, 36,* 321-51.

Többen, H. (1913). *Monatsschr. Kriminol. 9,* 449. Cited in Wilmanns, K. (1940). Über Morde im Prodromalstadium der Schizophrenie. *Z. Neurol. 170,* 583-662.

Többen, H. (1932). *Untersuchungsergebnisse an Totschlägern.* Berlin: Carl Heymann.

Todesursachenstatistik (1970). In *Das Gesundheitswesen der Bundesrepublik Deutschland,* vol. 4, 352. Mainz, Stuttgart: W. Kohlhammer.

Varma, L.P. & Iha, B.K. (1966). Characteristics of murder in mental disorder. *Am. J. Psychiatr. 122,* 1296-8.

Vervaeck, (1939). *Cours d'anthropologie criminelle.* Brussels. Cited in Werner, A. (1945). Die Rolle des Schwachsinns in der Kriminalität. *Monatsschr. Psychiatr. Neurol. 110,* 1-46.

Viernstein, A. (1914). *Z. med. Beamte 27.* Cited in Wilmanns, K. (1940). Über Morde im Prodromalstadium der Schizophrenie. *Z. Neurol. 170,* 583-662.

Vladoff, D. (1911). *L'Homicide en pathologie mentale.* Paris: Maloine. Cited in Schipkowensky, N. (1958). Manie und Mord. *Wien, Z. Nervenheilk. 14,* 2-3, 212-27.

Wanner, O. (1954). Schizophrenie und Kriminalität. *Monatsschr. Kriminol. 37,* 1-33.

Walsh, D. (1969). Mental illness in Dublin. First admissions. *Br. J. Psychiatr. 115,* 449-56.

Weber (1916). Der Familienmord in forensicher Beurteilung. *Arch. Kriminol. 67,* 269-98.

Weimann, W. (1957). Paralytiker als Mörder. *Arch. Kriminol. 119,* 67-77.

Weinberg, S.K. (1967). Urban areas and hospitalized psychotics. In *Sociology of Mental Disorders,* ed. S.K. Weinberg. Chicago: Aldine.

Weitbrecht, H.J. (1952). Zur Typologie depressiver Psychosen. *Fortschr. Psychiatr. Neurol. 20,* 247-69.

Werner, A. (1945). Die Rolle des Schwachsinns in der Kriminalität. *Monatsschr. Psychiatr. Neurol. 110,* 1-46.

West, D.J. (1965). *Murder followed by Suicide.* London: Heinemann.

Wetzel, A. (1920). *Über Massenmörder. Ein Beitrag zu den persönlichen Verbrechensursachen und zu den Methoden ihrer Erforschung. Abhandlungen aus dem Gesamtgebiet der Kriminalpsychologie 3*, Springer: Berlin.

Wetzel, A. (1932). Die soziale Bedeutung der Schizophrenie. In *Handbuch der Geisteskranken*, vol. 9, by O. Bumke. Berlin: Springer.

Wilmanns, K. (1908). *Über Gefängnispsychosen*. Halle: C. Marhold.

Wilmanns, K. (1940). Über Morde im Prodromalstadium der Schizophrenie. *Z. Neurol. 170*, 583-662.

Wing, J.K. & Brown, G.W. (1961). Social treatment of chronic schizophrenics. A comparative survey of three mental hospitals. *J. Ment. Sci. 107*, 847-61.

Wing, J.K. & Monck, E.M., Brown, G.W. & Carstairs, G.M. (1964). Morbidity in the community of schizophrenic patients discharged from London mental hospitals in 1959. *Br. J. Psychiatr. 110*, 10.

Winokur, G., Cadoret, R., Donzal, J. & Baker, M. (1971). Depressive disease. A genetic study. *Arch. gen. Psychiatr. 24*, 135-44.

Woddis, G.M. (1957). Depression and crime. *Br. J. Delinquency VIII, 85*, 26.

Wolfgang, M.E. (1958). *Patterns in Criminal Homicide*. Philadelphia: University of Pennsylvania.

Wynne, L.C., Ryckoff, I.M., Day, J. & Hirsch, S.J. (1958). Pseudomutuality in the family relations of schizophrenics. *Psychiatry 21*, 205-20.

Wyrsch, J. (1955). *Gerichtliche Psychiatrie*, 2nd edn. Bern: Paul Haupt.

Wyrsch, J. (1947). Über die psychiatrische Beratung im Strafvollzug. *Schweiz. Z. Neurol. Psychiatr. 62*, 1.

Wyss, R. (1967). *Unzucht mit Kindern. Untersuchungen zur Frage der sogenannten Pädophilie. Monographien aus dem Gesamtgebiet der Neurologie und Psychiatrie 121*. Berlin, Heidelberg, New York: Springer.

Wyss, W. von (1912). Verbrechen vor und im Beginn der Dementia praecox. *Z. ges. Neurol. Psychiatr. 10*, 245-80.

Zech, K. (1959). Die Kriminalität der Manisch-Depressiven und ihre forensiche Begutachtung. *Med. Sachverständige 55*, 1-8.

Zubin, J. (1967). Classification of behaviour disorders. *A. Rev. Psychol. 18*, 373-406.

Zubin, J. (1969). Cross-national study of diagnosis of the mental disorders: methodology and planning. *Am. J. Psychiatr. 125, Suppl.* 1-20.

Zumpe, L. (1966). Tötung und Tötungsversuche eigener Kinder durch psychotische Mütter. *Arch. Psychiatr. Nervenkr. 208*, 198-208.

NOTES

CHAPTER 2

(1) On 4 September 1913, after careful and secret preparations, Wagner killed his wife and four children and then went to the village of Muhlhausen where the following night he set fire to several places, shot nine villagers dead and injured eleven.

(2) At the present time the wording is as follows: 'If an individual has committed a punishable offence while he is not responsible for his actions (Section 51, para 1, Section 55, para 1) or is in a state of diminished responsibility (Section 51, para 2, Section 55, para 2) then the Court shall order his committal to an institution for treatment and care, if public safety calls for this. In cases of diminished responsibility committal is accompanied by punishment.'

(3) Crimes against life and limb, divided into homicide and manslaughter (Articles 111 and 113 of the Penal Code), murder (Article 112), manslaughter resulting from negligence (Article 117), infanticide (Article 116), abortion (Article 119), bodily harm, assault (Articles 123-126).

(4) In a study which is enquiring into the incidence of offences, the risks of offences being committed, and individual risk factors, it does not seem sensible to base case-finding on a single day's committals. By counting on one particular day the number of individuals with certain characteristics, e.g. the number of mentally abnormal offenders in the hospital, we obtain a prevalence rate. This is important for the planning of treatment needs and other administrative requirements. But 'administrative' prevalence rates determined in this way are affected by the proportion of patients committed because of a criminal offence and by differences in the duration of committal and therefore by differences in the course of illness and in decisions in regard to discharge. The offender-prevalence rate arrived at thus deviates to a certain extent from 'true prevalence'. Offenders who have died between the date of their crime and the case-finding date, perhaps because they have committed suicide, are also omitted, which must lead to a further error in findings based on one particular day. If we wish to examine crime risks and to test hypotheses it is therefore better to use incidence rates. In the light of these objections, the number of mentally abnormal offenders found within a fixed period of time in a defined population would be a more suitable basis on which to determine incidence rates.

(5) Second edition, Washington, 1968.

(6) The authors considered that their methods of selection left only two groups unrepresented: (1) those who because of their overt insanity had been committed by the courts directly to mental

hospitals (according to their estimate about 1.5%); and (2) those mentally ill patients who were transferred from prisons or remedial institutions to permanent confinement in mental hospitals (according to their estimate less than 1%). They thus claimed that their study covered about 98% of the men within the area surveyed who had been found guilty of a violent crime.

(7) Similar views were advanced by Pighini (1927), Mohr (1938) and Glaser (1934).

(8) In discussing this considerable discrepancy in the relative frequency of schizophrenia among offenders referred for psychiatric assessment in the same country and from the same cultural background, two factors must be taken into account. Maier excluded cases examined by military courts, while Wanner included them. The most important factor affecting the results was probably the marked increase over recent decades in the court's appreciation of the need for psychiatric examination of offenders. After the introduction of the Swiss Penal Code of 1942 the number of border-line cases examined, particularly those with personality disorders, rose considerably. This presumably led to a substantial shift in the diagnostic composition of the material assessed.

(9) At the Ciba Symposium on the Mentally Abnormal Offender in 1967 Kloek said that he and his colleagues used the diagnosis of schizophrenia with the greatest reserve, because of its 'magical element'.

(10) In severe mental illnesses, particularly if they seem to make the person affected 'unpredictable', it will certainly frequently be assumed that the offender thereby becomes a danger to 'public safety'. The chances of such offenders being committed to hospital are presumably therefore increased, while the chances of their being released are less, especially since it may be assumed that the illness is chronic or liable to flare up again. This may as a rule be regarded as applying to schizophrenics.

(11) More recent and precise figures are available, for example, from the Rhineland and from Baden-Württemberg. Thus Müller, Scheurle & Engels (1970) gave the proportion of schizophrenics in all psychiatric institutions in the Rhineland as 28.9% of the total in-patient population of 18 242. According to Schulte (1970) the percentages of schizophrenics in the eight regional mental hospitals of Baden-Württemberg were as follows: 27.5% of approximately 13 000 short-stay patients (in hospitals for less than a year), 59% of approximately 5600 long-stay patients (one year or more).

(12) In this connection mention should be made of a methodologically sound prospective study by Pokorny (USA, 1964), who determined suicide rates in various psychiatric disorders, using as his material 11 580 first admissions to the Veterans Administration Psychiatric Hospital in Houston, Texas, between 1949 and 1963. Over a period of 0 to 15 years he found that 117 of them (i.e. just over 1%) had committed suicide: 4 in hospital, 25 while on leave or after absconding from hospital, the remainder after discharge. Comparing these figures with age-adjusted suicide rates for male veterans in Texas (22.7 per 100 000 per year) he found that the suicide rate for the psychiatric patients, whom he divided into eight major diagnostic categories, was more than seven times higher. Depression headed the diagnostic list with a suicide rate that was 25 times higher.
Ciompi & Lai, whose follow-up study of depressives was published in 1969, found that suicide was the cause of death in 14.3% of

the 303 depressed patients who had died, which corresponded to a
suicide rate of 7.9% in the total number of 550 depressed
patients who had been followed up for an average of 20.5 years
from first admission to hospital.
Ciompi & Lai also reviewed the literature in regard to the
frequency of suicide as a cause of death in depressed patients:
Bond & Braceland (1937) reported suicide in 50% of 24 patients
who had died; Slater (1938) in 15% of 59 patients who had died;
Langelüddeke (1940) in 25% of the male patients and 10% of the
female out of 264 who had died; Lundquist (1945) in 15% of 119
who had died; and Kinkelin (1954) in 26% of 52 who had died.
Even although these figures are hardly comparable, because of
the very variable selective factors at work and the difficulty
of controlling them, they still demonstrate the general tendency
towards a high risk of suicide among depressives and this must
be taken into account when it comes to examining the frequency
of crimes of violence against other people in the sense of
extended as opposed to simple suicide.

(13) In order to form a larger group and for the reasons put forward
here, we included epileptic offenders within the category of
cerebral organic disorders. We subsequently drew a distinction,
however, between the nosological subgroups of 'epilepsy with
no demonstrable cause (genuine epilepsy)', 'epilepsy with
innate or early defects including mental deficiency (residual
epilepsy)', 'epilepsy with acquired cerebral damage (symptomatic
epilepsy)', and 'epilepsy with atrophic processes'.

CHAPTER 3

(1) The chances of identifying the offender depend partly on the rate
of crimes 'cleared up', which comprises the ratio of crimes by
identified offenders to the number of crimes reported, but
particularly on the ratio of crimes reported to the total of
crimes committed. The proportion of crimes not reported has been
called the dark figure. Since there is no way of knowing the
absolute number of offences, the dark figure is necessarily to a
large extent speculative. In this study, therefore, we can do no
more than draw attention to the problem. If we assume that the
dark figure for crimes of violence is high, then we have to accept
the possibility that the ratio of mentally disturbed offenders to
'mentally normal' offenders may be incorrect. Illness may affect
the ability of the mentally disordered to plan their offences and
avoid prosecution, so that they have more chance of being detected
than the 'mentally normal' offender. It may in any case be assumed
that the rates of offenders confirmed by us, and the risk of the
mentally ill and the mentally defective becoming violent offenders,
will be on the high rather than on the low side, taking into
account the possibility of a higher dark figure for comparable
criminality in the general population.

(2) Cf. the comments on methodological and technical problems of
investigations of the incidence of mental illness in Häfner & Reimann
(1970).

(3) Attack is here understood to mean a deliberately committed act,
inclusive of any emotional behaviour which must necessarily lead
to the same effect on the victim, regardless of whether the intention was achieved. By definition this excludes genuine acts of
self-defence and crimes of negligence. Sexual crimes, e.g. rape,
are then included only if the victim is killed or seriously injured
by a dangerous use of violence.

(4) Section 211 (murder): (1) The murderer receives a sentence of life imprisonment. (2) A murderer is someone who kills another person from a pathological urge to commit murder, for gratification of sexual drives, from greed or from some other base motive, insidiously or ferociously or using some means that endanger life or in order to further or conceal another crime.

(5) Section 212 (manslaughter): (1) Someone who kills another person by intent, without being a murderer, receives a sentence of not less than five years imprisonment. (2) In particularly serious cases the sentence may be life imprisonment.

(6) Section 213 (manslaughter in extenuating circumstances): If the killer is enraged through no fault of his own by maltreatment of himself or of a member of his family or by offensive behaviour on the part of the victim or if other mitigating circumstances are present, the sentence imposed is from six months to five years.

(7) Section 226 (bodily harm resulting in death): If the victim dies as a result of the bodily harm, the sentence is not less than three years.

(8) The attempt to commit a crime is defined in Section 43 as follows: (1) If a person puts into effect a decision to commit a crime or misdemeanour by taking action which constitutes the start of execution of this crime or misdemeanour, this person is, if the intended crime or misdemeanour is not brought to completion, liable to punishment for attempted crime. (2) Attempted crime is, however, punishable only in those cases which have been expressly defined by law.

(9) Section 216 (killing on request): (1) If a person is induced to kill because of an explicit or fervent request on the part of the individual killed, the sentence is from six months to five years. (2) Attempted killing of this kind is a punishable offence.

(10) Section 217 (infanticide): (1) A mother who kills her illegitimate child deliberately at or just after birth receives a sentence of not less than three years. (2) If there are mitigating circumstances, the sentence may be from six months to five years.

(11) Section 223 (minor bodily harm): (1) A person who deliberately injures another person physically or damages his health, is liable to a sentence of up to three years or to a fine. (2) If the victim is a relative the sentence is from one month to five years.
Section 223a (life-endangering injury): If the injury is inflicted by means of a weapon, particularly a knife or other dangerous tool, or by means of a deceitful attack, or if the crime is carried out by several persons jointly or by means of an action that endangers life, the sentence is from two months to five years.

Section 223b (physical ill-treatment of dependents): (1) A person who tortures or manhandles children, young people or those who are rendered defenceless by deformity or illness, who are in his care or protection or have been placed under his authority by welfare services or who are dependent on him in a service or work relationship, or who damages their health by wilful neglect of his duty to care for them, is liable to a sentence of from three months to five years. (2) In very serious cases the sentence is from one year to five years.
Section 224 (grievous bodily harm): If the injury results in loss of a limb, loss of sight in one or both eyes, loss of hearing, speech or the power to bear witness, or considerable permanent mutilation, or results in chronic ill-health, paralysis or mental illness, the sentence is from one to five years.

Section 225 (deliberate grievous bodily harm): If one of the aforementioned consequences is intentional and deliberately entered upon, the sentence is from two to ten years.

(12) For the period of the survey the following was valid: Section 51 (unfitness to plead and diminished responsibility): (1) Behaviour is not punishable if the accused at the time of the act is incapable, through disturbance of consciousness as a result of morbid disturbance of mental function or on account of mental deficiency, of appreciating that the act is forbidden or of acting in accordance with this insight. (2) If the capacity to appreciate the prohibited nature of the behaviour or to act on this knowledge is substantially diminished on one of these grounds at the time of the act, the provisions for punishing the attempt may be mitigated.

On 1 October 1973 Section 51 of the Penal Code was replaced by the following Sections. Section 20 (freedom from responsibility on grounds of mental illness): No blame shall be attached to a person who at the time of his crime was, because of a deep disturbance of consciousness, or because of mental defect or other severe mental abnormality, incapable of having insight into the prohibited nature of the crime or of acting in accordance with that insight. Section 21 (diminished responsibility): If the offender's capacity to have insight into the prohibited nature of the crime or to act in accordance with that insight is substantially diminished because of one of the grounds mentioned in Section 20, then the penalty under Section 49, para 1, may be mitigated.

(13) Our research population contained basically only those offenders whose crime was immediately associated with the illness, for instance because it was committed during a florid psychosis. Since, as has been mentioned, the practice in forensic psychiatric assessments is to assume that the offender is likely to have diminished responsibility if there is a previous history of endogenous psychosis or even of several attacks, such cases were also included. It must be remembered, however, that ascertainment of such cases is more unreliable the more time has elapsed since the illness, the smaller the number of the attacks, and the less florid their symptomatology. In mental defect and in chronic disturbances, such as degenerative cerebral processes, this factor is not important; on the other hand it may be of particular significance in endogenous depressions (periodic depressions or cyclothymias) with infrequent phasic swings.

(14) Zubin (1967) quotes an inter-rater reliability for psychiatrists of between 42 and 73% for the diagnosis of mental defect in the studies reviewed. For schizophrenia it is between 53 and 80%, for affective psychoses between 35 and 65%. For different groups of neuroses the rates varied more widely. For unspecified neuroses it was between 16 and 56%, for reactive depressions between 18 and 63%, and for anxiety states between 27 and 55%. Concordance of diagnosis for acute organic cerebral disorders (exogenous reaction types) and chronic organic cerebral syndromes was respectively 46 to 68% and 66 to 80%.

(15) According to Zubin (1967), concordance in assigning cases to the diagnostic group of 'functional psychoses' was between 71 and 80%; to the group of 'character or personality disorders' about 72%; and for organic syndromes in general between 85 and 92%. The level of agreement in these broad diagnostic categories varied between 64 and 84%.

(16) In the meantime Rangol published in 1971 a study on 'Lawbreaking by those who are not responsible for their actions' which provided a breakdown of offenders who were granted protection under Section 51, para 1 or 2, of the Penal Code.

(17) So far as patients who had already been discharged or had died were concerned the mental hospital authorities usually allowed us to look through the admission and discharge books in order to trace the files. In addition we called upon the memory of the relevant physicians and of the hospital records officer.

(18) The absence of refusals is associated with the fact that the data collected by the police, the prosecuting authorities and the courts, including the psychiatric assessment of the offenders, can if necessary be compulsorily acquired. As the assessment serves in the defence of the offender and is offered in a situation of psychological and legal pressure, active co-operation may usually be expected. It is true that this special situation is also a source of possible bias. But to counteract this there is legal provision for usually up to six weeks in-patient observation in a psychiatric hospital. This ensures that the assessment is made both on objective findings and on observation by outsiders. The majority of the offenders in our study underwent such a period of observation. This did not apply, of course, to those who took their own lives after their crime, on whom the only data available were those contained in the preliminary enquiry, supplemented in most cases by psychiatric findings dating from the time before the crime.

(19) In this connection a mistake crept in which has to be taken into serious consideration when evaluating our findings. Before the enquiry began we had anticipated that the two examiners would visit the psychiatric hospitals together and would record alternate cases. For purely practical reasons (difficulties in arranging dates), this rule quickly fell into abeyance. Except for cases from the regions of Hamburg, Bremen, Niedersachsen, Hessen (A. Schmitt) and Berlin, Saarland and Bavaria (W. Böker), which were all collected separately, the great majority of cases were covered in such a way that the two investigators each journeyed alone to neighbouring regions of the GFR. This meant that the allocation of cases to the two examiners was not random, but was governed by regional factors. The possibility cannot therefore be ruled out that concordance and discordance in certain vulnerable items assessed by the two examiners might have been affected by other, unknown variables.

(20) As the Federal Statistics of Convicted Offenders cover convictions for the previous year, and since as a rule a fairly long time elapses between crime and conviction, especially in the case of capital crimes, we based our comparison on the decade between 1956 and 1965. This postponement by one year, which is in accordance also with the practice of the Federal Statistical Bureau, ensures that the registered, convicted offenders had mostly committed their crimes in the decade 1955 to 1964, as had the mentally disturbed offenders in our study population.

(21) Of the total population 60.9% live in rural communities, 26.0% in medium-sized towns (10 000-100 000 inhabitants) and 13.1% in the large town of Ludwigshafen which has 170 000 inhabitants (see *Handbuch für den Regierungsbezirk Pfalz* (*Government Handbook for Pfalz*), 1962).

CHAPTER 4

(1) It is possible that the large city of Berlin, with its high rate of crime and its 12 area offices providing a close network of psychiatric hospitals and agencies for the treatment of the mentally ill, may have documentation on a higher number of violent patients than Saarland. The only case reported to us in Saarland came from the Regional Psychiatric Hospital of Merzig, an institution providing treatment and after-care for a large rural catchment area. It is conceivable that in such circumstances the recording and documentation of violent crimes by the mentally disordered might be incomplete.

CHAPTER 5

(1) In the GFR the mean age of the general population of legally responsible age was between 42 and 43 years on 31 December 1959. The mean age of the Landeck sample was 46.3.

(2) By limiting the control group to first admissions we could have avoided this distortion of age distribution by relapses and re-admissions. The resulting control population of non-violent psychiatric patients would, however, have been inadequate on other grounds. Basically we had to proceed on the assumption that violent crimes by the mentally disordered are not committed exclusively or predominantly in the early stages of the illness but occur throughout the illness, though their distribution during illness is not known. Illnesses of longer duration, including both chronic disorders and those which have a high relapse rate, must therefore increase the chances of concurrent violence and must presumably raise the age of the offenders above the average age of onset of the illness. For these reasons we considered that comparison with all psychiatric admissions (both first admissions and readmissions) was preferable to comparison with first admissions only.

(3) As opposed to inborn and early defects of personality and cerebral malformations which, in so far as they fell within our case-finding criteria, were almost always associated with mental deficiency and were accordingly placed in this category.

(4) The study of the incidence of mental disorders in the city of Mannheim carried out in our clinic by Reimann, Häfner *et al*. in 1965 also confirmed these differences in morbidity between the two sexes.

(5) In forming our control group from the admissions to a regional mental hospital we decided against taking only first admissions, because in our pilot study of abnormal offenders we found that the crime hardly ever took place in the early stage of a psychotic illness. On the contrary, a large proportion of psychotic offenders had already had several attacks of illness and perhaps several periods of treatment. It emerged subsequently that it would have been advantageous, for the purpose of some of our comparisons including those discussed here, if we had separated the first admissions from the readmissions in our sample: unfortunately this was not done.

(6) We must also bear in mind the possibility that the age shift is partly a reflection of the different age composition of the two populations at risk. The population of normal violent offenders at risk is the general population over the age of 14. The age composition of the population of abnormal violent offenders at risk is not accurately known: it consists of all those over the

age of 14 who are suffering or have suffered at least once from a
mental illness, from its date of first onset. Since the age of
first onset of several of the illnesses in question is on average
considerably higher than 14, the younger age groups are under-
represented in this risk group and therefore in the relevant
population. This must result in a raising of the arithmetical
mean and median age distribution of the abnormal as against the
normal violent offenders. As we do not know the age-incidence
rates of the illnesses studied, it is not possible to correct
this error statistically.
The age distribution of the mentally defective violent offenders,
unlike that of the other abnormal offenders, is much the same
as that of the normal violent offenders, a fact which might
strengthen the above objection. Mental defect is always apparent
by the end of the fourteenth year. From this point of view the
age composition of the two populations at risk - the mentally
defective and the general population studied - would seem to be
identical. Motivation is, however, also to a large extent
identical, as well as several other factors found in the criminal
violence of the mentally defective and in general criminal
violence, but not in the violence of the mentally disturbed.

There are other, more weighty considerations, again of a
statistical nature, which argue against the above view that the
age distribution of the mentally defective violent offenders is
similar to that of the normal violent offenders. The life
expectation of the mentally defective is considerably lower than
than of the general population, so that the older age groups must
be very much under-represented in the population of mental defectives at risk. To what extent this is so is again unknown, since
there were at the time of our survey no reliable data on the life
expectation of mental defectives. We must, however, assume that
the average age of mental defectives is markedly lower than that
of the general population of responsible age. This must have a
downwards effect on the age distribution of mentally defective
violent offenders, so that the 'true' average age must be
considerably higher than that of violent offenders.

CHAPTER 6

(1) Violent crimes which result in the death of one or more people,
    can, for example, be sentenced according to the motive or
    circumstances of the crime, etc., under the following sections
    of the German Penal Code:
    (* means: includes *only* fatal crimes; (*) includes *also* fatal
    crimes - in the rubrics of the German Penal Code attempted crimes
    are also recorded here.)

    178*   Sexual offence or sexual assault resulting in death
    211*   Murder
    212*   Manslaughter
    213*   Manslaughter in extenuating circumstances
    216*   Killing on request
    217*   Infanticide
    221(*) Abandonment of a child
    226*   Bodily harm resulting in death
    227(*) Brawling
    229(*) Administration of poison
    251(*) Robbery with violence, grievous bodily harm or death of
            the victim

307(*) Arson of a particularly serious nature
311(*) Causing an explosion
312(*) Deliberate flooding, endangering human life
324(*) Poisoning of water supply
330(*) Crime committed in drunken frenzy

Section 330 (refusal to lend aid) is also of some importance.
Under this section offenders are sometimes convicted who cannot
be proved to have caused death, for example because there are no
witnesses of the murder of a spouse or intimate partner, but
against whom the court can prove that they did not take any action
to prevent an avoidable death.

(2) From *The Health of the Federal Republic of Germany*, vol. 4, p. 352.
Kohlhammer: Stuttgart (1970).

(3) This comparison does not make allowance for the really essential
age correction, which could not be carried out for lack of
statistical reference data. In violent offenders the younger age
groups between 20 and 40 are very much over-represented. The
same is true of some groups of mental illnesses, e.g. schizophrenia: in other illnesses, such as degenerative disorders or
mental deficiency, the age distribution is very atypical. Moreover the age composition of the mentally abnormal violent
offenders shows a mean upward shift of about 8 years as compared
with that of the 'normal' violent offenders.

CHAPTER 7

(1) Since we matched not only the groups as a whole but also selected
diagnoses, we had to test whether these subgroups (schizophrenia,
manic-depressive illness, mental deficiency) were adequately
matched in sex and age, so that artefacts caused by these factors
should not be regarded as diagnostic differences. The matching
of violent and non-violent depressives was not so good in regard
to the item of sex. In other diagnoses both items were adequately
matched.

(2) With reference to alcoholism we cannot exclude the possibility of
a further bias: our control group came from North Baden, while
the violent offenders were drawn from the whole of the GFR.
Whether one may assume that drinking habits are the same in all
federal regions would seem doubtful.

(3) 'Broken home' was defined as incompleteness in the parent-family
through the disappearance of at least one parent, e.g. by death
of the father or by separation or divorce, from the family life
of the child before his eighteenth year. Our questionnaire had
made some provision also for details about the behaviour of the
family towards society (e.g. 'antisocial parents'). But as very
little information was available on this point in forensic assessments and particularly in case histories, we restricted our
analysis to the single item of 'broken homes'.

(4) We believed we were justified in taking the place of the crime as
the basis of regional classification, because the offenders for
the most part lived near the scene of the crime and because we
had not recorded where they were actually living at the time of
the crime.

(5) However, there is only limited comparability between our violent
patients and those studied by Macdonald, since he included also
patients whose mental illness was less severe.

(6) Example: Case no. 334: Mrs F., aged 40, ill for a year with a paranoid and hallucinatory schizophrenia, with delusions of sin and fears of catastrophe. A few days before the act she heard clear hallucinatory voices which repeatedly commanded her to kill her 2½ year old son. During the hours in which she struggled against the growing determination to carry out this deed, the voices threatened her with physical sufferings and punishments if she did not do as ordered.

(7) The idea that violence, even murder (and suicide), may represent a 'defence against psychosis', a primitive measure of self-preservation on the part of the ego apparatus in the face of severe disintegration, was also advanced by Menninger in his book *Das Leben als Balance (The Vital Balance*: 1968) and illustrated by him in several examples. Kloek and Diamond argued in a similar vein at the Ciba Foundation Symposium on The Mentally Abnormal Offender held in London in 1967.

(8) An analogy may be seen in the phenomenon of structural shift in the marriage of schizophrenics ('marital screw') described by Lidz and his co-workers (1957).

(9) To find out whether medical assessment of a high risk of violence is really reliable so far as hospital discharges are concerned - as our data would seem to suggest in a small subgroup - it would be necessary to conduct an investigation which started with a sufficiently large sample of patients who were judged medically to be high risk carriers and who were then discharged or absconded.

(10) To test this hypothesis the most suitable investigation would be a prospective one, comparing two matched cohorts with a high risk of violence after different forms of psychiatric committal in respect of rates of violence in the post-discharge period. The possibility of carrying out such a study is, however, very small, in view of the low number of patients involved and for various other reasons.

(11) Sixty-five per cent of them were housewives. Only 3% were employed as temporary or unskilled workers.

(12) There was no difference between the schizophrenic and mentally defective offenders in this respect.

CHAPTER 8

(1) In Chapter 9 we shall return to those abnormal offenders who were given the subsidiary diagnosis of 'chronic alcoholism'.

(2) This was an evaluation reported by Rangol carried out by the Federal Statistical Bureau in Wiesbaden of 185 sentences which were recorded by the Ministries of Justice in the German federal regions in trials for murder and attempted murder in the years 1959 and 1963 and which represented 77% of all convictions for such crimes in these two years. From the 185 sentences (193 'cases') 216 offenders were identified (including multiple defendants). For our comparison we have abstracted the analysis of victims and motives of 178 offenders judged to be fully responsible for their actions. The remaining 38 offenders were considered to have diminished responsibility.

(3) Thus a card index of murder and similar crimes kept by the police authorities in Berlin used a classification of motives which set the pattern for the whole of Germany before the war (1938). It distinguished between 14 groups of motives (sexual murder, murder with robbery, removal of burdensome persons, crimes committed from hatred, revenge, jealousy, etc.): third from the end, before the categories of 'murder, motive unknown' (no. 13) and 'border-line cases' (no. 14), came 'murder from mental illness' (no. 12) in a category of its own.

CHAPTER 9

(1) In the other patients, for whom a considerable defect in IQ was not demonstrated, the symptoms were as a rule at the level of impairment of higher intellectual functions and visuo-motor performance, a general organic psychosyndrome and/or changes in personality.
(2) Offenders in whom chronic alcoholism had already led to severe brain damage or cerebral atrophy are included under the main diagnosis of late-acquired brain damage.
(3) IQ 89 and below: ICD 310-315.

CHAPTER 10

(1) A factor which might influence the risk of violence in the mentally defective is their comparatively low expectation of life. It is conceivable that if this life expectation of the mentally defective were to rise, the proportion of violent offenders among them would also rise slightly.
(2) We proceeded from the assumption that relapses or exacerbations of the illness or mental crises of different kinds would play a considerable part in causing the mentally ill to commit violent crimes. Our hypotheses on the role of stress factors in causing violent crime therefore followed the lines of hypotheses already confirmed by research into the causes of functional psychoses and were formulated in accordance with the data available from the material studied.
(3) No central statistics exist for the decade 1955-64, either for the GFR or for nearly all the regions. Most psychiatric hospitals issued, and many of them still issue, statistics of patient movement covering their own records only.

NAME INDEX

Page numbers in *italic* type refer to the Bibliography

SUBJECT INDEX